Uses of
Epidemiology

For Galia

Uses of Epidemiology

J. N. MORRIS

C.B.E., M.D.(Hon.), D.Sc. F.R.C.P.

Professor of Community Health, and Hon. Director Medical Research Council's Social Medicine Unit

London School of Hygiene and Tropical Medicine

University of London

THIRD EDITION

CHURCHILL LIVINGSTONE

Edinburgh London and New York 1975

CHURCHILL LIVINGSTONE

Medical Division of Longman Group Limited

Distributed in the United States of America by
Longman Inc., 72 Fifth Avenue, New York, N.Y. 10011 and by associated
companies, branches and representatives throughout the world.

First edition 1957
Second edition 1964
  Reprinted 1967, 1970
Third edition 1975

ISBN 0 443 01106 0

Library of Congress Catalog Card Number 75–13512

Printed in Great Britain

PREFACE TO THE THIRD EDITION

I apologise for the book's late appearance and for any inconvenience so caused, and wish there were some respectable excuse. May I also be forgiven where events have overtaken a text that was so long in writing!

Epidemiology is the basic science of what is now called Community Medicine but, as before, the book is aimed equally to interest students and practitioners of clinical and laboratory medicine. The need for mutual understanding and collaboration between all of us never was greater and the book, I hope, can make a contribution to this.

The new edition is larger than the previous one but it is again a personal account and there is no attempt to be comprehensive. Indeed, a modern textbook of epidemiology, even excluding the infectious diseases, would be an immense enterprise — and beyond me.

It is a pleasure to thank the MRC Social Medicine Unit, and friends and colleagues at home and across the world who have helped me so generously. Three names I must mention: Miss Jane Cooper of the Department of Community Health who calculated many of the Tables and checked my sums; my Secretary, Miss J. Sullivan, for her infinite patience in preparing draft after draft; Mrs. M. Ong who so cheerfully and meticulously helped with the typing and references.

London, 1974   J. N. MORRIS

ACKNOWLEDGEMENTS

I am greatly obliged for permission to quote material to authors, editors of journals and reports, and publishers, as mentioned in the text: *Acta Cardiologica, Acta Medica Scandinavica,* American Heart Association, *American Journal of Public Health, Archives of Diseases of Childhood, British Journal of Preventive and Social Medicine, British Journal of Venereal Diseases, British Medical Journal, Bulletin of the New York Academy of Medicine,* Department of Health and Social Security, Her Majesty's Stationery Office, *Journal of the American Medical Association, Lancet, Medical Care, New Zealand Medical Journal,* Office of Population Censuses and Surveys, *Proceedings of the Royal Society of Medicine,* The Registrars General, *S. African Medical Journal, The Times,* Tobacco Manufacturers' Standing Committee, World Health Organisation, *Yale Journal of Biology and Medicine;* and others as specified.

J.N.M.

Contents

Introduction

During the nineteenth century death rates in middle age in England and Wales persisted high, but about the turn of the century sanitary reform and the rise in the standard of living began — at last — to show results in this age group. Death rates began to fall, both among men and women, and they continued to fall until the early 1920's. Then, rather abruptly (Fig. 1), there was a change. Mortality in women continued

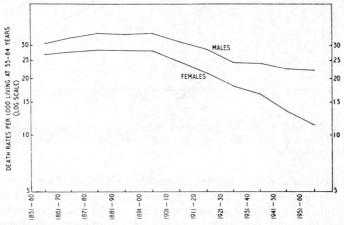

Fig. 1   History of mortality in middle age (55–64) 1850's to 1950's. All causes of death. England and Wales.
   Registrar General, *Statistical Reviews, Part I, Tables Medical.*

downward, but the improvement in men slowed and virtually stopped. A hundred years ago the death rate among middle-aged men was about 15 per cent higher than in women, after the first world war it was about 33 per cent higher, by the late 1950's the male rate was twice the female.

What was happening? The continued decline of mortality among middle-aged women was much as expected: the levelling of the male death rate occurred during years that saw more advances in medical science than all the rest of history. Middle-aged men have benefited from these; their mortality from pneumonia is under half of what it was before the sulphonamides were invented, from phthisis less than a quarter of that in 1946–7, the eve of streptomycin. Mortality from most cancers has fallen. Such gains, however, have been wiped out by other developments.

In particular, two conditions, both of them deadly and affecting men in middle age far more than women, have emerged from obscurity to become exceedingly common: ischaemic heart disease ("coronary thrombosis"), and "lung cancer" — cancer of the bronchus. Figure 2 illustrates the contribution of these to the recent course of mortality; without them, the sex ratio of the 1920's almost is regained. Coronary

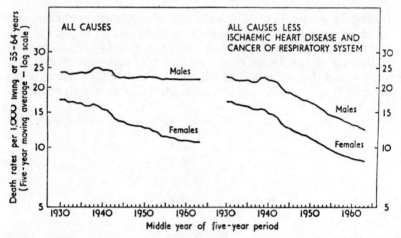

Fig. 2 Mortality in middle age (55–64) 1928–65; the contribution of ischaemic heart disease and lung cancer (the great majority of cancer of respiratory system). England and Wales.

thrombosis and lung cancer thus are modern epidemics. They exemplify the "chronic diseases" that have transformed morbidity as well as mortality and now dominate health-services and the practice of medicine.

Figures 1 and 2 illustrate one *use* of epidemiology, in *historical study,* and its basic method. The unit of observation in epidemiology is the group, or "population" as it is called. This may be the actual population of a country, as here, or any other defined group of people. Deaths, "cases" more generally, are studied only in relation to the group among which they occur. Studying disease, the epidemiologist sometimes starts with patients, then tries to refer them to their population. Characteristically, he starts with a population then seeks all those affected in it.

He has to reach a measure of $\dfrac{\text{cases}}{\text{population}}$, of all affected persons, as these are defined, in the defined population. By virtue of this, the epidemiologist can ask a special kind of question: he is concerned with frequencies, rates of occurrence. Thus all and particular fatalities occurring in the men and women of a specified age in the population of England and Wales, at one time and another, can be counted and the rate of death calculated to describe the historical changes of Figures 1 and 2.

This book is mainly about epidemiology as a way of learning, of asking questions and getting answers that lead to further questions. As a method of study, epidemiology may be contrasted with the clinical observation of patients, or the controlled experiment in the laboratory. In the main, epidemiology is employed in the *study of health and disease of populations.* This is the epidemiology of antiquity and of Farr and Snow, Hirsch and Goldberger; today it is the basic science of preventive and community medicine and is being applied to a variety of problems in health services as well as health. I shall be describing several "uses" of epidemiology in this book, and examples are given of results.

1. Historical Study

Historical statements in medicine are "epidemiological" (or ought to be): they relate to the frequency of events among populations at different points in time. Thus diseases wax and wane (tuberculosis, for example), new ones appear (encephalitis lethargica, asbestos poisoning, LSD psychosis), old ones are eradicated (smallpox), or just fade away (chlorosis, miner's nystagmus). The recent decline of many of the great infections has often been described, and the trends usually are very obvious — enough often in themselves to transform the picture of health and the pattern of health services in a few years. Each speciality has its own examples: ear, nose and throat surgery with scarcely ever a mastoid, GPI almost unknown, no more ringworm clinics, surgical tuberculosis wiped out, fever hospitals almost empty. It is difficult to convey to younger generations what it meant for mine that as late as the year 1941 2,400 children died of diphtheria in this country and there were 50,000 cases.[1][2]

Table 1.1 illustrates from rheumatic heart disease (RHD); alongside "coronary thrombosis", RHD provides a miniature of modern cardiology. It is a contrast in two respects — the steep fall in recent years,

TABLE 1.1

BEGINNING OF THE END? MORTALITY OF CHILDREN FROM RHEUMATIC HEART DISEASE*

Both Sexes ages 5–14 inclusive
Death Rates per 100,000 per Year

Population		1929–33	1946–49
England	County Boroughs	13·4	4·1
and Wales	Urban Districts	11·2	3·7
	Rural Districts	7·9	2·7
South	County Boroughs	17·9	4·2
Wales	Urban Districts	20·1	5·5
	"Rural" Districts	18·8	3·9

*I.e. all the deaths certified to heart disease, except congenital.

Many of the "rural" districts of South Wales are predominantly coal-mining villages.

From Registrar General (*Statistical Reviews,* Part I, Tables Medical) and local Medical Officers of Health.

References on page 285.

and the greater mortality among the poor. When it was common, compare the death rates in South Wales 40 years ago, this was the most "social" of diseases. By now there are too few of these tragedies to continue the comparisons of Table 1.1. During the ten years 1956–65, in fact, there were two deaths from rheumatic fever/heart disease in the children of the big towns of South Wales. The national rate in recent years has been under 1 per 100,000 children. Juvenile rheumatism is disappearing, and no longer can students routinely be initiated into clinical and social medicine, as they were for so many generations, with mitral stenosis and aortic incompetence (the other great cardiac infection also is now rare in this country).

Rheumatic heart disease is a good example of common historical puzzles: there is little doubt that the modern rise in the standard of living is a cause of the decline of "juvenile rheumatism", but this seems to have begun in the middle 1930's, during the Great Depression. It thus followed late in the wake of the decline in virulence of haemolytic streptococcal infection (beginning last century), and anticipated the mass use of sulphonamides beginning in the late 1930's. Latterly, penicillin prophylaxis of recurrent attacks has probably contributed, but I have been unable to get any facts on how often it is being used. In short, a little is understood.[3][7]

Pages 5-7 further illustrate the modern spectacular achievements in *Child Health*. Figure 1.1 includes one of the happiest manifestations of the decline of juvenile rheumatism: By 1957 the prevalence in London of such disability was a tenth of 1928 and London County Council's

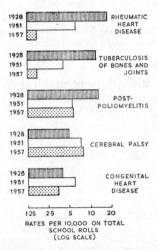

Fig. 1.1 Physically handicapped children in the County of London: prevalence rates in special schools over the period 1928–57. Total rate for all causes was 64 per 10,000 schoolchildren in 1928, 41 in 1951, 30 in 1957.

Palmer, W. T. & Pirrie, D. (1958) *Brit. med. J.* **2**, 1326.

special health and educational services which, before the 1939–45 war, provided a model for the world have been dismantled*. Glasgow has a notorious housing problem; I should have illustrated that also in Table 1.2 and the valiant if so far only moderately successful efforts to deal with it. But Glasgow is the right context in which to mention

TABLE 1.2
HEALTH OF GLASGOW SCHOOLCHILDREN, 1910–69

(1) Averages, per cent, ages 5–13/14 inclusive.

| | CLEANLINESS | | CLOTHING | | FOOTGEAR | |
| Period | Verminous | | Insuf-ficient | Ragged and dirty | Unsatis-factory | None |
	Heads	Bodies				
1910–19	20·3	2·8	1·3	5·9	2·3	5·2
1930–39	6·7	0·2	0·1	0·5	0·4	0·0
1960–69	6·5	0·1	0·04	0·1	0·1	0·0

(2) Average Heights and Weights
Inches and Pounds

| | Boys | | | | Girls | | | |
| Period | Aged 5 yrs | | Aged 13 yrs | | Aged 5 yrs | | Aged 13 yrs | |
	Ht	Wt	Ht	Wt	Ht	Wt	Ht	Wt
1910–19	40·4	38·5	55·2	74·5	39·7	37·7	55·5	76·8
1930–39	41·3	39·7	56·8	81·6	41·0	38·3	57·7	85·9
1960–69	42·6	42·4	60·0	96·6	42·3	41·3	60·2	101·8

Ewan, J. (1957) *The School Health Service*, Glasgow; Menzies, M. P., Glasgow, Public Health Department, personal communications.

another modern revolution in public health (I shall be using the term "modern" for the period since the second world war). Initiated by wartime policy, the virtual disappearance of gross nutritional deficiencies is as dramatic as the decline in infections. Rickets was epidemic in Victorian Britain and rife till the 1930's, particularly among the poor of industrial towns.[8] In the native child, rickets now turns up occasionally on the metabolic ward.[9] The record with childhood anaemia is almost as good. Part (2) on the growth of the children, another general "health

---

*In 1964 there were 76 such "rheumatic" children in all the special schools for the physically handicapped in England and Wales. Cerebral palsy in 1970 accounted for the largest number (2,944), but itself may be overtaken by the rising prevalence of children with spina bifida – 1,533 in 1970, a thousand more than in 1964 – before the wave of operations is over. There is of course growing pressure to send "handicapped" children to ordinary schools but this is unlikely to have affected the rheumatism figures by very much.

indicator", gives an overall view of the improvement in nutrition, though averages without the distributions, for example by social class, are of limited value. [10] [11]

I have intentionally let this stand from the last edition. "The reappearance of rickets in Glasgow gave rise to considerable anxiety. Rickets disappeared from the city in the post-war years, and only in 1959 did the number of (hospital-clinical) cases begin to increase again until in 1963 there were 10 cases of marked rickets, and in 1964, 38 cases (in native children). It is particularly in the poorer areas of Glasgow that rickets has occurred, where overcrowding and large families are common (and the smoke pall kept the sun out). In addition, many of these children suffer from anaemia due to lack of iron in their diets. Surveys have shown that in certain areas of the city many babies were being given liquid cow's milk as early as the second week of life. The results of these investigations led to a city-wide campaign." Since then a few cases have been recognised each year.

From *Annual Reports* of the Medical Officer of Health; and Miller, A. R., personal communications. [12]

HAS HEALTH IMPROVED?

By now I hope such a question will read as absurd as the "inevitability of progress". There are so many aspects of health; norms and expectations are redefined; people, behaviour and environment are always changing. [13] So many new adaptations have to be made. There were virtually no cigarettes or motor-cars last century. The first appearance can be dated of DDT in body-fat, of strontium-90 in bones. During the 1960's some 30 million women across the world took to the Pill. . . I wondered, Table 1.3, page 8, whether "sickness-absence", incapacity for work attributed to sickness, another of the established health indicators,* had fallen with the modern rise in living standards, decline of infectious disease, and remarkable fall of mortality at most working ages, part (1). When he advised the Beveridge Committee during the second world war, the Government Actuary forecast an increase in incapacity of $12\frac{1}{2}$ per cent because of improved social security benefits. He was writing before the antibiotics were discovered — yet proved uncannily right, part (2). Sickness-absence rates in men showed no improvement in the population-at-large or in special groups, like those illustrated, where employment, social-security and industrial-medical provision were relatively stable. Only in children (3) do the figures show the improvement I had hoped to find, and school-absence figures are particularly hard to interpret.

There are two main lines of explanation for what might have happened among the adults. Common everyday sickness is due mostly to conditions which as yet are little amenable to treatment. The figures moreover will reflect a multitude of communal pressures, the norms of the day about taking time off, unemployment often pushing the figures down, but full employment and high wages letting them rise.

*The term "health indicator" increasingly is employed to describe statistics on an important aspect of health and its trends that, possibly, also give some indication of what lies ahead.

TABLE 1.3
BEFORE AND AFTER THE THERAPEUTIC REVOLUTION

(1) *Mortality*

	Ages					
	15–	20–	25–	35–	45–	55–64
1927	2·6	3·3	3·8	6·6	11·9	25·0
1954–5	0·9	1·2	1·3	2·7	7·9	22·3

Death Rate per 1,000 men per year

Britain.

(2) *Sickness-absence*
Weeks of Medically Certified Incapacity for Work per Insured Man
(First six months only of such absences are included)

	Ages					
	16–	20–	25–	35–	45–	55–64
1927	0·8	0·8	0·8	0·9	1·2	1·9
1954–5	0·8	0·9	0·9	1·0	1·4	2·2

Estd. Britain.

London Policemen
Average Absent Because of Sickness, per 100 Men

	Ages				
	–25	25–	30–	40–	50+
1936–8	2·2	1·9	2·1	2·6	3·3
1955–7	3·1	2·8	2·7	3·1	3·4

Post Office
Days of Sickness-Absence per Man

1935–8	9·0
1946–9	11·8
1950–3	13·9
1954–7	12·6

Established staff, excluding registered "disabled persons". Britain.

(3) *Absence from school*
Average Absent in January of Each Year per 100 Children

	Infants	7–11 yrs		11–14/15 yrs	
		Boys	Girls	Boys	Girls
1936–8	16·0	10·7	12·3	10·6	13·7
1956–8	12·8	7·4	8·0	8·1	9·3

Birmingham.

Annual Reports of Ministry of Pensions and National Insurance (now Social Security), Metropolitan Police, The Post Office Medical Service, General Register Offices, Birmingham LEA; and personal communications.

RISE OF. . .

Historical questions whether there has been a rise in some disorders comparable to the decline of infectious diseases and undernutrition are often more difficult to answer. There was no doubt about casualties (e.g. head injuries) in road-vehicle accidents, though in fact the accident-rate per vehicle-mile, Table 1.4 overleaf, even in 1966 was less than the 1930's. There *was* little argument over epidemic polio, retrolental fibroplasia, asthma deaths[14] [15] (history moved fast), and today none about self poisoning in young women[16] [18] asbestos mesothelioma,[19] salmonella infections (large-scale food processing?). Many questions, however, interesting and important questions, for clinical medicine and for health services, are so bedevilled by uncertainties about nomenclature and diagnosis over the years that no categorical answer can be given. Consider these figures of sickness-absence, given by doctors about fellow doctors, and only fifteen years apart:

	No. of cases 1937	1952
Muscular rheumatism	18	7
Fibrositis	17	11
Lumbago, sciatica, sacroiliac strain	47	29
Prolapsed intervertebral disc	0	35
Total	82	82

Medical Sickness Annuity and Life Assurance Society Ltd.

This is a population among whom the vaguest (but perhaps most valid) diagnoses like "low back pain" are unwelcome. It is not necessary to believe that "discs" are a consequence of man's upright posture to question. . . John Graunt* certainly would have wondered — whether the "disease did first appear about that time; or whether a Disease, which had been long before, did then first receive its Name?" So can fashions in labelling distort the statistics (Graunt's law). "Myocardial degeneration" and "neurasthenia" are unacceptable terms today, which accounts for part probably of the recorded increase of "coronary thrombosis", some of the numerous diagnoses of "depression". Commonly, valid numerical estimates of the frequency in any period are lacking: among a thousand similar persons, how many cases *as defined* were found at one time and another. Or, and this is the crux of it, how frequently have new cases been arising (the "incidence")?

Each civilisation, Sigerist has said, makes its own diseases. But it has many ways of going about it: I will illustrate only with simple examples from modern changes.

*Graunt, J. (1662) *Natural and Political Observations made upon the Bills of Mortality*. London. See: Report of the Medical Officer of Health London County Council for 1957; Sutherland, I. (1963), *J. R. statist. Soc. Ser. A 126*, 537; Glass, D. V. (1963), *Proc. Roy. Soc. B 159*, 1.

TABLE 1.4

CASUALTIES FROM ROAD ACCIDENTS SINCE 1938

Both Sexes—All Ages—Britain

Year	Population (millions)	Index of Motor Traffic	Killed	Numbers Seriously Injured	Slightly Injured	Total Casualties
1938	46·2	100	6,648	51,000	176,000	233,000
1949	49·0	100	4,773	43,000	129,000	177,000
1955–7 (av.)	49·8	171	5,481	62,000	202,000	270,000
1961	51·4	263	6,908	85,000	258,000	350,000
1966	53·4	372	7,985	100,000	285,000	392,000
1967	53·6	391	7,319	94,000	269,000	370,000
1968	53·9	410	6,810	89,000	254,000	349,000
1970	54·3	444	7,499	93,000	262,000	363,000
1972	54·2	494	7,779	91,000	261,000	360,000*
1974						

*Under 15 years: 896 killed, 15,459 seriously, and 48,044 slightly injured.

"Breathalyser" tests for alcohol were introduced in Oct. 1967. Official estimate of lives saved 1967–70 is 3,815.

Road Accidents. Annually. HMSO, London; *Road Accident Statistical Review,* Royal Society for the Prevention of Accidents, Monthly, and personal communications; *Amer. behav. Sci.* (1970) *13,* 493; Feinstein, A. R. (1973). *Clin. Pharm. Therap., 14,* 462.

Relative Increase

This is the first thing to settle: Is the increase only relative? The death rate from congenital anomalies among male infants in England and Wales was 5 per thousand in the 1920's and a little under 4·0 in the early 1970's; the total mortality fell in the same period from 81 to 20 or so. Congenital malformation now accounts for about a fifth of the male infant death rate compared with about five per cent in the 1920's. The IMR from congenital malformation has in fact fallen; but this is not how it will look to paediatricians concerned with grave disease in infancy. Handicap from *congenital* heart disease among the children of London did not actually increase during the thirty years (page 5), but relative to *rheumatic* heart disease it did. Sorsby writes:

"Each solution brings its own problems. The latter end of the nineteenth century eliminated the residue of blindness due to such mass infections as smallpox and trachoma, bringing into relief the more individual infective causes of blindness such as ophthalmia neonatorum and congenital syphilis. These were being brought under control by public health measures in the first third of the present century, and the therapeutic revolution brought about by the sulphonamides and antibiotics in the 1930's and 1940's helped to reduce them to statistical insignificance. The consequences of these developments were the bolder relief into which the genetic and constitutional causes of blindness were thrown . . . cataract, glaucoma, the classical hereditary diseases . . ."[22]

Onion Principle. — Because some conditions have become less common others now are more important: this is responsible for much of the changing picture of community health, for many of our "new" problems. Killing diseases recede and the burden of non-lethal morbidity has now to be contained. Reduce physical disease in childhood and widespread maladjustment can no longer be ignored. As the "crowd diseases" have declined personal infections came to the fore. When environmental casualties are controlled genetic failures receive more attention. The lives of mothers and children are now protected, so public health activities can also be focused on old people. Abolish subsistence poverty and not merely widespread material hardship but widespread psychological impoverishment and other social under-privilege are exposed. A population that is preoccupied with physical survival cannot be much concerned with the quality of life. . . Problems solved surely are simpler than problems persisting; which is some consolation in our sea of troubles, in face of the open-ended demand for medical care.

Absolute Increase

Is the number of cases of. . . in fact greater? If so, is the disease commoner per head of population? Are new cases arising more often? The answers matter, if differently, to health and health services and to the understanding of both. Clinical impressions usually are the first indication, but they have to be tested in population statistics.

In Discovery But Not Disease. — Merely to find more of the cases there are, will swell numbers and rates. Including the coroner's as well the hospital cases of ruptured heart multiplied the rate for London several fold. The additional ECG leads increased the recognition of anterior infarcts. Energetic search in the population could readily double the known diabetics. Discovery of venous thrombosis at necropsy seems largely to depend on the search for it (newly important in assessing the risks of the Pill). We see the syndromes we are looking for — "battered babies", for example? Better diagnosis quite likely accounts for the evident increase of ruptured cerebral aneurysm or of phaeo-chromocytoma. . . New interest in an old condition, and the cases multiply. Hashimoto's disease — suddenly — was in the limelight, everywhere. . . A new description — prolapsed intervertebral disc, or school phobia — and the diagnosis is commonplace; no one thinks the actual syndromes are new, and it would be frightfully difficult to determine whether they are any commoner. . .Changing definitions will change the situation: labelling "hypertensive" the top third of the distribution instead of the top quarter, or lowering the nationally "recommend nutritional allowances". Officially, since 1 April 1971, *no* children in this country are "ineducable". "We can have as much or as little crime as we please, depending on what we choose to count as criminal".

In Disease, But Not Frequency. — Greater numbers of people-at-risk will by itself mean a real increase in the volume of disease. Every week in England and Wales two thousand are added to the population over 65 years of age, more liable to dementia, stroke, blindness, osteoarthrosis, fractured neck of femur,* poverty, loneliness, and the other afflictions of old age.

In Frequency, But Not Incidence. — Treatment can increase the number of survivors and thus the prevalence of a disease in the population; today this is among the most direct effects of medicine on society. Fewer with Down's syndrome are born (the incidence has fallen), but the total living at 10–14 years of age, their *prevalence,* is several times what it was in the 1930's before the sulphonamides were invented,[23-25] making difficult demands on clinical, special education, and social services (cf. Fig. 1.1).† Several hundred survivors with severe brain damage from head injuries, and unable to work, are added annually to the population.[26]

Modern Epidemics

Here are three measures from our own studies of the *increase in incidence* of ischaemic heart disease (IHD). They refer to men aged 45–64 and are per year:[27-29]

(1) *First clinical episodes per* 1,000 *London busmen, presentation as "sudden death":* the increase from 1949–52 to 1959–66 = 75 per cent.

(2) *First clinical episodes per* 1,000 *insurance salesmen, all presentations* of the disease: the increase from 1954–6 to 1958–60 = 83 per cent.

(3) *First clinical episodes per* 1,000 *physicians: all presentations* increased between 1957–60 and 1961–5 by 23 per cent, *presentation as "sudden death"* by 26 per cent.

These rates have been standardised, adjusted, to allow for differences over the years in the age composition of the populations-at-risk. In each study, the data were collected in a uniform way throughout.

Figure 1.2 presents indicators rather than accurate measurements of the history of ischaemic heart disease and mortality provides only a blurred picture of incidence. But the consistency of necropsy records in many hospitals impresses;[30] and the continued increase in these certified death rates anyhow until the late 1960's, long after IHD became widely known among certifying doctors. In the end, however, the kind of "hard" evidence presented in Figures 1 and 2 of the book may be the most convincing. As a result of much study, it has to be

*However, female "admissions" over 65 years of age for this to NHS hospitals were 327 per 100,000 in 1961, and 547 in 1972, an increase not simply explained by the age-structure. Treatment fashions and opportunities?

†Cf. also *patients aged 55 years plus in mental subnormality hospitals:* 1954—5,341; 1963—10,934; 1972—13,340. England and Wales.

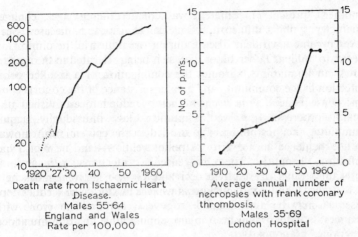

Fig. 1.2 Two indicators of the rise of ischaemic heart disease in middle age.
Registrar General (log scale); and Morris, J. N. (1951) *Lancet* 1, 1, 69.

postulated that there has been a true rise in incidence of IHD during
this century: apart from the decline of cardiac infections, exceeding
medical alertness to the condition, the spread of electrocardiography,
the broadening of the clinical picture, the ageing of the population;
apart from all these possible confounding factors. Such a proposition
obviously raises fundamental questions. The rapid rise of a mass
disease must be due to mass changes in life-style, the introduction of
widespread new pathogens, maladaptation to social change. How have
these, and ineffectual population defences, been translated into biology,
metabolic disorder, lethal disease, epidemics?

Lung Cancer: Mid-century Outbreak. — The issues are the same, if
clearer.[31] The diagnosis of lung-cancer has become easier, of course,
as the true nature of "mediastinal sarcoma" was appreciated, confounding pulmonary infections declined, X-rays and bronchoscopy
multiplied. The contrast in the statistics between the mortality of
men (who began mass-smoking of cigarettes during the 1914-18 war,
and even earlier in the century) and women (starting later and smoking
less) disposed of lingering doubts. The more it is found in men, of
course, the more will be the inclination to seek and diagnose it in them;
but this could scarcely be responsible for so large a sex differential in
the modern increase. (N.B., because of the case fatality-rate of lung
cancer, mortality is near enough the same as incidence.)

Even more modern epidemics, too recent to possess a history, is the
business of the next chapter.

CHANGES IN NATURAL HISTORY

Diseases wax and wane. They also vary in severity from one period to another, "present" in different ways or at different ages, change in character: syphilis, influenza, dengue and cholera, to name a few. Scarlet fever became a virulent disease during the industrial revolution, then began to milden. Tuberculous disease is being relegated to the aged, and to Asian immigrants, through the combination of a smaller pool of infection in the community and greater resistance of the cohorts coming on: consequences of new chemotherapy added to established public health progress. Improved sanitation, less individually acquired immunity, and postponed exposure led to the epidemic shift upwards in age-incidence and severity of poliomyelitis — and now of Type A infectious hepatitis. The emergence of infections with antibiotic-resistant strains of staphylococci and Gram-negative organisms are new hazards, and goodness knows what is in store: the term "hospital disease" may be appropriated from last century. The mode of life changes; so do organisms; so do populations, their immunity and reactions.[32-34]

Coronary Artery Disease

Occlusion, and massive coronary *thrombosis* have become commoner during the present century,[29][30] but there is no evidence of any corresponding increase in the underlying and long well-known coronary *atheroma,* Table 1·5. (In close to 100 per cent of the 530 serial, unselected, necropsies of deaths from injuries, etc. some mural lesions were reported . . . and so on.) The disappearance of "ossified", "pipe-stem" arteries from routine necropsy experience confirms that calcification of the intimal lesions is less common. The character of the *modern* epidemic of coronary disease can be postulated more specifically in terms of occlusive not merely "arterial" disease.

Mental Disorders

There is no evidence of any overall increase of insanity as "civilisation" advances, a controversial issue since the French Revolution. [20] Historical questions on the frequency of the psychoneuroses are particularly hopeless of direct answer, and what clues there are come mainly from imaginative writers and the social historian. The diagnosis, what is regarded as "neurotic" behaviour, depends so much on contemporary norms, the attitudes to mental illness and the availability of treatment. But changes in incidence could also mean no more than a difference in presentation because society no longer responds to a particular way of asking for help. So other psychological defences are raised, and there is a new pattern of symptoms, though the underlying conflicts may remain the same. Swooning girls are fewer than in Victorian times; but more may be depressed, drug-dependent, try to poison themselves, get pregnant, drop out. Sixty years ago in the East End of London unruly boys threw stones at horses, before the 1939–45 war they stole cycles, now they "take and drive away" motor cars. "Shell-shock", motor hysteria and effort syndrome, were epidemic in the

TABLE 1.5
RECENT HISTORY OF CORONARY DISEASE: TWO PROCESSES

Men aged 45–59
Rates per Cent

Coronary Arteries (n)	Deaths from Injuries, Infections Cancer, etc.*		Deaths from Hypertension, Cerebrovascular Disease, etc.†	
	1908–13 (530)	1954–6 (1,394)	1908–13 (87)	1954–6 (292)
Mural atheroma				
Some/little	c.100	c.100	c.100	c.100
Moderate	} 53	} 34	36	32
Much			40	30
Calcification present	19	10	26	22
Lumen stenosis	4·2	13	10	28
Including occlusion of a main artery	0·8	2·1	1·1	5·5
Ischaemic myocardial fibrosis				
Reported present‡	1·3	4·4	3·4	17

1908–13, London Hospital. 1954–6, National Necropsy Survey; the modern London Hospital data are similar. (Number of cases in brackets.)

*Not specially associated with atherosclerosis/coronary disease.

†Specially associated.

‡Average annual number of necropsies with fatal *ischaemic heart disease* (recent coronary thrombosis and/or myocardial infarction) in males aged 45–59, the London Hospital: 1908–13 = 1·2, and 1954–8 = 4·2.

Morris, J. N. (1951) *Lancet 1*, 1, 69; Morris, J. N. & Crawford, M. D. (1958) *Brit. med. J. 2*, 1485; (1961) *Lancet, 1*, 47.

first world war; anxiety-depression, "battle fatigue" and dyspepsia in the second. A new public sophistication, different community expectations during World War II — some behaviour abnormalities even were regarded sympathetically — these provide some explanation of how people reacted, and broke down, in different ways.[21] [35] As well as estimates of "rise" and "fall", the useful model for historical study will allow for varieties of expression of disorder and the exchange of one for another.

The "unchanging human heart"? It is hard to believe that neurotic disorders are merely changing in style, in the choice of language that will communicate distress. Surely, enough social and cultural, including familial, changes are under way to alter the character of psychological disorder? Male/female roles are in flux; the age, frequency and standards of marriage have shifted; society is child-centred, children are reared more permissively and less confidently and in the West far fewer are grossly deprived. Religion is in retreat; attitudes to work are softening;

sexuality is little repressed by comparison with last century; aggression, whether there is more of it or not, in crime, politics and everyday life, is more openly acknowledged, with prolific expression in public fantasy. We've scarcely a clue to how television is conditioning people.[36-40]

Health Services

Patients with psychotic illness are now regarded differently, allowed to take care of themselves as much as they can, isolated less; social relationships are encouraged and return to community life outside. The new drugs are a great help. The patients respond to the more therapeutic "moral" environment, withdraw less, are not so liable to deteriorate — thus changing the clinical picture. Psychotic illness is becoming milder and quieter, there is less catatonia and violence in schizophrenia, less apathy, hostility, loss of identity.[41 42]

Health services are altering the character of many chronic conditions which are not cured but may be dragged into a more or less steady-state despite the grossest tissue destruction; Addison's disease, for example, and pernicious anaemia, Graves' disease, severe hypertension, chronic bronchitis and emphysema, ulcerative colitis. Extended survival now superimposes the natural process of growth on spina bifida, of ageing on severe subnormality — producing new clinical pictures.

REMARKABLE HISTORY OF DUODENAL ULCER

In Victorian England, peptic ulcer commonly took the form of acute gastric ulcer in young women, a condition rarely seen nowadays. Since the turn of the century, duodenal ulcer (DU) has become common as a chronic disease of men, and it reached epidemic proportions in the 1930's and 1940's.[43-46] A survey just after the war, mainly in London, showed that by the time they reached age 55, about 6 per cent of men have suffered from DU.[47 48] Since the middle 1950's, however, and as mysteriously as it arrived, DU has been receding, Table 1.6.

An improvement, evidently. But is there a fall in the *frequency* of ulcer (in proportion of the population contracting it), or a reduction merely in *severity* among those affected — a change brought about possibly by better treatment? Mortality is falling (1), but improving medical care makes this a poor indicator of secular trends in a disease that anyhow kills few of its victims. The burden on hospitals, the rate of perforation, haematemesis and melaena (2) also have fallen, if not impressively, but mass partial gastrectomy in the 1950's* may have freed many from the risk of complication. Sickness-absence in industry is lower (3): judging by the long average spells of incapacity, victims of ulcer now are "signed off work" only in serious circumstances, so this could be a clue. There is no means of settling the question in the

---

*During 1953-9, about 20,000 elective operations for ulcer were done annually on men, two-thirds of them for DU.

TABLE 1.6
RECENT HISTORY OF PEPTIC ULCER
Rates per 100,000 per Year   Men Aged 45–64

(1) Mortality

	Gastric ulcer	Duodenal ulcer
1922–4	16·9	9·1
1930–2	26·3	14·1
1940–2	33·2	19·2
1950–2	17·1	17·8
1960–2	7·5	9·2
1970–2	4·2	5·6

Registrar General, England and Wales.

(2) Admissions to Hospital

	Total Peptic ulcer	Perforation GU	DU	"Cold" surgery GU	DU	Haematemesis and Melaena GU	DU
1956	478	16	55	84	126	—	—
1959	412	16	40	70	78	58	66
1962	428	13	32	64	105	54	70
1966	362	9	32	44	100	37	54
1972	299						

Hospital In-patient Enquiry. England and Wales. HMSO, London; and persona communications.

(3) Sickness-Absence

	Spells of sickness GU	DU	Gastritis etc.	Days of incapacity GU	DU	Gastritis, etc.
1954/5	600	450	1,310	38,000	30,000	29,000
1956/7	520	380	1,260	27,000	23,000	25,000
1966/7	430	340	1,210	23,000	19,000	23,000
1968/9	410	360	1,070	23,000	20,000	20,000
1970/1	350	300	930	24,000	15,000	18,000

MPNI & Dept. of Health & Social Security, *Annual Reports* and personal communications. "Gastric" ulcer in these figures is probably used sometimes as a general term for "peptic" ulcer.

absence of population rates over the years of *new* cases, *first* attacks, first spells, i.e. of the *incidence,* the basic and critical figure in all epidemiology and about as difficult a fact to pin down in DU as in any of the chronic diseases.

A study among doctors has shown a sharp reduction in *first spells of incapacity from duodenal ulcer* since the late 1940's:[49]

Ages	Annual Rates per 1,000 Men		
	1947–50	1957–60	1961–5
35–44	1·9	1·3	0·7
45–54	2·5	1·0	1·0
55–64	2·0	1·7	1·3

Spells of sickness-absence lasting at least 6 days.
SMU and Medical Sickness Annuity and Life Assurance Society Ltd.

That there has been a true decline in incidence is the most interesting possibility. This would suggest to anyone in sympathy with "psychosomatic" theories, and there are none better for mass DU,[49-51] that the type of personality disposed to the disease is less common — unfortunately not a testable proposition; that the environment is less of a strain — which is scarcely conceivable; or that under stress men react differently. Have other functional disorders that might be "equivalent" taken over? Overt anxiety? The ubiquitous depression? Migraine? Spells of sickness-absence, however labelled? Alcohol? Pill-taking,* one or several of these? As coronary thrombosis is so widespread there will be smaller gain from mere ulcer "sick role". For many, as said, the current pace of culture change may be far too fast for comfort, so changes in the incidence and presentation of psychosomatic disorders, too, should not surprise.

HISTORY OF POPULATION; AGEING

A basic fact in any diagnosis of changing medical and social needs is the ageing of the population, and this is only to be understood from history. Two movements have to be distinguished.[52-55]

1. During the second half of the nineteenth century the number of liveborn children in England and Wales rose steeply, from about 550,000 a year in the 1840's to about 940,000 a year in the early 1900's. In general, there was no worsening of death rates; so during the present century the *number* of old people in the population has risen steeply.

2. After the early 1900's the number of births fell, reaching their lowest point, about 580,000, in 1933 and again in 1941; as it moves up the age scale, therefore, the great Victorian and Edwardian cohort is being replaced by far smaller families. So during the present century the

---

*Prescriptions for hypnotics, tranquillisers, etc., issued by general practitioners increased from 2·3 millions monthly in 1962 to 3·8 millions in 1972. There are no earlier data.

proportion of old people in the population has risen steeply — from under 5 per cent to nearly 13 per cent.

I have referred to the number of births. This is what matters here, not the "birth rate" per thousand of the population (or of the women aged 15–44). With the spread of birth control, the birth *rate* in fact stopped rising in the 1870's and it began to fall in the 1880's; but this was not reflected in a fall in the actual *number* of births till after the turn of the century.

Foresight

Catastrophes apart, the first of these two movements, the growing number of old people, may be expected to continue till 1981 and 1991, as shown in Table 1.7. The future of the second movement, literal meaning of "ageing" of the population, cannot be forecast with such confidence — there are no simple figures to extrapolate. The proportion of old people is now rising very slowly and, very likely, will so continue during the 1970's to reach 13 per cent. What happens then will depend mainly on what happens meanwhile to births. Table 1.7 has to be based on predictions about the future of births, deaths and migration, that are safe only on deaths and virtually speculation on births. After the postwar peak of just over 880,000 live births in 1947 (birth rate, 20.5 per 1,000), the number fell to about 670,000 in 1955; B.R., 15·0. Then, in

TABLE 1.7
RECENT, PRESENT AND "FUTURE" POPULATION OF ENGLAND AND WALES

Thousands

Ages	1971(1) M	F	1981(2) M	F	1991(2) M	F	2001(2) M	F
0–14	11,764 (100)		11,192* (95)		12,170* (103)		12,711* (108)	
15–44	18,754 (100)		20,962 (112)		22,116 (118)		22,914 (122)	
45–64	11,765 (100)		11,012 (94)		10,885 (93)		12,112 (103)	
65–74	1,712 (100)	2,388 (100)	1,938 (113)	2,568 (108)	1,889 (110)	2,465 (103)	1,792 (105)	2,249 (94)
75+	705 (100)	1,516 (100)	881 (125)	1,873 (124)	1,005 (143)	2,094 (138)	1,020 (145)	2,123 (140)
All ages	48,604 (100)		50,426 (104)		52,624 (108)		54,921 (113)	

(1) *Census 1971, Advance Analysis.* HMSO, London.
(2) *Population Projections No. 3, 1972–2012.* HMSO, London.
Proportion of 1971 in brackets. Projections in *italics*.
*Many or all unborn in 1971.

one of the phenomenal turnabouts of the mid-1950's, births again began to increase, reaching 876,000 by 1964, a rate of 18·6 per 1,000. Since then, the number has been falling again to an estimated 641,000 in 1974 (B.R., 13·0 per 1,000). The Pill? Fading hope of a home? Concern about over-population? Other countries with enviably better economic records are having a similar experience. The indications are that the 1955-64 boom in births was due mostly to earlier marriage, and more rapid child-bearing — "borrowing" from the future — quite little to an increase in the size of families (to an average of 2·4 or 2·5 children), so unlikely to last. Now there seems to be a postponement, anyhow of first births. The peak post World War II birth cohort have arrived at their fertile twenties; but birth rates are falling among them also, so that the larger number of women is not in fact bearing more children.[56]

Age Structure of the Population

Here are the main facts:

Population of England and Wales, 1871–1971

	TOTAL	–15 years	65+years			
			Nos.		Per cent of total population	
			M	F	M	F
1871	20,066	7,150	423	509	2·1	2·5
1901	32,528	10,546	661	857	2·0	2·6
1931	39,952	9,521	1,273	1,691	3·2	4·2
1971	48,604	11,764	2,417	3,904	5·0	8·0

(Thousands)
Census figures

Numbers of old people have more than quadrupled this century. We are the oldest population ever, the presence of a large army of the retired is something new in history. For health administrators, as distinct from pensions, the main fact is of the over 75's, the age of disability and the increase in their numbers from 1901 is even greater: fourfold in men, fivefold in women. Since 1939 the number of these "old-olds" has more than doubled, to more than two millions now, Table 1.7; and the number will continue to grow, as "projected" in the Table, with inevitable increase in multiple physical and mental infirmities in the population, in the number of old folk we may expect to be poor, dependent, housebound, bedfast. Their own children, now in middle-age, who will be looking after these old-olds have increased less than half as much (reflecting the fall in the size of families) and their numbers are unlikely to increase in the rest of the century. The not quite five per cent of the population aged 75+ occupy close on 25 per cent of hospital beds at any one time and just over 75 per cent of the places in local authority Communal Homes. Yet most of the serious disability in the old-olds is contained at home, by the family. A change in familial attitudes, scattering of families, and a rise in effective demand from the greater numbers-to-be could overwhelm the services — as is already happening in the retirement towns round the coasts ("political arithmetic").

Death Rates and Population

The course of mortality also has varied and, at the least, I must consider its *decline among young people*. In the second half of the nineteenth century there was a substantial reduction in their death rate from tuberculosis and alimentary infections, results of higher living standards and sanitary reform. This improvement has continued; here are some illustrations (together with recent figures for completeness):

Average Annual Death Rates

Per 1,000 Males in the Population of Specific Ages

	IMR*	5–9	15–19	25–34
1851–70	168	8·4	6·4	9·8
1891–1900	168	4·3	3·8	6·8
1906–10	129	3·3	3·0	5·3
1921–5	86	2·6	2·7	4·1
1966–70	21	0·42	0·96	1·0

*Infant mortality rate: deaths before the first birthday per 1,000 live births occurring in the year. The IMR averaged just under 160 from 1871 to 1890.

Up to now, the improvement of death rates at younger ages has had little effect on the age structure of the population. However grand an achievement, a decline of mortality in children, on these statistics, can increase only be little the number of survivors who will live, most of them, to old age. The near 50 per cent drop in the death rate at 5–9 years of age from 8·4 to 4·3 per thousand, reduced the number of deaths in a thousand boys by four, and increased the number of survivors by four, from 991·6 to 995·7. That is to say, the size of the cohort moving onward has hardly been affected. Big gains in the number of survivors from falling death rates were not achieved till after the turn of the century when *infant* mortality, a different order of magnitude, began — at last — to improve; and it is only now that these saved infants are reaching old age. The decline of mortality in the 19th century has been a factor in the twentieth century's growing number of old people, but it matters less than the increase of births.

Expectation of Life

Looking at these mortality figures a slightly different way, to provide another health indicator, there has been a spectacular increase in the *expectation of life* of young people during this century.[55] At birth the increase is as much as 20 years, to reach an average expectancy now of 68·9 in men and 75·1 in women. For age 35, the average future lifetime at the beginning of the century was 31 years (male) and 33 (female); by 1970–2 these figures have become 36·6 years and 42·2. The figures for the middle-aged have also risen, only by little in men, however (cf. pages 1–2).

For example:

Expectation of Life at 60

On Mortality Experience of	Men	Women
1901–10	13·5 years	15·0 years
1920–2	14·4	16·2
1970–2	15·3	19·9

Because of the decline in death rates, among the young in particular, more people are surviving to old age. Having "arrived", longevity is changing little. A hundred years ago, life expectancy at three-score and ten was 8·4 years in men and 9·0 in women, fifty years later, in 1920–2, 8·8 years in men, 10·0 in women; the corresponding averages now, fifty years on, plus the golden age of scientific medicine, plus considerable social achievements, are 9·4 and 12·5. The small gains at this age are often extended survival, snatch victories by antibiotics and the rest, setting medicine and society intractable ethical and practical problems in caring for the partly living. There is little support in such figures, for the notion that old people are now appreciably "healthier", more vigorous.* Of course many now reaching old age formerly would not. A hundred years ago in England and Wales a quarter of those born reached 70; on current experience, a little over half the males

---

*How much is realistically to be expected at this period of life? The control of cancer (by immunology?) and the prevention of coronary heart disease (by more sensible behaviour?) would each add some years overall. The approximation (downward) of male to female death rates would transform the quality of life in old age. There may be little improvement in *health*, however, until radical discoveries are made in slowing the processes of ageing through the mode of life and/or medicines, or (SF) in artificial organs and transplants.[45] Meanwhile, the control of hypertension looks promising for the prevention of cerebrovascular disease; treatment of disorders in the elderly before they lead to a crisis beyond repair is a sensible hope; and the wisdom that exercise of faculties, physical, mental and social, is needed for the *health of old people*, as of everybody, too often remains to be applied. In England and Wales, a lifetime of deprivation is unlikely to be so common in the future, and this should reduce the inequalities in local death rates.

and close on three-quarters of the females will do so; many, most of them, surely, already carrying some significant pathology if not yet handicapped. An epidemiologist of health must also point out without being able to explain that, as at many ages, male death rates among the elderly in Scandinavia are substantially lower than ours. For example: in 1970, the standardised rate at ages 65 and over (not a very good statistic) per 1,000 in men was 59 in Sweden and 63 in Norway (65 in the Netherlands), but 78 in this country. As expected, the female rates were closer, ranging only from 39 in Sweden to 45 here. Within England there are substantial differences: in 1958–64 for example, at 65–74 years, the rates were 50(M) and 28(F) per 1,000 in Reading, 69 and 36 in Middlesbrough.

Sex Ratio

Where mortality, including losses in wars, strongly affects British demographic patterns is in gender, the sex ratio as it is called. The death rate is higher among males at all ages*, the greatest excess being at 15–19, motor-cycles mainly, and 55–64, for very different reasons. Male conceptuses greatly exceed female, this is the biological rule; but by birth the sex ratio of the population, M;F, is just over 1. The ratio falls gradually, and the numbers of men and women equalise at the middle forties. Throughout the usual marrying ages, therefore, there is a slight excess of males. The sex ratio then falls steeply, and over 75 years of age is less than 0·5:1 As many as a sixth of the very old ladies have never married (the slaughter of young men in the 1914–18 war will be recalled) and three-quarters of the remainder are widowed; together these women are at the greatest risk of needing institutional care, for example, and they occupy nearly half the places in communal homes.[58-60]

So I must leave this historical introduction to population and to the social policy of old age, the largest of all "client groups". If only for thinking ahead, it is necessary to identify the inderlying historical trends. A few things, at least, are certain.

NUMBERS AND MISERY

After this glance at our own recent history, I must mention if quite inadequately, what is the world's biggest problem in population, mankind's biggest problem it could be said. The example chosen, an island and not among the most backward (as exemplified in the quality of its statistics), is a miniature of the "population explosion" — and the other problems facing the new nations, mass poverty, malnutrition, the drift to towns (the squatters and the shanties), the need for racial and religious tolerance, etc., etc.[61]

*Till 97, anyhow. After that the balance is redressed.

Malaria was hyperendemic in Mauritius and DDT spraying was started in 1949. The attack quickly succeeded and the principal vector *Anopheles funestus,* in fact almost "eradicated", a history that is less complicated and more successful than in many developing countries.[62-64] This was the record.

Vital Statistics of Mauritius[65]

	1939–45	1946–8	1950	1960	1970
Infant mortality	156	147	76	70	57
Death rate, all ages, per 1,000	27·7	24·4	13·9	11·2	7·4
Population (thousands)	418	433	465	645	815

A drop in infant mortality which in England and Wales took nearly half a century was compressed into very few years. But the people of Mauritius did not adapt to the new situation — that far fewer children die — until the mid-1960's. Then the birth rate began to fall, from around 40 per 1,000, as it was, till now in the mid-1970's it is around 24. The rate of "natural increase", i.e. the surplus of births over deaths, is of course greater than before the antimalaria campaign. The *age distribution of the population,* and consequently the burden of dependency, is very different from ours.

	PER CENT	
	Under 15	Over 65
Mauritius	41	3·7
England and Wales 1970.	24	13

The 0-4 year olds are the largest age group of Mauritius and the population profile truly is a "pyramid": it is a "young country". As the great wave of children moves up the age-scale thousands more have to be educated, then found jobs, though already under — and unemployment is very severe; figures of 15 and 20 per cent are common in such countries.

The population of Mauritius has been growing by about 2·5 per cent a year, rather more than the average for the developing countries. On a conservative projection, world population, at the beginning of 1974 about 3,800 millions, will reach 6 or 7,000 millions by the end of the century, depending on the fertility decline — one side of the "ecological crisis". Numbers are multiplying as the children whose lives have been saved in turn bear their own.[66 67]

Triumph of Medicine and Public Health

General measures, in maternal and child health and improvement of the environment are progressing in many places, besides specific preventives like DDT and vaccination for smallpox. And an array of therapies has become available for "tropical" infections and infestations, including mass-killers like cholera, as well as antibiotics for pneumonia, meningococcal meningitis, tuberculosis (and for venereal disease). The results are not only as intended. The poverty of nations and the misery of mankind may yet prove to be their numbers, and medicine and public health in one sense are responsible.[68-70]

Population, Food, Standard of Living

Half to two-thirds of the world is wretchedly poor by typical Western standards, and despite some real achievements in the 1960's the gulf between the haves and the have-nots is widening. In the "undeveloped" countries, with average incomes below £1 a week, agriculture and economic growth is barely keeping pace with population. In some countries like Mauritius the standard of living actually is falling. By FAO norms of 2,400 calories daily needed per head, perhaps 15 per cent of the world's population is underfed. Protein-calorie malnutrition, mineral (Fe, I) and vitamin (A, B_2) deficiences — stunted growth, marasmus, kwashiorkor, goitre, anaemia — and associated infections — are the lot of many millions, and there is growing anxiety about the long-term mental as well as physical effects of infantile malnutrition.

The United Nations has declared the 1970's the Second Development Decade, with the aim of increasing economic growth of the low-income countries to 6–7 per cent annually, well above the rate of population increase, and so to move towards the "take off" to prosperity; food production is to rise by 4 per cent annually. Such campaigns in the 1960's often made little headway; during the mid-1960's in fact the food situation deteriorated, though by its close there were some remarkable if localised advances, and the "green revolution", with fertilisers and new high-yield varieties of wheat and rice gives a "breathing space" and intensive farming of the sea for protein-rich fish is now getting under way.[71] [72]

The hope for the low-income countries is that *everything* that is needed will happen: more up-to-date agriculture and land reform; irrigation (N.B. *its* threats), diversification of the economy (Mauritius has one export, sugar); industrialisation, in its turn; an increase in purchasing power — goodness knows how the world rise in commodity prices will balance out. Living standards may then begin to rise; and the improvement in health, particularly of children, the provision of new sources of economic security and the growth of education, hopefully will raise aspirations and provide the climate of opinion for population control as public policy and for individual acceptance of planning of families.

During the 1960's there was an upsurge of interest in birth control by modern methods (apart from the widely prevalent abortion). The World Health Organisation (WHO) dedicated from the start to the needs of the developing countries and since 1955 to the "eradication" of malaria, at last began to play its proper role. Public health is adjusting to the challenge of family planning. It has an ideal base (mothers are specially receptive) and much relevant experience in nutrition and family health; epidemiological observation and experiment could more often be used. Pharmacology may help with more effective agents (prostaglandins?), and plastics and metals with less troublesome intrauterine devices. Inventions to match those which started the population explosion are needed, and the cultural and economic incentives to use them. The behavioural sciences here have their great opportunity (and even before them, the 3 Rs).

It all sounds too slow, and how much misery there will be before a new balance is achieved, with low fertility as well as low mortality, numbs the imagination.*[73]

Whatever happens in the future to the size of families, the population explosion is already a fact, and further vast increase of numbers is inevitable.[54] [75] The rest of the world can give much technical aid aimed at self-sustained growth and the emergency food without which some of the new countries could not survive: quite small nutritional and medical measures may make the difference between life and death. Including more "private" than public effort, we in Britain devote only about 0·8 per cent of our gross national product (GNP) to helping the developing countries. The UN target, reaffirmed as "enlightened self-interest" by the Pearson Commission, is one per cent, which we show little signs of reaching. In the long run of course the problem must be their own, but current Western disillusionment with aid to the poor countries can only pile tragedy on tragedy.[76]

*   *   *

LOCAL VERSION

It is poor taste, to say the least, to return at this point to the current growth of population at home. Public agitation about it has been mounting, sparked by the rising birth rate 1955–64, by high (coloured) immigration in the early 1960's, by the world debate — and by the increasing prolificacy of official estimates of the population to be expected by the end of the century. Between 1959 and 1964/5 these "projections" on current trends rose from 52½ to 66 millions; since then of course the computers have been backtracking hard, Table 1.7 (the snares of forecasting). We are already among the most populous

---

*A few countries, e.g. Hong Kong, Singapore, Taiwan and Korea have achieved a substantial decline in their birth rates to 30 and less per 1,000, though it is not clear how much is due to family planning campaigns. These are examples of simplicity and ease in the context of India, Latin America, etc. In Mauritius, with Hindu, Moslem and Roman Catholic populations, an eclectic family planning campaign under government auspices, and supported by Britain, Sweden, USA and the International Planned Parenthood Federation,[74] is now showing results, as indicated.

of developed countries, and our adaptation to the post-war baby boom as it progressed foreseeably and foreseen through school and university was painful indeed.

Health of Towns

During the 1960's our population expanded about 7 per cent, less than the rate in the second half of last century but not negligibly. Malthusian anxiety over numbers is conflated with widespread discontents at life in metropolitan-industrial-mobile-high consumption Britain. For example: (a) the more affluent the society (and nearly everyone wants some of that), the more do people demand space, goods, medical care, schools, to see the sun (on inactive service). Between 1971 and '72 motor-car licences increased by 5·5 per cent, population by about 0·5 per cent. (b) Technology is generating multiple effluent, indisposable waste, noise, dirt, stink. So numbers are only part of the ecology-environment-resources-quality of life question. We think of *crowd diseases* in terms of population density and infection, but wonder if there is more to it in *social pathology*. The prospect of bigger aggregations of people, even worse congestion, wearier commuters, more loneliness (though not solitude or privacy), greater pressure on services, even longer queues for the shrinking countryside — our own versions of New York, Tokyo or California — understandably dismays, though regrets for a lost England are often merely sentimental. Through the 1950's and 1960's, population increased mainly in the outer suburbs of the cities and by "overspill" into smaller towns and villages beyond; dereliction of city-centres is already evident.

Meanwhile, population growth is slowing down. As seen, the number of births has been falling since the end of 1964 and shows no signs of levelling off (early 1975). Immigration is quite strictly under control and overall there is a net loss now from migration. The movement to conserve the best of the old and to stop cars from fouling/wrecking the environment, is having some success. A less apocalyptic debate is under way, acknowledging also the benefits of science, technology and economic growth, the bonus of living in cities. There is still time for planning acceptable population densities; local government reform has produced more sensible relationships between town and country; public-service transportation looks like having a new lease of life, further motorway devastation is less likely. The pioneer "urbanised" country, we showed the way again in the New Towns; now the first new city is being built, and we are learning how to "grow" more successfully on to old ones. Moreover, many, perhaps a third, of the children in this country still are conceived unplanned and unwanted: in theory this could solve the problem.

Population Control

"Family planning" and birth control services, educational and practical, often do not match individual wants or expressed demand, still less what the community widely accepts as needed. Thus about 8 per cent of all births are illegitimate and a further 9 per cent extra-maritally conceived then legitimised; nearly half this 17 per cent, say 7 per cent of all live births, are to teenagers . . . But about 13 per cent of live births in England and Wales are fourth or later children; to reach a "norm" of 2·1 or 2·2 children per family, on present mortality rates this would produce a steady-state in the population, there would scarcely be room for any of these large families, and there will also have to be fewer third children who constitute about 15 per cent of live births. Public opinion is only beginning to move this far and the Government's not at all, though about a quarter even of third children are said to be "accidental". Abortions are being performed at the rate of 100,000 per year. [77-83]

POSTSCRIPT

In these overheated times, the anxiety is reversed now – over the dangers of a *falling* population. Viz. these recent figures on the natural increase in England & Wales.

Totals in Year: First 34 Weeks

	Live Births	Deaths
1973	459,000	387,000
1974	433,000	385,000
1975	409,000	386,000

OPCS *Monitors.*

2. Community Diagnosis: Community Health

Using epidemiological methods we can describe and try to diagnose the *condition of the people*. Indices are produced of health and wellbeing and the character and dimension of problems are charted. Illustrating again from sickness-absence, in the year 1970/71 the $16\frac{1}{4}$ million men now insured for benefit (close to 100 per cent of men at ages 16-64) recorded $6\frac{1}{2}$ million spells of certified incapacity attributed to sickness and injuries, resulting in 245 million days lost from work. Thirty million days were certified to bronchitis, 11 million (an unusually low figure) to acute upper respiratory infections including "influenza". Ischaemic heart disease, hypertension, etc., accounted for 28 million days lost; rheumatic disorders, arthritis, prolapsed intervetebral discs, etc., for 19 million; psychoneurosis, anxiety symptoms and the like and labelled as such, for 13 million. Virtually all the absences included in these figures lasted four days or more.[1]

Such facts are sketchy and rather suspect. How accurate the labels are,[2] and what may lie behind them, often is hard to assess, often no more readily than for death certificates when Farr began his work. GPs cannot spend time in categorisation of minor troubles; at the other extreme, they are reluctant to "certify" cancer (or pox) — with all that it signifies — to patients, their families, sundry third parties. The information moreover is about fitness for work, a special and social way of looking at health, and this limits its value as a measure of disease-prevalence for example. Another shortcoming is that most of the data is about "*spells*" of incapacity, which does not tell us how many *persons* are incapacitated. (This is a difficulty throughout administrative statistics, which usually require information about "events", and in this instance the volume of incapacity, rather than how many individuals are involved, which is also essential for a picture of health.) But such figures, with their complete coverage, do provide crude indicators of the burden of ill-health on the community, and the load on general practice. For economic reasons, sickness-absence figures are reported very quickly, and by virtue of sheer size and numbers, the earliest warning of a "flu" epidemic may be an abrupt increase in the volume of absences from work, regardless of the "diagnoses" on the certificates (cf. the "plague"). The public, too, which composes the figures can be informed about particular issues; the figures on "chronic rheumatic disorders", for instance, and on their money-cost have aroused widespread concern.

References on page 287.

Sometimes the distribution among the population gives clues to causes: pioneer observations by Halliday and his colleagues on the high prevalence of "rheumatism" in miners led to the research that was so rewarding on occupational disc-degeneration and other syndromes.[3] The figures *should* have aroused concern about bronchitis and pollution, but the 1952 smog was necessary for that. To those working in hospitals the figures provide up-to-date background and perspective, some idea of the importance in the people's health of the patients they are and are not meeting. (Community medicine and clinical medicine.) And such figures are essential of course for Government: on average, for example, in 1970/71 just over 900,000 (M+F) of the labour force of 25 million drew sickness-benefit, costing the country directly over £7 millions weekly — and how many times that in personal losses and lost production?

Prevalence of Chronic Disability

How new facts can be "discovered" in such data is illustrated by *chronic disability*.[4] This is defined (operationally) as the proportion continuously incapacitated for work for more than three months on account of ill-health, and it accounts for about two-thirds of all sickness-absence. Comparing 1967 with 1957 (Fig. 2. 1), this rate had fallen as expected among younger men — the antituberculous drugs, tranquillisers, the continuing decline of rheumatic heart disease, etc. — but it was substantially higher during middle age. Ischaemic heart disease and chronic bronchitis are known to be much involved in this: as seen, incidence of the former has probably been rising; in chronic bronchitis

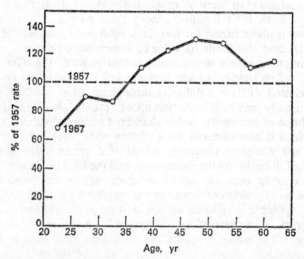

Fig. 2.1   Prevalence in men of absence from work for over 3 months. Rates in 1967 are compared with those for 1957 (corrected). Britain.
Department of Health and Social Security.[4]

lives are being saved, so raising the prevalence of chronic sickness. And again psychological and social factors may well predominate: disengagement by not-so-healthy men because of productivity drives and the intensification of industrial work, changing attitudes to "fitness" for work as a result of occupational pensions, more wives are "gainfully employed". It is urgent to investigate this peculiarly unpleasant bit of contemporary history; judging from clinical experience, many of these men never find a job again. The *prevalence* of disability today is much influenced by health and social services; but rehabilitation often is inadequate. We must also expect such national averages to conceal big local differences. A considerable social problem — in the "quality of life" — may have crept up on us unawares, worst in communities least able to cope. Simple sums show that the marginal improvement in life expectancy of middle-aged men during the 1960's was largely absorbed in higher sickness-absence*. Or, composing a "health indicator" from the Figures on pages 1 and 30, it could be said that during the 1960's middle-aged men deteriorated in health.

MORBIDITY IN MIDDLE AGE

Table 2.1, overleaf, provides different pictures of ill-health according to the level it "presents". And how they differ! Straightaway, it must be said that the selection of "diagnoses" and their grouping are arbitrary: the main point is to make sense at the particular level, however awkward this proves for comparison. "Middle age" is defined more widely than before.

By way of introduction (rather ancient data by now, but they make the point), the Table starts with the kind of information obtained by *Social survey* interviewers, "knocking on the door" of samples of the population and asking about their health. In reply (1), they were told of many vague symptoms, producing minor inconvenience, as well as a little about more serious trouble. The value of the labels attached to such complaints is dubious. Thus, less than 2 per cent of these middle-aged women's very many troubles were recorded as "gynaecological", which more likely reflects reticence with a lay person than any other kind of fact. (N.B. the legend: about two-thirds of the men and three-quarters of the women reported some such "sickness" in a *month,* the other rates in the Table are per *year.*)

Next (2) gives the "leading causes" of sickness during one year in a study by 171 *general practitioners* in 106 practices of the National

*These data on middle-aged men were first dug out of the official statistics more than 10 years ago, but little analysis by cause, occupation, region, etc. is possible yet (see the new *General Household Survey* however). Social security is a fabulous store of information, but it wants a lot of retrieving. Such "chronic disability" during middle age increased still further till 1969, when the proportions reached 5·6% in men aged 55–59, and 11·5% at 60–64 (16·43% actually in men aged 64). Between 1969 and 1971 the rates fell a little.

TABLE 2.1

BURDEN OF DISEASES IN MIDDLE AGE

IMPORTANCE OF DIFFERENT CONDITIONS AT DIFFERENT PRESENTATIONS   AGES 45-64

PRESENTATION	MEN CONDITION	MEN PROPORTION OF TOTAL CONDITIONS %	WOMEN CONDITION	WOMEN PROPORTION OF TOTAL CONDITIONS %
In Population-at-Large[1]	"Symptoms", often vague including headache and nervousness, constipation, etc.	20	"Symptoms", often vague including headache and nervousness, constipation, etc.	29
	"Rheumatism", etc.	13	"Rheumatism", etc.	17
	Acute upper respiratory infections and influenza	10	Acute upper respiratory infections and influenza	7
	Gastric trouble	10	Gastric trouble	7
	Bronchitis	6	Bronchitis	3
			Varicose veins	2
To General Practice[2]	Acute upper respiratory infections and influenza	14	Acute upper respiratory infections and influenza	12
	Injuries	8	Rheumatism, etc.	8
	Bronchitis	7	Psychoneurosis, and symptoms of nervousness, etc.	8
	Rheumatism, etc.	7	Injuries	6
	Disorders of stomach and duodenum, including ulcer	6	Menopause; and menstrual disorders	5
	Psychoneurosis, and symptoms of nervousness, etc.	5	Bronchitis	5

Admissions to Hospital[3]			
(All cancer	10)	Gynaecological disorder	21
Injuries	9	Prolapse	3
Ischaemic heart disease	8	Fibroids	4
Hernia	7	(All cancer	11)
Bronchitis and Pneumonia	5	Injuries	7
Cancer of bronchus	4	Cancer of breast	3
Peptic ulcer	3	Disease of gall-bladder	3
		Varicose veins	2
Causes of Death[4]			
Ischaemic heart disease	34	Ischaemic heart disease	16
Cancer of bronchus	13	Vascular lesions of nervous system	11
Vascular lesions of nervous system	7	Cancer of breast	11
Bronchitis	6	Cancer of bronchus	5
Cancer of stomach	3	Cancer of ovary	4
Injuries	3	Chronic rheumatic heart disease	3

(N.B., all data refer to ages 45–64)

[1] 670 men and 780 women per 1,000 interviewed reported such sickness, per *month*. Britain, 1950. Logan, W. P. D. and Brooke, E. M. (1957) *The Survey of Sickness 1943 to 1952.* HMSO, London.

[2] 604 men and 667 women consulted the doctor per 1,000 on his list, in the *year*. On average each man had 1·9 "conditions", each woman 2·1. England and Wales, 1955/6. Logan, W. P. D. and Cushion, A. A. (1958) *Morbidity Statistics from General Practice.* HMSO, London.

[3] There were 91 male and 80 female admissions per 1,000 of the national population to "general" (i.e. other than mental) hospitals in 1970 in England and Wales. These are figures of the "principal condition treated". In addition, and not shown in the Table, 3·9 men and 5·5 women per 1,000 of the related population were admitted to mental hospitals in England and Wales in 1970. *Hospital In-patient Enquiry* and Statistical Report Series on *Psychiatric Hospitals and Units,* Dept. of Health and Social Security, Annually. HMSO, London.

[4] 13·7 men and 7·3 women per 1,000 of the population in England and Wales died in 1970. These are figures of the main, or underlying, certified cause of death. Registrar General. (*International Classification of Diseases,* 8th revision, WHO, Geneva.)

Health Service; the figures aren't up-to-date, but this is about the most comprehensive picture of morbidity that we have. The close on 400,000 patients in these practices may have been representative enough (though the doctors, so interested in recording their work, probably and alas are not). Sixty per cent of the middle-aged men consulted the doctor during the year (604 per 1,000) and were given 1,149 separate "diagnoses" that resemble those already quoted for "incapacity to work". Fourteen per cent in men were for acute respiratory infections, which, with injuries at 8 per cent, make up the majority of acute troubles. Comparing the rates in parts (1) and (2) of the Table it is evident that most "trouble" with health is not presented to doctors (i.e. not expressed as a demand for medical care, in the jargon.) General practice, too, is a great potential source of information on the people's health. But there are limitations to these data. Thus, there is nothing in (2) to indicate whether emotional difficulties account for an important part of the general practitioner's work. The Social Survey's data suggest a prevalence of "nervous" symptoms — including presumably the quite trivial — of about 13 per cent in men (20 per cent of 670 interviewed) and 23 per cent, characteristically more, in women. In fact, general practitioners nowadays prescribe a "sedative" of some kind at about one in four or five of their contacts with adults (cf. p. 18). Moreover, the diagnoses often seem to be rather forced and specifically medical for the kind of complaints and problems that are so often "presented" to the GP.

Since *Uses* is much concerned with *cardiovascular disease,* details are given of its *prevalence* during middle age in the second national general practice morbidity survey (of 1970–1) for a change. There were close on 70,000 individual patients aged 45-64:

Patients Consulting, per 1,000 on Practitioners' Lists, Ages 45–64

DIAGNOSIS	MEN	WOMEN
Coronary heart disease	33	13
Hypertension, etc.	31	44
Cerebrovascular disease	6·2	3·9
Peripheral arterial disease; other "arteriosclerosis", etc.	8·1	5·1
Varicose veins, phlebitis, etc.	15	31
Haemorrhoids	13	10
Rheumatic fever and heart disease	1·5	3·3

Adding up, about 10 *per cent* of the men, and 11 per cent of the women, consulted their GPs for "cardiovascular" disease during the year. Some patients surely had more than one "diagnosis", so these are overestimates.

Continuing this simple "shop arithmetic", the conditions taking the middle-aged into *hospitals* (3) are very different from those bringing them to general practitioners. Colds, rheumatics and nerves are left outside, but bronchitis persists and, indeed, it is the only condition important at all "levels" of the Table. There is a considerable scatter of diagnoses in hospitals, nothing to compare with the load of upper repiratory infections in general practice or ischaemic heart disease in mortality. Chronic diseases preponderate, though often of course in acute exacerbation. Again, however, the statistics are incomplete; again, they represent *spells* in hospital (the load on the service) not *individuals* admitted, so can only occasionally provide estimates of incidence or prevalence of disease in the population. The figures on perforations, page 17, are a good example of how useful the data on persons could be; one spell/one man is a reasonable assumption about perforation — but what about the bleeding?

Finally, the Table (4) gives the leading *causes of death* in middle age. The two "modern epidemics" are prominent, and the contribution of cerebrovascular disease in both sexes.

"Soft" as many of them are, and with all their limitations, the implications of such facts about community health, avoidable and unavoidable misery, extend widely into the doctor's image of his job, medical education, the strategy of research, social policy, planning and priorities of health and welfare services: at each "level".

CONDITION OF THE PEOPLE

Table 2.1 illustrates the variety of community health, and how difficult it is to describe it other than by mortality![46] "Morbidity" is what we choose it to mean. Particular *symptoms,* e.g. angina on effort, or poor (as defined) human relationships. Measurable *abnormality of function or structure:* ST-T depression on the electrocardiogram, or an intimal plaque. *Social incapacity,* e.g. in parental roles. In the chronic non-communicable conditions, special questions arise of how to define when "morbidity" begins, and how long it lasts — maybe the lifetime; how to grade severity and disability (and therefore "need") and how to measure their fluctuations and crises. The study of morbidity has to become a leading activity of community medicine.[7] Mortality is useless for describing the "mental health" field, for example. The thousands of coronary deaths tell us little about the tens of thousands of years spent "living with a coronary". Vast numbers in the population could be laid low by prolapsed "discs" or miserable from psoriasis, without a flicker in mortality rates.

"Morbidity" provides but one illustration of the modern community's need to know itself, a need whose recognition, afresh, represents a striking change in public consciousness. From the condition of the recruits in the Boer War to the thalidomide calamity, and not forgetting

the orphan boy whose death precipitated a new service for Child Care. . .
society evidently is prone to be caught by surprise, and not in all
instances inevitably . . . First are the outbreaks that make News.
In this country in recent years we have had the 1952 smog disaster,
1963 cold-weather deaths, motor-bike accidents, heroin addiction,
Xmas-drink road slaughter, motorway pile-ups, race riots, aerosol
deaths from asthma, Aberfan . . .

Humdrum by comparison, we want current, fact-finding surveys. How
much obesity? Functional disorder — insomnia, amenorrhea, eating
too little? Physical unfitness? Allergy-prurigo-asthma states? How
common is truancy?, drop-out?, "school phobia"? (And whence has
that surfaced?). Miseries like hernia, varicose veins, genital prolapse?
Little strokes? Alcoholism? Dependence on psychotropic medicines?
Troublesome enlargement of the prostate? How much treatable but
untreated depression in the aged? Hypothermia? Osteoporosis? How
many disrupted families are there locally? Young-marrieds without a
home? Families carrying senile dementia? Single-parent families?
. . . For (new) health-services: How many with complete heart
block? Developing chronic renal failure? Rh-negative mothers bearing
rh-positive children? Thinking ahead, can we begin to make appropriate "community diagnoses" for amniocentesis?

We are only just beginning to get a usable inventory of local citizens
with recognised major chronic disabilities, and I don't know a single
community in the UK that has an up-to-date account also of the very
old and their living conditions. Far too little has been learned from
Public Health, with its long experience of *notification* of acute specific
fevers, and *registration* of chronic conditions, of tuberculosis (since
1911), rheumatic heart disease, the blind. Apart from cancer and
hospitalised major mental disorder, there are few usable data, even on a
national scale, on the prevalence of the chronic diseases and disabilities
that dominate the practice of medicine in a society like ours — with its
(physical) problems of maternal and child health largely solved and
serious infections largely under control.[8][9]

The more complex the society, the more it needs to be inquisitive, to
seek trouble — and try to prevent it. Of course, success cannot be
guaranteed for any line of enquiry, still less that action will follow;
but that does not excuse mere waiting on events to react to (and be
shocked at). In the 1960's the academics redefined and rediscovered
poverty.[10] In 1961, the shameful increase of homeless families in
London roused the public conscience (10 years later the situation was
worse).[11] In the 1970's "revelations" are no way to learn about conditions in long-stay hospitals. The growing number of over 75's and
the conditions under which many of them live, is warning of a coming
winter "emergency". . A steady increase year by year in the national
average of calories taken from fat till now it is close to 45 per cent of
the total (Fig. 2.2), half the fatty acids saturated, makes no sense in

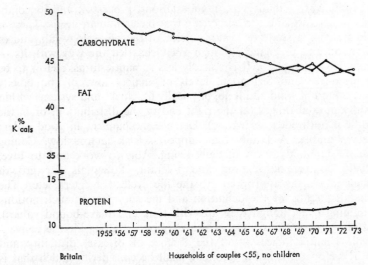

Fig. 2.2 Proportion of calories from carbohydrate, fat and protein. National Food Survey 1955–73.
Marr, J. W. (1973) *Health Trends* **5**, 37.

terms of any hypothesis about needs for health — or about the origins of atherosclerosis and heart disease. . What are the implications for Community Health of the relaxing of the forces of natural selection and the passage of deleterious genes? Fibrocystic disease, achondroplasia and the rest (consider the demand on services of even small increments). . The USA, as said, is a caricature of man's future: technological unemployment already is hitting us also, and at the same weak spots, (coloured) young people and the over 45s; some of our inner city neighbourhoods are beginning to resemble their ghettoes.[12] [14]

Diagnosis of the state of community health must be dynamic. In a world of change, epidemiologists have a special duty to observe the impact "upon the people" of the way we live, to diagnose where wellbeing is increasing and where losing out, to probe for unintended consequences, to identify trends and to think ahead.*

Epidemiology of Health

Because of training and environment, we more readily think of disease and morbidity than of what is normal, of *health* — adaptability

---

*On change: "Health is an expression of fitness to the various factors of the total environment. Any change in the environment demands new adaptive reactions, and disease is the consequence of inadequacies in these adaptive responses . . . 'It is changes that are chiefly responsible for disease', wrote Hippocrates in Chapter XV of *Humours*, especially the great changes, the violent alterations both in seasons and in other things".[15]

and fulfilment — its degrees, manifestations, processes; and its conditions in heredity and a mode of life that meets human needs. There is little systematic study of health outside of the physiology lab. and of childhood and pregnancy, though WHO has led the way with its — romantic — definition. It is scarcely less romantic to ask: How to be symptom-free and feel good, levels of anxiety low, of spontaneity high? Sound of wind and limb, physically fit, clocks and systems within healthy normal ranges (at the right end of the distribution, or in the middle if both ends are wrong). Defence mechanisms in good order; reserves ample. A family that supports. Risk factors low. Coping with the ups and downs of daily living. Able to work and to love, socially competent, relating and tolerant. Potentials for growth actualised. All as appropriate to the life cycle. (Et cetera, etc.) The demand mounts for the definition and measurement of such notions (brimming over though they are with time and place-bound values), and of the conditions under which they occur, alongside the conventional "health" indices — of the absence of disease, disability and death![16] Hopefully, in the book we shall be considering much that is relevant and may help; this is likely to be a next thrust for epidemiology. The approach is obvious only when we extend systematic study from the clinical or "diseased" end to the whole distribution of bodily functions, including the healthy end. Who are the blessed, with plasma cholesterol under 200 mg, whose blood pressure does not rise in middle age?

Table 2.2 gives some measurements of physical fitness during middle age, in relation to exercise habits. Figure 2.3 describes a relation to the environment: the contrast in the aggregate amount of physical activity entailed in these two jobs on London's double-decker buses (dietary calories per kilo, 38·9 in drivers and 43·8 in matching conductors) is

TABLE 2.2
PHYSICAL FITNESS IN HEALTHY MIDDLE-AGED MEN
Volunteer Samples — Mean Values

Physical Activity (mainly in leisure-time)	n	Mean Age	Vo_2/max (c^3/kg/min)	Heart Rate at Rest
Sedentary	16	48	32·0	78
Light No running	34	50	35·5	77
Vigorous exercise: Moderate Regular running	60	51	38·0	71
Vigorous exercise: Heavy Regular running +	34	53	37·7	69

Seattle, U.S.A.
McDonough, J. R., Kusumi, F. & Bruce, R. A. (1970) *Circulation*, *41*, 743; Bruce, R. A. (1971) personal communication.

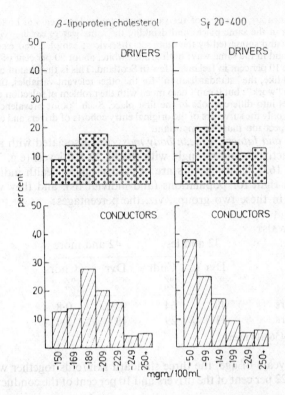

Fig. 2.3 Blood lipid levels in samples of London busmen aged 50–59 free of clinical or electrocardiographic evidence of coronary heart disease. Groups of 94–168 men. Means, β-lipoprotein cholesterol: *drivers,* 201 mg per 100 ml, and S_f 20–400, very low density lipoprotein, 148 mg per 100 ml; *conductors,* 188 and 92 mg per 100 ml.
    Courtauld Institute of Biochemistry, Middlesex Hospital, Mills, G. L.[42]

postulated as part explaining the significantly different shapes of the distributions of the "low density" β lipoprotein, and also of the pre-β molecules Sf 20-400, rich in triglyceride. More conductors have enviably low levels, many drivers high levels carrying, at the least, a known greater risk of future trouble. Sample studies[17] show that both groups are eating the same, surely excessive, proportions of saturated fat, 22 per cent of total calories, and of sugar. The conductors plainly are tolerating the average ("normal" in that sense) diet better, they have greater absorptive capacity, or their metabolism is "set" at lower levels; we don't know. Here are two quite ordinary groups of working men, but one plainly is healthier, more normal (in that sense) than the other. (What is "physiology"? Corresponding groups in the poor countries would have lower levels and, in that sense, be healthier men.)

The busmen are of course of the same age; similar long years in London Transport; living in the same places and drinking the same water; earning virtually the same wages and supported by the same social services; sampled and examined the same time and in the same way; both groups white, about 90 per cent of them born in England, 10 per cent in Ireland, a few in Scotland. This is the kind of comparison of like with like, the "standardisation" for the other relevant variables, that permits focusing on "work"; but it can't help much with the problem of selection of different personalities into different jobs in the first place. Such "point prevalence" surveys can include only the survivors of the original entry cohorts of drivers and conductors, and this aspect too must be important.

Weight and fatness, so *lean body mass,* are associated with aggregate physical activity, and strongly with the Sf 20-400 levels (e.g. 7 (a) and (b) on p. 163). These factors are of course major health indicators in their own right for populations (and individuals), and they vary substantially in these two groups, viz. the percentages:

TROUSER-WAIST inches	32 and less		42 and more	
	Dvr %	Cndr %	Dvr %	Cndr %
25–34 years	48	64	3·1	0·8
55–64 years	11	29	18	5·4

Samples of 456-814 men.

At 50–59 years of age, the three standard skinfolds together were over 60 mm in 22 per cent of the drivers and 10 per cent of the conductors.[17][18]

Notes on Procedures

I can say little in this book about practical matters, on how epidemiologic surveys actually are carried out. But some illustrations will be given of the issues that arise.

Populations

The first thing to determine in studying a chosen population is: who in fact is present? The Table shows for an ordinary general practice we wanted to study the true membership, and not merely those officially registered:

Composition of a General Practice

No. registered in the Practice	3,611
Persons actually found on search to be present	3,037
Missing persons	574

The deficit was eventually made up thus:

Registered more than once	53
Previously died	59
Transferred to another doctor's list	178
No trace on other local doctors' lists or in the district	284
Total	574

To check all 3,611, account for the 574 "dead souls", and produce the correct figure of 3,037, involved much shoe-leather, hundreds of home visits and other enquiries. But only discharging this elementary duty to scrutinise the data gave us an accurate population base for study and for any sampling that might later be done. (Though that was not the intention, it also had implications for the administration and financing of the recently established National Health Service.)[19] [20]

To proceed: all populations are "biased", and "Who is present?" must be followed by the questions "How did they get there?" and "Who got away?". That is to say, it is necessary to ask about *selection*. Ødegard[21] found an excess of schizophrenia in merchant seamen and showed it was due to selective *entry*, the choice of this occupation by persons with manifest personality disorder, precursor possibly to the disease. Schilling showed that the deficiency of byssinosis in female cotton workers reflected their selective *exit* from the mills because of the disease and not immunity to it.[22] A lot of work had to be done to make sure that the excess of ischaemic heart disease found in bus drivers was not an artefact produced by the departure of conductors with early symptoms. Studies of whole communities are also liable to selective bias. Factors favouring emigration to New Towns — in age, family structure, occupation, health, temperament and so forth — will affect morbidity rates in these towns; and in the towns that have been left. During the 1930's, assessment of the effect of the Depression on health was bedevilled by the impossibility of dealing accurately with migration: to what extent, for example were the high rates of rheumatic heart disease, or phthisis, in the young women of the North of England or South Wales the result of the escape of the healthier to more prosperous parts?[23] [24]

POPULATION MEASUREMENTS[25] [29]

Definition of the relevant biological and social variables is the next task. What are the characteristics of the population being studied? Studying *morbidity* it is often necessary to describe, in terms of particular symptoms and signs, every subject in a population, or sample from it. What will constitute a case must be agreed; definitions, whether "quantitative" or "qualitative", will usually only be adopted after pilot tests.

Measurements can be discussed under three heads [30] (and I might add a fourth, *acceptability*). The first is *simplicity,* and therefore cheapness, the utmost consistent with the level of study ("cost-efficiency"). Thus in mass surveys a single breath can be very informative about lung function. To screen for psychoneurosis among recruits, the US Army in World War II used 15 tests; later it was found that one of these — a brief questionnaire dealing with psychosomatic complaints — identified 93 per cent of those identified by the entire battery.[31] The electrocardiogram in population studies of ischaemic heart disease meets this requirement to be simple enough for application on a large scale.

Such observations have then to be assessed for *reproducibility,* the second requirement: i.e. whether they give the same result again in the hands of the same, or other, observers [32] recognising, of course, that the subject can change very quickly, e.g. in blood pressure (in contrast, say, with height). The traditional clinical history and physical examination are difficult to "reproduce", *repeat.* But the individual case-study of clinical practice gives opportunities for multiple examinations, is concerned anyhow with the "total picture" and to reach a main diagnosis. Variation due to human or instrumental error, as well as systematic differences between observers, matters far more in focused, "one-shot" epidemiological surveys.* So, in the frequent absence of objective signs on clinical examination, and because the clinical history is so important, Fletcher and colleagues developed the Medical Research Council's standard questionnaire which yields a reproducible diagnosis of "chronic bronchitis", as this is defined in terms of cough, sputum and record of chest infection.[33] In the case of the electrocardiogram,[34] epidemiological studies have progressed from its clinical inspection by eye, to measurement in a standard way and the definition of specific patterns; next for the measurement to be done by a single, trained observer so avoiding *inter-observer variation;* and, now, to the recording of the curves on magnetic tape with analysis by computer to eliminate *intra-observer variation.* Reproducibility, however, is not enough.

Validity

In ad hoc survey, but especially if it is the preliminary "screening" stage of a definitive survey, the *validity* of the indicator has also to be assessed: i.e. how well in fact it measures what is intended to be measured, the third requirement. This is done by comparing the indicator in action with the "reference" standard or "norm", the best method of making the particular diagnosis or measurement. Biopsy, for example, when screening by mammography for breast cancer, or the specialist's clinical examination to validate questions on hearing and vision. It can then be estimated in how many the "disease", or whatever, as defined, is wrongly found to be present (the *false positives*) and how many cases

---

*Nevertheless, what has been learned in epidemiology about observer – variation has much implication for clinical work – and for other activities, including the marking of exam papers, selection of students, the sentence of the Court, or the counting of chromosomes.

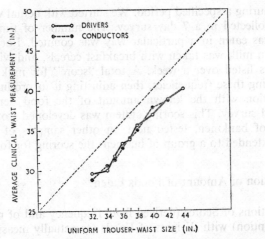

Fig. 2.4 *Survey methods*: Validation of uniform trouser-waist size by clinical measurement of waist. Comparison of the two measurements in a sample of 365 busmen aged 40–64. London Transport, 1956–8. On average, the clinical measurement was about 2 inches smaller than the tailors' — throughout the range of nine sizes, and equally in drivers and conductors.

Brit. J. prev. soc. Med. (1961) **15**, 143.

are being missed (the *false negatives*).* The numbers misclassified, in relation to the frequency of the condition being investigated, will decide whether the indicator is good enough for the question being asked. In some situations, false positives could be calamitous (e.g. in the diagnosis of pregnancy), could affront (e.g. on the breathalyser), or swamp the service and defeat the objective. In others, false negatives are what matter (e.g. in screening for early cancer, or for phenylketonuria (PKU), or by failing to identify high-risk mothers for delivery in hospital).[35]

Here are two examples, from our own work, of validation of simple methods against more refined. Figure 2.4 shows how adequately the trouser-waistband of their uniforms can assess *physique* in these busmen; the trouser-size was simply copied from tailors' stores records for a sample of men whose girth had previously been measured clinically.

It has been exceedingly difficult to produce simple and valid methods of assessing *individual diets* which are suitable for large-scale field surveys. With big numbers, to organise the weighing of the food eaten during sample days, under free-living conditions (probably the best method, is impracticable.[18] [36] [37] Our approach used menu records which permit the counting of the frequency with which various *foods* are

---

*If there are few false positives, the indicator is said to be highly "specific"; if few false negatives, highly "sensitive". Master's two-step test for angina is highly specific, but poorly sensitive (many false negatives). Simple tests on vision that we are now piloting for a screening instrument among the elderly typically are reasonably sensitive, but not specific enough (too many false positives) to be useful.

eaten during a specified period. We started with actual weighed dietary data, collected in a 7 day survey. The number of times a particular food was eaten in a particular way was counted. For example, each occasion milk was taken with breakfast cereals, and with cups of tea, etc. was listed over a week. A total "score" for milk was produced by adding these frequencies, then adjusting it to produce a maximum correlation with the known amount of the food derived from the weighed survey. This scoring system was developed from data on one group of bankmen, tested next on other samples of bankmen and later, extended to a group of busmen: the scoring for foods was about

Estimation of Amount of Foods Eaten

Correlations of Scores (derived from frequency and of mode of consumption) with Weights of Foods (as actually measured)

		In initial group of Bankmen (44)	Drivers (27)	Conductors (26)
Milk	r	+0·95	0·91	0·85
Meat	r	+0·95	0·74	0·60
Butter	r	+0·78	0·92	0·88

Number of men in brackets.

as good (or as bad) in the independent group of metropolitan manual workers as in the original sample of provincial white-collar men. The patterns of consumption were in fact similar. To assess *nutrient* consumption, it was necessary to combine the scores obtained for foods; which proved much more difficult.

(Note: Instead of reproducibility, "*reliability*", a nicer word, is often used. But sometimes it is used also for validity: " . . . this deduction from the not very reliable results of a not very reliable questionnaire."[38] *Et tu!* Better stick to the jargon.)

The main point, sometimes overlooked in these struggles with method is to state a sensible question that will elicit information worth the effort entailed. This, of course, is where the investigator tells — his imagination, experience, familiarity with the subject-matter, judgment.

Surveys of Mental Disorders

The greatest difficulties at present are met in psychiatry, in producing satisfactory indicators where subjective symptoms are so important and often all. Here are the results of a special study of a four-doctor *general practice:*

Prevalence of Psychiatric Disorder During One Year

	Proportion of "Population" Aged 15+
1. Patients referred to consultant psychiatrist	1%
2. Patients with disorder in specified psychiatric categories of International Statistical Classification of Disease (WHO)	5%
3. "Conspicuous psychiatric morbidity", as defined	9%
4. ls 3. + other patients with obvious psychological illnesses, or with illness where physical factors were not considered significant in causation	27%
5. ls 4. + other patients with "psychosomatic" or "stress" conditions	34%

Kessel, W. I. N. (1960) *Brit. J. prev. soc. Med.* **14**, 16.

The estimate of "mental health" in this population obviously depends on the criteria adopted. Provided the definition is stated, it is just as sensible (and far simpler) to suggest that in about 10 per cent there was conspicuous psychiatric morbidity as that about a quarter or a third had psychological troubles: each figure would have to be validated. In obtaining proportions beyond the order of 5 and 8 per cent of page 32, information from ad hoc study of the patients was also included, so the pictures are scarcely comparable. The observation over a year allows for the great personal variability. Overall, the fraction selected to be seen in hospitals, a fortiori in teaching hospitals, evidently is minute: compare the 1 per cent with any of the other rates. And these figures presumably are under-estimates, because about a third of the persons registered with the practice did not consult their doctors during the year and, the safest thing to do technically, it was taken that none of these had "psychiatric disorder".

Individual doctors were not very reproducible in their diagnosis of category (3), mostly neuroses, ranging from 4·2 to 12 per cent in fact of their samples of the population-at-risk (an illustration of the kind of problem involved in estimating the levels of anxiety and depression in populations for grading their mental health). *Chance* error apart, there would be *systematic* observer-variability among the doctors in their "feel" for psychological mechanisms, conscious and unconscious, and in their attitudes to them, which will produce different numbers of "positives" and "negatives". Moreover, the condition of such patients is likely to vary because the observer influences the subject (makes him feel better or worse) merely by the act of studying him, an analogous situation to taking of the blood pressure. Such "interaction" may also operate more subtly through selection of mutually sympathetic doctors and patients, or because of the social distance between middle-class doctors and working-class patients. These problems are far from

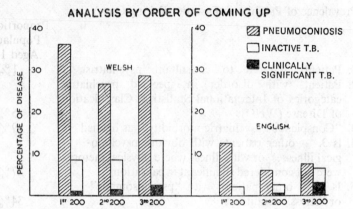

Fig. 2.5 Per cent with disease found in volunteers, analysed by order of coming up for examination.

Cochrane, A. L. (1950) *The Application of Scientific Methods to Industrial and Service Medicine*. HMSO.

solution; the most hopeful approaches at present are in the use of validated standard questionnaires, and multiple recordings of the same subject.[39][40]

A Joint Enterprise

To close for the present: the essence of the epidemiological method is that the same information must be obtained about every member of a defined "population". Only thus can numerator appropriate to denominator be produced. So many, x, in the population smoke, y don't; $x/(x+y)$ gives the frequency, or proportion, of smokers. But not everyone of a long-suffering public will come forward straightaway for examination. Those who don't "play" are likely to be different from those who do, reluctant participants from the eager. Figure 2.5 illustrates.

We made the same kind of observation when a sample of families in a local general practice was invited to act as "healthy" controls to match a series of 49 patients with duodenal ulcer.[41] This is how these ordinary families co-operated, and how they were later assessed on the basis of all the information available to the practice:

Family Response		No. Eventually Found to Have a Major Social-Psychological Problem
"Good" co-operation	20	3
"Fair" co-operation	12	5
"Unco-operative"	17	11

The trend of these small numbers, and the contrast between the families who agreed at once to participate and those who were unwilling throughout, is striking.

The bias introduced by a high refusal or failure rate may be serious — every research group will have its own (often horrible)) examples. How serious will depend, of course, on the nature of the question, and on the range of difference being observed. By now it is "professional" to try to persuade 90 per cent of the subjects to participate, analyses then can readily be done on the worst interpretation of the missing 10 per cent, and there will be little temptation to make up the desired sample-size by further sampling. In our survey of London busmen [42] it took as much trouble — this by now is an iron law of epidemiology — to win the cooperation of the final 15 per cent as of the 77 per cent of men who agreed at once to join us. A final failure-rate of 8 per cent, however, cannot matter very much in describing anatomical and biochemical distributions of drivers and conductors since the 60 or so individuals, out of about 750 concerned, were fairly equally spread between the two occupations and over a span of 25 years of age. (Everyone has a height, weight, blood cholesterol level, etc.; the — unknown — value of these, moreover, is unlikely much to affect willingness to co-operate.) But a failure rate even of this size could be serious in a study of disease incidence (or mortality) where small differences are begin sought, since it is highly probable that the affected individuals will decline or are missing. One way and another, however, a lot can often be discovered about those who "fail" to cooperate* and it is usually worth trying to do so.

REGISTRATION OF ISCHAEMIC (CORONARY) HEART DISEASE

"There is a quite unacceptable lack of knowledge about the occurrence of IHD in the community and on its human, social and economic costs . . . Registration of major conditions, by notifying, then follow-up of cases ("surveillance", "dispensarisation") is an established health public practice in the field of chronic disease. Linkage of records about all coronary cases is needed for defining the scale and nature of the community problem, and in helping to keep track of individuals, their fate and how they fare. These community-wide information systems (e.g. for an area health authority) would measure local needs and how local services compare. By study of the outcomes in representative patients under different regimens, some evaluation would be possible of new and old methods of care of IHD. Registers would provide sampling frames for therapeutic trials. Estimates could be made of the *economic cost* of IHD in medical services and social-security benefits,

---

*"Failures (to take part in the survey), where they occurred, were attributable in Scotland either to greed of time or to superstition; in Ireland to carelessness or to political feeling; in Wales to suspiciousness; and in England to stupidity."[43]

TABLE 2.3

MODEL ABSTRACT FOR A "REGISTER" OF CLINICALLY PRESENTING CORONARY HEART DISEASE

Experience of 7,000 Male Medical Practitioners
Ages 40–64
Part A: Total Episodes, Deaths, and Men Affected: Average in One Year
Britain – Early 1960's

STAGE IN NATURAL HISTORY		TOTAL CASES: CLINICAL PRESENTATION		INCL. DEATHS	
First clinical episodes starting in year (incidence)	"Heart attacks"	Fulminant ischaemic attack (FIA)	12	Sudden deaths	12
		Acute myocardial infarction (AMI)	36 } 61	Later deaths	8 } 20
		Angina pectoris (AP)	11		
		Other	2		
Second, third, etc. clinical episodes starting in year*	"Heart Attacks"	FIA	10	Sudden deaths	10
		AMI	13 } 34	Later deaths	4 } 14
		AP	6		
		Other	5		
Men continuing ill into year from previous year		AMI (etc.)	53		
TOTAL men ill in year (active prevalence per 1,000)**			148 (21·1)	Sudden deaths	22 } 34
				Later deaths	12 (4·7)
Men affected in previous years, not active in current year***			170?		

The "Register" is compiled from the episodes of CHD. causing absence from work for at least a week, or death, in a "population" of 7,000 doctors insured against sickness as well as death. The average experience in one calendar year is derived from the experience in 5 years, 1961–65.

*The first episode may have occurred in any year.

For this Table, the actual nos. of cases and deaths have been "standardised" on the age-structure of the population of England and Wales for 1966. Rounding off to nearest whole number.

"Sudden death": i.e. occurring on first day of episode (mostly in first hour apparently) and, therefore, before clear picture of acute infarction .

**The few men who made more than one appearance in the same year have been counted each time for simplicity.
(Figures *in brackets* are *rates for year per 1,000* e.g. $(61+34+53)/7,000 \times 1,000$ gives *Period Prevalence per 1,000* for the year of 21·1)

Of the total of 12 "later" deaths, four occurred during the remainder of the first week of the episode, eight after that.

Angina pectoris: i.e. uncomplicated angina.

***Incomplete, because only a limited retrospective search was made for first attacks occurring before 1961, so some cases which were "silent" throughout the study-years will have been missed.

MRC Social Medicine Unit and Medical Sickness Annuity & Life Assurance Society, Ltd. *Brit. med. J.* (1952) **1**, 503; (1968) **3**, 701; *Am. J. Med.* (1969) **46**, 674.

from sickness-absence and loss of life. Coronary registers of all cases, wherever and however they present and are cared for, would assemble a more complete clinical picture of the natural history of the disease than is obtainable in hospitals or by any clinic or individual practitioner, and patterns that are outside any clinician's experience might be discovered. Hopefully, by having a "population laboratory" on tap, such registers could facilitate systematic study of the aetiology, in particular of the pathogenesis and premonitory symptoms of the most terrible of all cases, the large number with fatal outcome very soon after onset of a presently recognisable attack.

For success, registers must depend on a high degree of professional support, and this will require considerable public and professional education — how considerable is exemplified by the fact that in many countries little serious attempt is made to establish the cause of naturally occurring "sudden deaths".

Pilot schemes should at the least:
1. ascertain and classify all suspect cases of "heart attack" in the defined population;
2. record all care given;
3. measure progress, medical and social, short and long-term, by cumulative personal files;
4. schedule cases for periodic review.

Adapted from the *Report of a Working Group Convened by the Regional Office for Europe,* WHO. 1968.

An Illustration

Pages 48, 49 sample what might be drawn from such a register. There would be 15,000 men of this age in an "average" E & W population of 100,000; so, if the figures in the Table are typical, and can be transferred to a notional community of that size, there might be 150 men, i.e. 1 per cent, who suffer a heart attack during the year (12 + 36 first attacks, plus 10 + 13 later, × 15/7 because there would be 15,000 not 7,000 men). This total includes close on 50 (12+10×15/7) "sudden" deaths in fulminant attacks, presumably ventricular fibrillation, and occurring mostly within an hour, and even within minutes, of the onset of presently recognised symptoms. These "electrical" deaths are the epitome of the modern epidemic and in scale recall the great plagues of the past. They constitute about 60 per cent of all IHD deaths in middle age (in this instance 22 of 34 during the year) and since, overall, IHD apparently is responsible for close on a third of male deaths in middle age (Table 2.1), we are dealing now with a sixth or more of the total mortality. Most of these victims do not — cannot — reach the hospital and its facilities alive; they are dealt with by the family, the public, GPs, the Coroner, his pathologists. (I well remember the incredulity with which *hospital* based clinician-friends greeted such figures when they first emerged 20–25 years ago from the early *population* studies).

Social costs of ischaemic heart disease for the country as a whole can be roughly estimated for 1970. The expenditure on social services was over £60 million including: NHS hospital costs (£15M); sickness benefits (nearly £20M) and widows' payments (nearly £30M). The loss of production from incapacity to work and premature death must represent a much larger sum. This is territory for value-judgment as much as anything; for example, after 65 years of age, loss of life could be regarded — economically — as a "saving". But about 250,000 years of future *working* life were lost by the deaths from IHD in 1970 (page 68). There must also be something like half-a-million coronary widows under 75. To anticipate, the kind of data in the Table straightaway gives some idea also of the scale of emergency service that needs to be provided for the immediate treatment of heart attacks. A good illustration of two practical purposes of the Register: to help *individuals* and to inform decisions on *services*. What is being done in the reader's own community in the treatment of the fulminant cases? And what discernible benefit is there in *community* death rates?

HEALTH AND THE MODE OF LIFE: SOCIAL MEDICINE

Epidemiology may further be defined as the study of *health of populations in relation to their environment and ways of living*. First

TABLE 2.4
HEALTHY AND UNHEALTHY DISTRICTS

England and Wales
Men Aged 45–64   Ave. Ann. Rates per 100,000
1958–64

Lowest Rates		Cause of Death and Mean Rate	Highest Rates	
Solihull	1,061		Manchester*	1,828
Ipswich*	1,096	All causes	Merthyr	1,855
Oxford	1,175	1,524	Salford	1,987
Ipswich	277		Swansea	527
Wolverhampton	283	Coronary heart disease	Wallasey	541
Exeter	314	421	Halifax	598
Ipswich	53		Oldham	234
Bath	63	Bronchitis	Manchester	251
Oxford	76	140	Salford	270

County Boroughs.
The ranges for females, and at ages 65–74, are similar.
From Registrar General's Tables and 1961 Census.
*Ipswich in best two and Manchester in worst two since 1920's (at least).
I.e., very roughly, 20 per cent of the men in Solihull die in middle age (between 45 and 65), 40 per cent of the men in Salford.

an old-fashioned analysis (Table 2.4) — as old as *Airs, Waters, Places* — which may return to favour with the new interest in "urban renewal" and in "positive discrimination" to help disadvantaged areas. It was surprising to find such disparities in middle age, though the general situation and the particular towns at both ends are familiar enough from studies of infant mortality. The distributions of deaths from "all causes" and from bronchitis make sense in terms of industrial history and contemporary poverty, the map of coronary heart disease was quite unexplained until recently (but in the 1970's no prizes can be offered). Table 2.5 is community diagnosis that again points ahead to needs for services.

Social Class

Table 2.6 is a simple social analysis of the first reproductive cycle in Aberdeen, a Scottish city with close on 200,000 inhabitants. The team are concerned with the efficiency of the physiological process — Farr's "laws of vitality", the "epidemiology of health" again. The value of a scale like *social class* is evident.

This method of analysis was devised early in the century by Dr Stevenson, one of Farr's successors as Chief Medical Statistician at the General Register Office.[44] He based "class" on occupations, their level of skill and role in production, and their "general standing" in the community. The former is more objective, the latter involves also what people feel about "status". The population is divided into five classes as follows:

Social Class	Description	Examples
1	Leading professions and business	Medical practitioner, Stockbroker
2	Lesser professions and business	Teacher, shopkeeper
3	Skilled workers: non-manual	Most clerks
	manual	Engineering craftsman
4	Part-skilled workers	Machine minder, most agricultural workers
5	Unskilled workers	Porter, builder's labourer

At the census of England and Wales in 1971 the proportion of "heads of household" in the various classes was: 1, 4·8 per cent; 2, 19·9 per cent; 3, 49 per cent; 4, 18·7 per cent; 5, 7·6 per cent. Close to a third of S.C. 3 were "non-manual"; two-thirds, manual. Married women are allocated to husband's occupation, children to father's. Broadly, the main divide and the main continuity of social life in Britain, classes 1, 2 and the non-manual "white collar" grades of 3 (about 40 per cent of all) are commonly regarded as the *middle classes,* the manual workers of 3 together with S.C. 4 and 5 as the *working classes* (about 60 per cent).

TABLE 2.5
INDICATORS OF THE "CONDITION OF THE PEOPLE"
RANGES IN LARGE COUNTY BOROUGHS OF ENGLAND

County Borough[1]	Sickness–Absence[2]	Mortality[3]	Old People[4]	Social Conditions[5]
St. Helens	166	12·7	102	2,448
Merseyside	131	12·1	104	2,188
Stoke	129	12·0	95	2,039
Middlesbrough	122	11·5	85	2,225
Sheffield	91	13·1	118	1,531
West Midlands	90	11·5	103	1,427
Reading	78	11·5	127	1,013
Leicester	77	12·4	125	1,322
Southampton	76	10·9	112	1,158

[1]"Merseyside" and "W. Midlands" are the C.Bs. of these conurbations.

[2]*Report on An Enquiry into the Incidence of Incapacity For Work 1961/62.* HMSO, 1965. Males 16–63 years, standardised for age. Figure for England = 95. Number of days of incapacity. "Merseyside" and "W, Midlands" give the experience of the whole of these conurbations for this item only.

[3]From Registrar General 1961. Both sexes, all ages; crude rates per 1,000.

[4]Proportion aged 65 + per 1,000 population. Census 1961.

[5]Crawford, M. D., Gardner, M. J. & Morris, J. N. (1968) *Lancet, 1,* 827. Overcrowding, unemployment, proportion in lower social classes and so forth. The higher the figure, the worse the social conditions. Data mostly for 1961 and around it.

TABLE 2.6
REPRODUCTIVE PERFORMANCE AND SOCIAL CLASS: ABERDEEN
Married Women Bearing a First Child
1970–2

| Findings in Primiparae | Social Class of Husband | | |
	1 & 2	3	4 & 5
Annual Rates per 100			
Age:			
–20 years	14·3	25·1	37·5
30+ years	9·3	4·3	3·8
Physique:			
Height under 5 ft. 1 in. (155 cm.)	13·1	21·9	24·6
Education:			
Left school above the minimum age	59·7	26·9	15·6
Reproduction: *Annual Rates per 1,000*			
Prenuptial conception	23·8	36·0	44·8
Low Birth Weight	49·0	66·4	106·5
Perinatal Mortality*	10·9	14·2	28·6

MacGillivray, I. Personal communications.

2,590 single children. Booked + Emergency.

*Perinatal mortality = S.B. + Deaths in 1st week of life per 1,000 related births.
Corresponding rates for Scotland in 1970–2 were:

| | 19·3 | 24·5 | 30·3 |

Since occupation is so highly correlated with income and living standards, the classification represents these also: "social class" is a model of prosperity/poverty, gratification/deprivation; of advantage/ disadvantage, privilege/under-privilege; the distribution of power and of "life chances" in society. The whole mode and style of life evidently are implicated in social class: income and wealth, financial security; physical environment; size of family and birth spacing; how children are reared; mean IQ levels, educational opportunity, parental interest and ambitions for children; language codes and way of speaking; the self-image, horizons and long-term goals; expectations of health and attitudes to illness, the utilisation of services. It is not surprising that compendium though it is, and withering at the edges as subsistence poverty is eliminated, jobs are upgraded, professions unionise, status deference declines, and some patterns of consumption converge — TV, home-ownership, Marks & Spencer, women's mags, the motor-car, holidays abroad, youth culture — this distinction by "social class" continues a powerful tool for the exploration of the levels of health that people enjoy, the troubles they suffer, and how they cope with these.[*45 50]

Inequality of Opportunity

To return to Aberdeen, Table 2.6 shows some exceptionally low perinatal mortality *rates* but the *range* between the classes is substantial. Inequalities in infant mortality in fact continue marked, if less than 60 years ago when this particular mode of analysis was first used. In the Scotland of 1951-2, infant death rates were 21·1 per 1,000 live births in classes 1 and 2 and 45·1 in 4 and 5. In 1971-2, the corresponding figures were 13·5 and 24·8. Multiple explanations have been proposed

*Social Origins of Students Entering Medicine. England and Wales 1955–6
  Social Class

1 & 2	78%
3 Non-Manual	8%
Manual	12%
4 & 5	2%

Kelsall, R. K. (1957) *Applications for Admissions to Universities.* London. For males the figure in classes I and II was 76 per cent, females 85 per cent. The Scottish rates were little better, doctors' children accounted for only a part of the inequality. The maldistribution in other faculties was not quite so gross. Needless to say, such figures do not reflect the talent in the population or even the proportions from different classes completing grammar school, though they do still reflect working-class horizons and aspirations. (Occupations ≡ social class, social class ≡ occupation, Tawney.)

So 80–90 per cent of the future doctors were middle-class, about 70 per cent of their patients — the general population — then were in lower classes. Such social distance may produce real difficulty. The doctor must not expect the majority of his patients to share *his* assumptions (or even to be at ease with him). To communicate effectively and get a good history, to be able "to take the social factors of the case" into account, he must study the *patients'* attitudes and ways of living and learn about them as the good physician does through experience and sympathy.

why so wide a gap persists despite the advances in the standard of living, in social services and in medical knowledge.

First, as said, work is being upgraded, average living standards rising, and class lines to some extent being redrawn; in Scotland about 31 per cent of infants were born into classes 4 and 5 in 1951–2, about 27 per cent in 1971–2 (and some of these must have been recent coloured immigrants). Likes are not quite strictly being compared and, anyhow, the unfavourable mortality gradient that persists affects somewhat smaller numbers.

The second explanation can be dismissed: that class differences in mortality are importantly due to difference between them in the ages at which mothers bear children or in the numbers borne. For example, *infants of young mothers who already have large families* are particularly vulnerable, and of course there are more of these infants in the lower classes. But historically (Table 2.7) such families (30 years of age is a convenient break) had a higher post-neonatal mortality in class 5 than class 4, in 4 than 3, and so on. This kind of order can be imposed on a vast range of infant mortality statistics — or could when the data were available.[51]

TABLE 2.7
POST – NEONATAL MORTALITY RATE: MULTIPLE CAUSES
Large Families; Social Class; Maternal Age

England and Wales
1949–50
Rates per 1,000 Live Births

Social Class	PNMR All Children All Causes of Death	PNMR Fourth and Later Children			
		Mothers – 30 years		Mothers 30 + years	
		All Causes	Infections*	All Causes	Infections*
1	4·8	} 15·0	6·5	9·2	3·6
2	5·7				
3	10·3	21·9	12·6	14·3	7·3
4	13·7	26·4	} 15·6	17·6	} 9·4
5	17·0	29·1		18·1	
All	10·8	23·7	13·4	15·0	7·7

*Respiratory and alimentary, 1950.
Deaths at 4 weeks–1 year. Single, legitimate infants. Both sexes.
M.R.C. Social Medicine Unit and General Register Office, Joint Enquiry.[51]

Third, and most direct: persisting unequal death rates between the classes reflect multiple persisting social inequalities. Money wages of many of the poorest have improved with modern affluence. But the gaps between lower incomes and higher have narrowed less. Moreover, as Aberdeen data illustrate, gross differences between classes remain in what may be regarded as their health "capital". Thus, the women vary in physique, which is related very likely to inequalities in their own childhood nutrition. There are far more tall women in classes 1 and 2, in classes 4 and 5 far more who are short, resulting in added risks of caesarean section and birth trauma for example. "Prematurity", if not the very smallest birthweight, shows the same social trend. Perinatal mortality is strongly associated, in the expected direction. The poorer education of the "lower" classes is a factor, too, in their lesser utilisation of available health services. At the outset they report pregnancy later, which may be related to the "wantedness" of children and knowledge of family planning; middle-class women more often "book" for confinement in hospital, so benefitting more fully from advances in treatment (habits and attitudes lagging behind incomes). The "physiological" failures reflected in *perinatal mortality* reflect the lifetime experience of the mother. It is a problem also in "ecology". Pockets of poverty persist, replenished by downward drift of the chronic handicapped in some way, and social differences as said remain gross. Thus, Victorian thunder still is needed to mobilise the public, which is beginning to despair of ever solving the housing problem of the cities.

At the census of 1971:

Unfit Housing

POPULATION	PROPORTION OF HOUSEHOLDS		
	Without hot water tap (%)	Without fixed bath or shower (%)	Sharing WC (%)
Glasgow	16	22	10
Aberdeen	9	22	20

The abolition of 19th century misery . . .

The current environment with its deprivations — exemplified in large families when the mother is young, less expert, and the births crowded, too — is specially powerful after the perinatal period, in relation to infection in infancy, for example, and to the mysterious cot deaths. And so in the overall persistently unsatisfactory class trends of *post-neonatal mortality*.[51][55]

It is not only the class trend. The post-neonatal mortality rate didn't fall throughout most of the 1960's; why, is not yet clear. The succumbing of weaklings salvaged during the neonatal days? Bottle-feeding in unsanitary homes? A reflection of the contemporary poverty debate? — that during those years there was little closure of the gap in the standard of living between the well-to-do and the poorest. "Auditing" of such infant deaths will provide an immediate indicator of how well local health and social services are being deployed.[55]

Standard of Living

The modern improvement can be expressed in many ways: e.g. cars, home ownership. Table 2.8 provides a baseline. Allowing for the rise in prices and population, compared with the mid-1950's there was, in the early mid-1970's, about half as much again more money to *spend personally* (goods and services people buy for themselves), and (b) over twice as much money spent in *social consumption* (publicly purchased goods and services, like the NHS). Combining these two,

TABLE 2.8
AFFLUENT SOCIETY
BRITAIN

Indicator	1938	1948	1956	1964	1970	1972
Average Weekly Earnings[1]	£3·11s.	£7·1s.	£12·4s.	£18·13s.	£28·18s.	£35·16s.
	(50)	(100)	(173)	(264)	(410)	(508)
Cost of Living: retail prices index	50	100	145	180	235	275
Expenditure on Social Services: millions[2]	£600	(£1,934)	£2,924	£5,668	£9,145	£11,399
National Assistance/Supplementary Benefits[3]	£1·11s.	£2	£3·7s.	£5·4s.	£8·10s.	£10·13s.
Personal Disposable Income, per head[4]		£278	£334	£418	£440	£505
Unemployment rate per cent	13	1·8	1·3	1·8	2·6	3·8
Married-Women Working: per cent at ages 15–59[5]	?10	28	35	40	39	41
Home Ownership: per cent "owner-occupiers"	32	32	32	44	49	51
Family/Household Amenities: per cent with						
washing machine	?1	3·6	19	50	62	66
TV set	(0)	1	40	80	90	93
car	?16	15	24	40	54	55
Hire-Purchase Debt: millions	£?	£105	£376	£1,115	£1,350	
Expenditure on Advertising: millions	£100	£120	£300	£550		£700

Several of the figures in Table 2.8 are estimates only; in some instances they are not for Britain but for United Kingdom (i.e. including also N. Ireland).

[1] Adult males in manufacture.. Before deductions for income tax and social security. These are averages of wide ranges. Moreover, workers in "services" often are paid less; in September 1970 the *average* weekly earnings of NHS male ancillary workers were £21·7 and of those in the *lowest decile*, £15·3.

[2] Central and local government, capital expenditure and current; including social security, health, welfare, education, housing. U.K.

[3] Basic regular payment for old-age pensioner couple, excluding rent, (£10·13s = £10·65).

[4] At 1963 constant prices.

[5] Paid employment outside the home; including part-time.

Peacock, A. T. and Wiseman, J. (1967) *The Growth of Public Expenditure in the United Kingdom.* London. *National Income and Expenditure; Social Trends; Report of Family Expenditure Survey.* HMSO. Annually.

Before the Deluge!

(a) + (b) is a useful shorthand for the average S o L. Fig. 2.6 illustrates the main gain in children's nutrition. Only during the 1939-45 war did Simon's dictum of 1890 begin to lose its force: "How far the poor can be made less poor. In the whole range of questions concerning the public health, there is not any one to be deemed more important than the question which these words raise."[56] There is no doubt that the poorest have been lifted since the 1930's — there's nothing more eloquent than bare feet (p. 6) — it is no longer the mass denial of elementary human needs, though hardship and severe if not subsistence poverty persists. The distribution has moved up. But Plimsoll lines need constantly to be reset once subsistence, absolute, physiological poverty is overcome. "People are poverty-stricken when their income, even if adequate for survival, falls markedly behind that of the community. Then they cannot have what the larger community regards as the minimum necessary for decency; and they cannot wholly escape, therefore, the judgment of the larger community that they are. . . degraded for, in the literal sense, they live outside the grades or categories which the community regards as acceptable. . ."; "people judge themselves by their relationship to what seems average".[57] Today there is a wide awareness of such "relative deprivation".[58] [59] That is to say, the poor will always be with us, the lower end of the distribution; the debate on poverty is merging with the debate on equality, on persisting inequality in shares of rising living standards. The Victorians were emphatic also about the *corollary* to Simon's dictum that poverty begets disease: *disease → poverty → disease,* one of mankind's vicious cycles.[61] [62] This, too, is a lesson that has to be relearned in each generation. But, of course, British poverty, and the powerlessness of our poor, are incomparably less, of another quality altogether, from the absolute poverty of the third world.

From sundry official and unofficial studies it may be estimated that in the early mid-1970's approximately half a million children, 1 in 20 or 25, were living close to the official poverty line defined by "supplementary benefit" ("welfare"). Mostly, of course, they were in the families of low wage-earners, many of them coloured, in social classes 4 and 5 scattered widely through industry and "services" (including shamefully local government and the hospitals of the National *Health* Service). The number of families with three or more children grew in the 1960's by about 350,000 to one-and-three-quarter million, only lately attracting allowances and supplements enough appreciably to make up low wages. Such a family, however stable, with less than about £25 per week, will spend 40 per cent and more of its income on food. If not in protected housing it is liable to be overwhelmed, especially in the inner cities, to become homeless, break up altogether as a family, its deprivations associated with multiple problems: a checkered history of multiple infections, low birthweight, infant mortality, inferior physical growth and mental development, school failure and wasted ability, juvenile delinquency, maternal apathy and depression, an insatiable demand for health and social services. The main *group in poverty* of course are the elderly: about 1 in 3 probably are around the supplementary benefit level, and mostly receiving this; i.e. they are very poor. The other groups for the doctor to bear in mind are the chronic sick, and the mentally and physically disabled. They are often chronic unemployed, with their multiple deprivations and incapacities; and one-parent (fatherless) families. It is now abundantly clear that the fate of such

MILK
pints/head/week

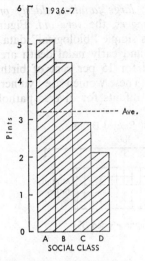

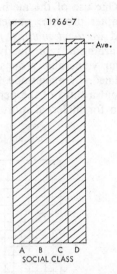

Fig. 2.6   1936–7: Proportions of population, class A (highest income) = 5 per cent; class B = 20 per cent; class C = 60 per cent; class D = 15 per cent. (Crawford, W. & Broadley, H. (1938) *The People's Food.* London.)
1966–7: A, 10 per cent; B, 35 per cent; C, 35 per cent; D, 20 per cent. (*Annual Reports of the National Food Survey Committee, Household Food Consumption and Expenditure,* HMSO, London.)

vulnerable groups cannot be left to the general improvement of living standards. Late 1973, with still high unemployment, food prices outstripping wages, inflation accelerating out of control, and now the energy crisis on top is a bad time to be writing. And now the economic recession is looming. [60 63-65]

INDIVIDUALS AND POPULATIONS

Such analysis of the phenomena of health by social class, civil state, sex and age, by standard of living and culture pattern, is the stock-in-trade of epidemiology. Within groups, or "populations", there will obviously be individual variation; but summing the group experience, and the demonstration of difference beween groups, tells something that could not be known before. Often it will provide the first indication that a problem exists. Since Farr's day the exposure of unfavourable group experience has been a powerful weapon in educating the community to the need for action. This is often the beginning of the search for causes — to analyse why infant mortality differs in the social classes, what ways of living are involved?

Vulnerable Groups

One use of the method is to identify those at special risk and the chapter provides numerous examples: *large families, elderly primips* and *worn-out multips, poor kids, teenagers,* the *very old.* Figure 2.7 returning to reproductive wastage uses simple "biological" data only. Four vulnerable groups for stillbirth and early natal death are here defined. In magnitude they accounted for 15 per cent of births but about a third of the perinatal deaths. (These women are "vulnerable" also for maternal mortality and their infants for diverse pathology.)

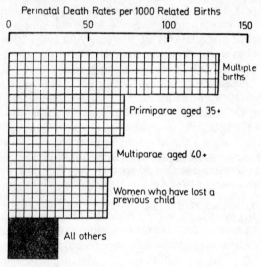

Fig. 2.7   Four vulnerable groups for perinatal mortality. 1950. England and Wales. *Brit. J. prev. soc. Med.* (1965) **10**, 97.

Groups at high-risk have long been the concern of public health, in the school medical service and in maternity and child welfare. They have led to action against accidents and other industrial hazards. New opportunities for giving support at vulnerable periods are being recognised, for example in losses such as bereavement.

The "epidemiological imagination" uses such social/biological group regularities to illumine the clinical instance. The child under multiple deprivation is at risk of multiple trouble. Delinquency is likely to mean something different in boys from social class I and social class 5. Alcoholism is one thing in an Irishman, another in a (orthodox) Jew. "Illegitimacy" in our terms is no stigma to a Jamaican. Tuberculosis is more likely in the Asian immigrant; venereal disease in uprooted men. Workers will not wear safety boots if it is the norm not to. It's hard to relax in a competitive high-pressure milieu. The cigarette-smoker taking inadequate exercise urgently needs help.

MODERN WORLD

Table 2.9 now fills the gap between (2) on page 8 and the figures at the opening of this chapter (p. 29). Consider the last column; the underlying trend evidently is upward. But how much could be acute respiratory infection which so strongly affects sickness-absence rates? Column (1) extracts the months when this matters least, and Col. (2) those when it prevails: if 'flu, indeed, is responsible for the upward drift of Col. (1) it is an "epidemic distemper" proceeding from a quite "inexplicable alteration of the air" (Sydenham). More likely the Table is, or was, a sign of the times: rising wages and sickness benefits, more wives "in gainful employment" — and the general retreat from work and rising expectations of the Age of Leisure throughout the affluent Western world. Since the middle 1950's, average working hours in industry have fallen by over two hours a week, some industries have very high " absenteeism" rates and strikes. (The jobs so often are boring, more can now afford to be "alienated"?; dilemmas for the certifying doctor.) The greatest increase is in short absences of less than a week, which add up ordinarily to only about 12 million lost days per year but are a nuisance out of proportion. "Psychoneurosis" and nervous symptoms, together with minor injuries, are the certificated causes showing the greatest increase. In the late 1960's the picture changed, with mass unemployment, economic stagnation and inflation. Whether it is about a patient or a prevalence, people and the way they live have to be studied, not merely diseases. This is to consider the multiple physical, mental and social manifestations and causes of health. The terms "whole-man medicine" and "ecology" try to express the principle, and a "multidisciplinary" or "systems" approach hopefully will help in achieving it.

TABLE 2.9
SICKNESS-ABSENCE: NEW CLAIMS FOR BENEFIT PER WEEK

Britain
Thousands

Year	May–September	Rest of Year	Annual Average
1949–53	99–105	147–177	127–145
1954	108	160	138
1956	115	175	149
1958	114	179	152
1960	127	178	157
1962	130	205	173
1964	141	196	173
1966	156	242	206
1968	159	235	204
1969	165	258	219
1970	156	240	205
1972	149	209	184
1974			

YOUNG PEOPLE

The post-World War II baby "boom" in due course became the adolescent "bulge". Mere increase in numbers of the "population-at-risk", without any rise of incidence, must mean more of their sundry troubles, dysmennorhoea and "appendicitis" in girls, asthma — and osteosarcoma, epilepsy, schizophrenia. But well-nourished for a lifetime, and with phthisis in retreat, young people today are among the healthiest in the population, make little demand on conventional medical care and have remarkably low death rates. At the same time, young people are in the van of the changes now under way in society, and since they are maturing earlier and passing through their own

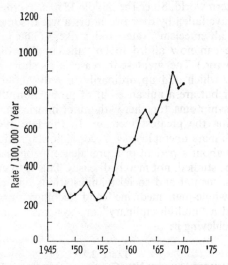

Fig. 2.8 Breaking and entering. Males 17–20 inc. England and Wales. 1945–70. *Criminal Statistics* and *Supplement*. Home Office. Annually. HMSO. London. Power, M. J.

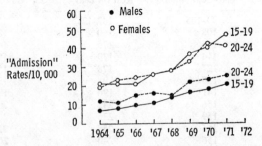

Fig. 2.9 Poisoning in young people. "Admissions" to hospitals, England and Wales. *Hospital In-Patient Enquiry*. Annually. McLaughlin, C. See also, Alderson, M. R. (1974) *Lancet* **1**, 1040.

TABLE 2.10
CASUALTIES IN ROAD ACCIDENTS; YOUNG RIDERS OF MOTOR-CYCLES, ETC.
Killed and Seriously Injured
Britain

Year	Casualties
1951	1,371
1953	1,710
1955	2,624
1957	3,601
1959	6,579
1961	7,834
1963	8,827
1964	10,835
1965	10,642
1967	8,729
1969	7,373
1971	7,061
1973	

Ages 16–19 incl.; both sexes. The greatest increase by far is at 16 years.
Road Accidents. Annually. HMSO. London.

uneven physiological and emotional development and identity crisis, they are likely to be mixed-up and vulnerable. It is not surprising that behaviour among young people changes so rapidly that concurrent monitoring is necessary.

Motor-cycle, scooter and such accidents (above) have risen steeply, casualties of the craze to get about fast; fashion is switching to motor-cars and, however aggressively driven, almost any cars are safer, so there are hopes this epidemic is abating . . . Everywhere in society is uncertainty, but on nothing more than on sexual behaviour.* There are some 50,000–60,000 births a year in teenagers, illegitimate or legitimated by the marriage, (Table 2.11, overleaf) . . . The increase of anti-social behaviour is particularly clear at 17–20 years of age, of serious stealing (Fig. 2.8) as well as joy-riding in "borrowed" cars, of vandalism and — often — mere senseless violence . . . There is an epidemic of self-poisoning (Fig. 2.9), and drunkenness offences also are rising steeply. Again, there is too little by social class, still less by the numerous other groups to which the young people belong.

In the mid 1950's young people "entered" into society and "youth culture" was born. *Epidemiology of health:* there ought to be statistics of vitality, independence, freedom from sexual guilt . . . Plainly,

---

* "The fundamental changes in society will force changes in some of the sexual rules; but the scepticism and conflict about some as being "arbitrary", once set in motion, tend to undermine all of them and thus to paralyse regulation in general. The absence of clear and enforceable rules apart from the peer group leads to many wrong decisions and personal tragedies. To an unusual degree, each young person must fend for himself by a costly process of trial and error".[66]

TABLE 2.11

MATERNITIES CONCEIVED OUTSIDE MARRIAGE

Rates per 1,000 Unmarried Females
England and Wales

Age	1938	1952–5	1956	1960	1964	1968	1972*
15–19	11·8	15·7	19·0	24·0	30·3	37·2	36·9
20–24	32·6	42·8	48·6	58·0	68·0	65·9	62·7
Total							
15–44	18·6	25·3	28·9	35·5	42·5	46·7	43·2

*Of females aged 15–19, 91 per cent currently were unmarried. About 60 per cent of these conceptions at 15–19 are later legitimated by marriage; the remainder are born illegitimate; 50,000–60,000 live births are involved. About 70 per cent of all births at 15–19 are so conceived out of wedlock.

The Abortion Act became operative in April 1968. The rate at 15-19 in unmarried girls in 1971 was 12.6 per 1,000, and at 20-24 years 22.1.

From Registrar General *Statistical Reviews,* Tables, Part II, Population; Annual *Supplements on Abortion;* and personal communications, OPCS.

TABLE 2.12

ESTIMATES OF GONORRHOEA

England and Wales.

Age	1957	1967	1969	1971	1973
Males					
–19	828	2,918	4,055	4,669	
20–24	4,171	9,427	11,524	12,544	
25+	10,309	18,285	20,785	21,818	
Females					
–19	939	3,252	4,661	6,143	
20–24	1,377	3,931	5,248	6,665	
25+	1,816	3,898	4,859	5,630	

No. of attacks of diagnosed fresh infection during the year at venereal disease clinics. British Co-operative Clinical Group (1962). *Brit. J. vener. Dis. 38,* 1;Willcox R. R., personal communications; *Annual Digest of Health and Personal Social Service Statistics. Brit. med. J.* (1971) ii, 602.

No estimate is available of cases dealt with in general practice, etc.

"Gonorrhoea out of control", WHO, 27 Jan., 1971.
"All God's children got de clap . . . the legitimate new freedoms are being bank-rupted through criminal selfishness . . ." Neville, R. (1970) *Oz, 31,* 4.

Population of E. & W. at ages 20–24 in 1971: M, 1,869,000; F, 1,848,000 (but an unknown number of foreigners are included in the estimates).

medicine by itself is powerless to comprehend let alone control the sources of health and ill-health in this generation. Granted, but what services ought medicine now to lead in providing? For what needs? The absence of interest-groups in young people's health, not to say of of the emergence of a specialty, is puzzling.[67-71]

Is Health Improving?

On the information presented in Chapter 1 as well as this, Yes and No can be the only answer. As a postscript[4], Fig. 2.10 brings the mortality picture forward.

Connecting with pages 1 and 2 of the book, notice in Fig. 2.10 that death rates now are falling little also in middle-aged women — and very generally. The trends are similar in Scotland, and U.S whites; at higher levels in U.S. non-whites, at lower in Sweden.

Evidently we are not dealing with anything particular to the condition of Britain, or any simple failings of our National Health Service; these disappointments must be the product of very general forces. The parallel improvements in the rates among countries at several levels of mortality, and in various social circumstances, suggest that

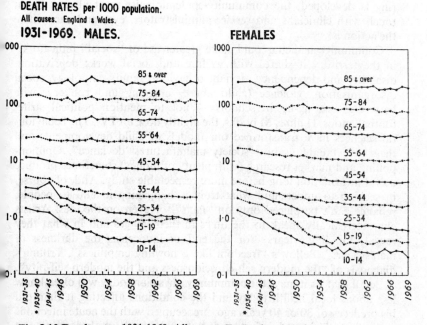

DEATH RATES per 1000 population.
All causes. England & Wales.

1931-1969. MALES.   **FEMALES**

Fig. 2.10 Death rates, 1931-1969. All causes. England and Wales.
*1940 to 1949 Civilians only.

the great wave of scientific discovery between the late 1930's and late 1950's, particularly in overcoming infectious diseases, was being efficacious. However, this does not appear to be enough to take us much further. Diseases, accidents, and ageing, mostly incurable by "medical care," predominate now. It looks like the end of the road for present policies on health, based as they are so largely on treatment, and there is a new interest in the possibilities of prevention through changing the mode of life.

COMMUNITY DIAGNOSIS

The conditions of existence are altering rapidly (though some things seem unassailable — the social origin of medical students, for example, didn't change through the 1960's). Technology can be extrapolated more easily than the biological. However, under strain, the organism has a limited recognisable repertory of reactions: mutations, malformation, inflammation, blood dyscrasias, neoplasm, sundry functional disorders, neurosis, violence. So we could try to monitor these, and if there are signals of something untoward seek the origins. Routine computer-surveillance of cause-of-death statistics,[72] and, to seek possible adverse effects, linking hospital diagnoses with drug treatments, are established information systems by now.[73] However fast more systematic monitor-ring is developed, the community-epidemiologist must always be in touch with clinicians and service-administrators, eyes and ears where the action is.

Community medicine could make greater use of "social" indicators[12] in the territory it shares with welfare and social work: deprivation, disability and dependency, deviant behaviour, family-pathology, social disorganisation, violence (child abuse, mugging and robbery, wife battering, beating-up in schools — not to mention political strife, football mobs, H films, M books, the nightly dose on TV). The behavioural sciences have transformed our models of child development; and they have taught us how society manufactures 'deviance". Opinion-polling and market research (with plenty of money) sometimes produce useful information long before more respectable study. And, of course, in seeking to understand what truly is happening in and to people, reliance can't be placed only on "facts", or even on theories. Artists characteristically speak to the times in their images and in what they reveal: Golding's tears "for the end of innocence, the darkness of man's heart", Bellow's "freedom like a howling emptiness", Trilling's diagnosis of "the modern self-consciousness and the modern self-pity".

Be all that as it may: the community physician today will often know less about local health today and the conditions affecting it than did his predecessor 30 or 40 years ago, preoccupied with the acute infections and tuberculosis and infant and maternal health, with squalor and undernutrition. *New measurements* have to be developed, to give current substance and reality to "community medicine", for the clinician and the medical teacher as well as the health-service administrator — and the public. Hopefully, in these first two Chapters some examples have already been given of useful information on the people's health from the most local to the national, and Tables 2.13 et seq. add a few more.

TABLE 2.13
CLEARING THE AIR OF LONDON

Winter Averages

Winter	Smoke		SO_2	
	(a)	(c)	(b)	(c)
1954–6	51		11·5	
1956–7	45		10·2	
1958–9	43	309	11·9	340
1960–1	24	200	9·7	277
1962–3		173		365
1964–5		126		276
1966–7		87		214
1968–9		67		221
1970–1		61		176
1971–2		61		180
1972–3		55		145
1973–4				

Inner London.
(a) Milligrams of smoke per 100 cubic metres of air.
(b) Parts of sulphur dioxide per 100 million parts of air.
(c) Micrograms per cubic metre.
Average daily reading, seven stations.
   Annual Reports of the Medical Officer of Health, London County Council; Stewart, A. B. (1973) personal communications; *Annual Abstract Greater London Statistics*. London.
The Clean Air Act became operative in 1956.
   ". . . Now not only do the wild flowers rampage over every bombed site, but window boxes in the flats are gay with flowers, and the charming little 'parklets' that have been opened up have real herbaceous borders, and roses thrive there, too." "Stepney To-Day", a tribute to the Act. *The Listener,* 27 January, 1966.

TABLE 2.14

MORTALITY IN TRANSPORTATION ACCIDENTS, USA

1969-71

Mode of Transport	Death Rate of Passengers Per 100 million passenger-miles per year
Automobiles	2·10*
Scheduled domestic flights	0·10 ⎫
Buses	0·19 ⎬ **
Railroad passenger trains	0·12 ⎭

Drivers are included as "passengers".

*In 1970, number of deaths of *passengers* = 34,200; death rate = 1·9 per 100 million passenger-miles (the British rate was about 2·9). 10,600 (estimated) *pedestrians* also were killed in the USA in all motor-vehicle accidents in 1970.

**In 1971 number of deaths of passengers = 320.

Accident Facts, 1972. Chicago, National Safety Council; and personal communications. *Road Accident Statistical Review*, ROSPA, Monthly, London; and personal communications.

TABLE 2.15

FUTURE YEARS OF "WORKING LIFE" LOST PER 1,000 AND PER YEAR FROM DEATHS OCCURRING IN 1970-71

England and Wales

Cause of Death	Future Working Years Lost Per 1,000 population aged 0-64 years in 1970-1	
	Males	Females
All Causes	71	45
Coronary heart disease	11·8	2·8
Accidents	9·8	3·3
Bronchitis, Pneumonia	7·0	4·6
Cancer of bronchus	4·0	—
Cancer of breast	—	2·7
Other cancer	7·6	7·9
Other infant mortality	13·9	10·3
etc., etc.		

Years of working life lost from each death at ages 0-64 are added; "Working Life" is taken to be 15-64 years of age, inclusive. Averages based on the 2 years 1970-1 were calculated.

Registrar General, *Quarterly Returns*, June, annually; and personal communications. Gardner, M. J., personal communications.

TABLE 2.16
"DISEASES OF MEDICAL PROGRESS"*

England and Wales

Condition	Estimated Numbers
Therapeutic misadventures	
Number of deaths reported as possibly due to medicines during 1964–71, approx:**	
Oral contraceptives	332
Phenylbutazone	217
Chlorpromazine	102
Etc.	
Spina Bifida	
Seriously disabled mentally or physically which are being added to the population per year***	200
Casualities in road accidents	
Surviving and being added to the population per year with serious brain damage, unable to work****	700
Residents aged 75+ in mental hospital for more than 1 year	
1954	14,345
1963	18,826
1972	19,631

*Moser, R. H. (1969), Springfield, Ill. The title of his invaluable American compendium. See also: *Adverse Drug Reactions* (1972) Ed., Richards, D. J. & Rondel, R. K., Edinburgh.
**Girdwood, R. H. (1974) *Br. med. J., 1,* 501.
***Lorber, J. (1968) *Med. Offr., 119,* 213.
****Lewin, W. (1968) *Br. Med. J., 1,* 465. London, P. S. (1967) *Ann. R. Coll. Surg., 41,* 460.

TABLE 2.17
ESTIMATES OF STROKE IN THE COMMUNITY

Age Group	Standard USA Million Population		Annual Incidence		Point Prevalence**	
			Estimated incidence per 1,000 Per Year	Expected New Cases Per Year	Estimated Point Prevalence Per 1,000	Expected Total Cases in Community
0–34	582,083	(59%)	0·00	0	0	0
35–44	113,561	(11%)	0·25	28	0	0
45–54	114,206	(11%)	1·00	114	20	2,284
55–64	91,464	(9·1%)	3·50	320	35	3,201
65–74	61,155	(6·1%)	9·00	550	60	3,669
75+	37,531	(3·8%)	30·00	1,126	95	3,565
Total	1,000,000	(100%)		2,138*		12,719

*Total of first and later attacks is approx. 2,500.   **Cases surviving one month,
Stallones, R. A., Dyken, M. L., Fang, H. C. H., Heyman, A., Seltser, R. & Stainler.
J. *Stroke, 3,* May-June, 1972.

TABLE 2.18
ESTIMATES OF (1) MORBIDITY ⟶ (2) NEEDS ⟶
Sample Survey, Great Britain, 1968–9
BOTH SEXES   AGES 16+

	%
(1) Prevalence of Lesion – "Impairment" in population*	7·8**
(2) Proportion of (1) Disabled by the Impairment	
Severely (24% of them living alone)	11·6
Very Severely (5·2% of them living alone)	5·1

*Outside institutions.
**Ranging according to age from 0·9% at 16–29 years to 38% at 75+.
  Harris, A. I. (1971) *Handicapped and Impaired in Great Britain.* HMSO, London;
and personal communication.

3. Working of Health Services

From health to health services. How to describe them? How are services working in reality, as distinct from laws, plans and pronouncements about them? How are they adapting to the changing pattern of health and disease? To what extent is new knowledge being translated into medical care? How are services coping with the manifold needs illustrated in Chapter 2? How are the community's specialist resources and emergency facilities mobilised to reduce perinatal death? At the start of the National Health Service, we found that only two of four needs-priority groups that could so readily be defined (p. 60) had high rates of hospital confinement. Elderly "multips" and mothers who had already lost a child were delivered in hospital less often than the majority of mothers who were not at particular risk. These were some of the figures:

High-risk Group	Perinatal Mortality Rate per 1,000 Births, 1950	Proportion of Mothers Confined in Hospital
Multiple pregnancies	131	85%
Primiparae aged 35+	72	88%
Multiparae aged 40+	65	49%
Women who had lost a child	62	51%
All others	31	60%

Such facts are insufficient for the community physician: *vital statistics* can state the issue and outline distributions, the short Table just quoted is an example. To provide a basis for planning local service programmes social medical investigation would have to be on several levels. Population statistics again will describe outcomes of the services in morbidity and mortality. Ad hoc *social surveys* could help: to characterise the important groups of mothers; and on such questions as the demand for hospital facilities, local housing conditions, the availability of home-helps, prevailing attitudes (rational and irrational) including the doctors'. Representative *case studies* ought also to be made to bring the statistics to life, to provide pictures in personal-domestic-clinical terms how obstetric need and advantage are balanced against other values and priorities: what, in the event, decides whether particular mothers are

References on page 289.

confined in hospital. Informed at all these levels, the correct decisions are more likely to be made and local campaigns to change the kind of situation shown in the table will stand more chance of success. The reports of the Chief Medical Officer show rapid progress, nationally: thus, under half the women aged 35+ bearing a fifth or later child were confined in hospital in the mid-1950's, 90 per cent in the early 1970's (a few, though, not in beds directly 'covered' by a specialist obstetrician). Insistence on the special needs of such groups has to be distinguished from the general issue of hospital confinement; short-stay "early discharge" schemes obviously are relevant to every aspect. The decline in the birth rate has provided unexpected relief, and by now there often are empty obstetric beds.*

Operational research, may be defined as the *systematic study,* by observation and experiment, *of the working of health services with a view to their improvement.* Slow to get started, it has suddenly become fashionable, under the banners of "management" and "efficiency". Of course, the epidemiological is not the only method of study; economics and ethics, systems analysis, mathematical models, work-study, and various behavioural-science disciplines increasingly are being used. The "chronic" ward, old people's welfare committee, any social-work agency, the juvenile court. . . provide plenty of opportunity for clinical observation of the workings of health services. But medical population studies are essential: of the people's needs and demands; how these are being met; and the success of services in lifting the burden of disability and improving health. It is in the context of these that the various disciplines and viewpoints concerned in medical care have to be reconciled. Epidemiological methods at present often are primitive, but they will not improve of themselves. The remainder of this chapter asks some elementary questions about health services, beginnings of an *epidemiology for administrators,*[1-4] looking at patient-care, a little on health and prevention, but not on education.

"MEDICAL POLICE"

The simplest sums can be worthwhile. How do the million schoolboys under 16 get hold of the 100 million cigarettes they smoke per year?[5] Only a quarter or third of front-seat car occupants wear seat-belts even on motorways (though nearly all cars are fitted).[6] In how many local factories are safety, including fire, precautions below the legal minimum?

---

*The issues are changing again. In recent years there has been a sharp increase in the induction of labour, from *c.* 15 per cent in 1965 to almost a third in 1972 (CMO's Report, 1973), and, judging by comment among clinicians and service-administrators, the rate is still rising. Mothers at low-risk are being induced (because of shortage of staff resources round the clock?), as well as those manifestly at high-risk. What is happening in the reader's own community? Can local information systems provide the necessary data?

WHAT IS GENERAL PRACTICE?

General practice, primary care, is no longer the most "difficult" area of the National Health Service: that distinction belongs to the long-stay hospitals. But we began this study back in 1950 because of the contemporary crisis in general practice, a crisis of identity, role-definition, status, professional satisfactions (1948 model). In the quite ordinary practice observed, as typical as a sample of one can be,[7] [8] 60 per cent of the "nuclear" families were wholly registered with it; the frame at least was there for the GP to be a *family doctor:*

Definition of "Family"	Proportion of such families who were completely registered with the practice
Mother and children	96%
Parents and children	60%
Parents, children and relatives living at the same address	27%

Utilisation of the services of the practice was quite unequal. About a quarter of the "population" had no contact with the doctor during the course of the year (next page). 16 per cent, on the other hand — about 500 persons in far fewer families — had 10 or more consultations, accounting for half the total work. Plainly, there was plenty of opportunity for the GPs and these patients to get to know each other.* Of the problems dealt with, 16 per cent were readily definable as serious, affecting life or livelihood. Simple "shop arithmetic" again, but novel when the sums were done, and the vacuum had been filled with generalisations that "the GP is a specialist in the trivial", an "expert in minor illness", and so on. Of course, there was a good deal of that (cf. Table 2.1), much of it, doubtless, the emotional difficulties and ups and downs of daily living that are perceived as important by the public and, in today's climate of opinion, regarded as the doctor's job. Anyhow, when so much is "serious", the general practitioner requires a good knowledge of internal medicine, to be up-to-date in relevant clinical technology. About a third of the work involved helping patients and their families to cope with chronic disease and disability. The GP, member now of a team, has to provide continuing care with realistic objectives, to be concerned in rehabilitation and resettlement at work including housework, mobilising personal and familial resources — and the appropriate community nursing, welfare, income and other services in aid.

*The concentration was not confined to the year under review. Such numbers recall the limitations of data about "spells" of sickness for describing the heatlh of the population.

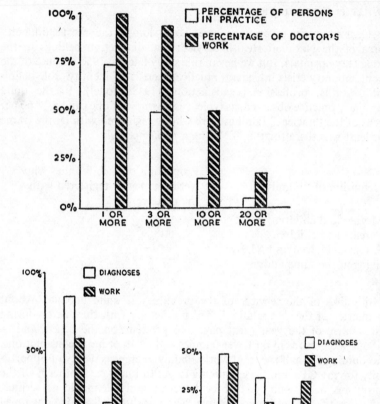

Fig. 3.1 Work of a general practice in one year. Outer London, 1951/2. *Upper figure:* 72 per cent had 1 or more consultations; 28 per cent had none; ave. = 5; 49 per cent had 3 or more consultations in the year and accounted for over 90 per cent of all the work. *Lower left figure:* 16 per cent of the diagnoses were of "serious" problems, accounting for 43 per cent of the work. *Lower right figure:* 18 per cent of the diagnoses were of "chronic" conditions, accounting for about 33 per cent of the work (and, not shown, over twice these proportions after 65 years of age).
Brit. med J. (1954) **1,** 109.

The impact of the aged on this (one) practice (at that time) may be stated thus: the 300 persons over 65 made up rather fewer than 10 per cent of the doctors' lists, but they were responsible for about fifth of the total activities, a quarter of the home visits, a third of all the "serious" work and half that with chronic disease. Table 3.1 is an abstract of

TABLE 3.1
GENERAL PRACTICE IN THE NATIONAL HEALTH SERVICE

Contact during One year Between the Average General Practice of (approx.) 2,500 Patients and Other Branches of the Health Service
1971
England and Wales

Hospital Contact		
Admissions		249
including Psychiatric	10	
first Psychiatric	3	
on Waiting Lists for Admissions		26
Outpatients Clinics Attendances		1,721
new attendances	413	
Accident and Emergency Departments Attendances		686
new attendances	412	
Use of Diagnostic Services		
Pathology requests by G.P.		263
Radiology requests		204
Mass Miniature Radiography referrals		18
Domiciliary Visits by Consultants		15
Community Services		
Cases attended by *Health Visitor*		223
Home Nurses		55
Domiciliary midwives		26
Home Confinements	5	
Early Hospital Discharge	21	
Home Helps		23
Chiropodists		49
Meals on Wheels		
main meals provided per week		25
Women attending (Hospital & L.H.A.)		
Ante-Natal Clinics		41
Ante-Natal Classes		7
Post-Natal Clinics		11
Children attending		
Infant Welfare clinics		101
(during first year of life)	33	
School Health Service		315
medical inspection	89	
dental inspection	226	

Composition of Practice

Age	-14	15–44	45–64	65+
Male	297	474	282	120
Female	281	474	302	196

In a year:		
births	40	
deaths	29	
marriages	22	
divorces	3	

Number of old people living alone   80 (1966 Census)
Persons on Supplementary Benefit   143
    of whom, elderly are   95

DHSS *Digest of Health & Personal Social Services Statistics* 1972; DHSS *Annual Report* 1971; *Social Trends* 1972. HMSO. London.
Garraway, W. M. Personal communications.

official information to complement this "case study" in the field. There are about 3,000 contacts in the year between a practice and the hospitals alone, 60 a week, a staggering feat of organisation. No wonder many believe that communication at the interface between the hospital and the world outside is the key to success of the whole of the Health Service.

NEEDS ⇌ DEMAND ⇌ SUPPLY ⇌

The first merit of an "epidemiology of health services as well as of health", is that the idea of *the people's needs* will not be forgotten. Community diagnosis provides the elementary information for comprehensive planning of services. How much of the misery of these middle-aged men, (p. 30) could be prevented by higher quality general practice and industrial rehabilitation? What about national priorities for coronary care; local implementation of the Clean Air Act (p. 51)? Matching provision in general (Table 3.2)? or, in your district, for the handicapped (Table 3.3)? About half the survivors in page 70, c. 6,360 individuals in the population of a million (1 in 20 of all the "old-olds") have more than minor handicap/disability on account of stroke — and, therefore, special needs. What was the impact on general practice of the increase of sickness-absence between the mid-1950's and the late 1960's? Targets for health education services are indicated clearly enough on pages 37, 40, and 63. Et cetera, etc.

"Morbidity", the impairment, abnormality, has first to be perceived as discomfort, pain, disability, "need", then expressed in demand for help. Little is understood yet about the individual and social factors involved in *need→ demand*. Consider the 60 per cent increase in spells of "sickness" during the summer months (p. 61); the clinical variability of angina — or of depression; the protection of matrimony against hospitalisation; differences between Lancashire cotton operatives and Welsh miners in their endurance of chest trouble; the national cultures of the "stiff upper lip" or beating the breast. Needs are changing — what is regarded as psychological "illness" and what as the human condition, what old people "would rather put up with". Many medical and social "needs", moreover, and especially in the fields of health and prevention, are defined by society and its professionals when it is believed that something should and can be done about them. And epidemiology is opening up a new world of the non-patient, as needy often as those under care. [14-18]

We visited a sample of 101 "ordinary" families in our general practice to obtain a more complete diagnosis of "needs" and found that during a period of six months, over a third of 813 *manifest health problems*

TABLE 3.2

SERVICES IN HEALTHY AND UNHEALTHY DISTRICTS

Selected County Boroughs of England

General Practice[1]	Home Nurses[2]	Home Helps[3]	Social Workers[4]	Communal Homes[5]	County Borough
35	18	54	12	17·6	St. Helens
41	16	49	8	15·6	Merseyside
37	14	51	6	19·8	Stoke
38	13	31	7	32·1	Middlesbrough
40	18	75	9	11·2	Sheffield
38	15	51	8	18·1	West Midlands
44	12	67	9	21·6	Reading
36	21	75	8	25·5	Leicester
39	15	31	11	16·5	Southampton

Cf. page 53.
[1] GPs per 100,000 population. 1965. Ministry of Health, *Annual Report*.
[2] Per 100,000 population. 1965. *Health and Welfare. The Development of Community Care*. HMSO, London.
[3] *Do*.
[4] *Do*. Local Health and Welfare Authority only.
[5] Places per 1,000 population aged 65+. *Health and Welfare*.

TABLE 3.3

ESTIMATES OF (2) NEEDS ———→(3) DELIVERY OF SERVICES———→

Both Sexes, Ages 16+
Sample Survey, Great Britain, 1968–9

	%
(2), Proportion of (1) Disabled by The Impairment	
Severely	11·6
(24% of them living alone)	
Very Severely	5·1
(5·2% of them living alone)	
(3), Proportion of Severely and Very Severely Disabled and Living Alone (2) Who were Provided with	
Home Help	50
Nurse	23
Health Visitor	10
Social Worker	13
Meals on Wheels	17
None of These	29

Cf. Table 2.19, page 70.
Population outside institutions.
Harris, A. I. (1971) *Handicapped and Impaired in Great Britain*. HMSO, London; and personal communication.
See also: Warren, M. D. (1974) *The Canterbury Survey of the Impaired and the Handicapped*. University of Kent.

(as we defined these — not just any symptom) were not being treated by the practitioners or other local health services:[19]

	All Health Problems Diagnosed		"Mental Health" Problems	
Treated by National Health Service				
GP alone	360⎤	(62%)	18⎤	(24%)
Otherwise	144⎦		5⎦	
Not treated by National Health Service	309	(38%)	73	(76%)
Total	813	(100%)	96	(100%)

The "untreated" included a good deal of serious difficulties, in particular psychological. The family seemed to be coping effectively much of the time, helped often by relatives and friends and occasionally by pharmacists and sundry social agencies. But to us many children were clearly in need of further help; there was no *demand* for it.

Needs and Demand Usually are Relative

Much of this trouble should have presented to the Health Service. What we thought we knew about thresholds of complaint, the role of Medicine in the relief of anxiety, the public image of the doctor's job — and the facilities widely provided — made these findings surprising. Such figures may in fact represent working class illness-behaviour; expectations and demands rise with education, people have to learn about all except a few basic needs. Here is another area awaiting illumination by the social sciences, with their concern for the subject's point of view, for the irrational in behaviour, for folk-notions of ill-health, for the consequences of declaring illness and the sick-role to different kinds of people. The assessment of *need* as any basis for planning, for priorities and rationing, then, will be a formidable enterprise, even if restricted to the clinically manifest. Among the bewildering assortment of psychological troubles, page 45 for example, it is out of the question for psychiatrists to treat other than a tiny fraction; a challenge to find new ways of helping? How much for general practice or social work? "Counselling"? Meanwhile, for the first time, systematic information is to be sought of the public perception of their own needs as a guide to service.[20]

Needs often are declared in *demand* only when help is offered, services *provided;* whence the notion that both need and demand are "elastic". The "fit" between Table 2.5 and page 77 is loose indeed, a kind of iron law of the social services: Leicester, the booming town, provides substantially more domiciliary services than Stoke which, despite its age-structure, managed to have rather more hospital admissions, 95 per 1,000 against 88 — surely to do with the number of beds inherited locally, not needs (or accessibility). Doctor-consultation rates among women, most of them previously not "insured", rose far more when the National Health Service began in 1948 than among men who previously were "covered", by 12 per cent against 2·8. As mental hospitals open their doors, people are less afraid of stigma; build attractive Communal Homes and more old people will want to live in them. "Neurotic" illness, it is postulated, will be brought more often to more sympathetic GPs. The new Abortion Act and the 2,000 operations carried out every week is the latest illustration. How supply can usurp altogether the role of demand is evident in public housing, or child guidance, or swimming facilities; commonly the supply is hopelessly short of clamant demand.

Provision for Industrial Health. — Who does the work of the industrial medical officer in the great majority of factories employing the great majority of workers which have no occupational health service of their own? Do these factories, they are very often small, produce a disproportionate amount of industrial disease? During 1930–61, less than 10 per cent of the 370 cases of industrial lead poisoning in accumulator manufacture occurred in the group of large factories making 90 per cent of the product — and provided with fine industrial medical services.[21] What was the statutory appointed factory doctor of the day up to in these small factories? Does he spread know-how from the large ones? In the context of the National Health Service what "industrial medicine" ought generally to be supplied? What job — and skill — analysis of it has been done? Should there be more doctors in industry? Where are they to come from anyhow? On what social accountancy? Now we are to have another beginning.[22]

New Knowledge

These *death rates of males aged* 20–34 *from diabetes* suggest that social classes 1 and 2 benefited more or sooner from the introduction of insulin than classes 4 and 5, and this was true throughout "juvenile-onset", insulin-sensitive diabetes:

Social Class	1921–3	1930–2
1 and 2	64	26
3	50	25
4 and 5	46	35

Rates per million per year. England and Wales

By 1949–53 mortality in all classes was much lower, but the social disparities of 1930–2 had grown.

Today, for example, we ask about *coronary care*: continuous monitoring of blood pressure and the electrocardiogram, ventricular defibrillation, correction of acute metabolic disturbances and the prevention of thromboembolism; many advocate that every district general hospital has facilities for "everything" — drawn from where? Page 48 gives some idea of the size of the problem, and of the stakes. On these doctors' experience, a hypothetical district of 100,000, as said, would have about 150 "heart attacks" in a year. Numbers might double to 300 or so when women are included, and age limits are lowered as well as extended to 70. (And there might be an equal number of false alarms.) Table 2.3 however, doesn't give enough "diagnosis" for community action.

Thus, most of the truly sudden ("electrical") deaths, half of *all* coronary deaths, occur in the first hour of the attack and mostly apparently in the first minutes. How many could be prevented through resuscitation by the family, a faster tempo throughout the service, and/or by attaching flying squads to the coronary-care unit? So we need information on a community basis about the early minutes and hours of local heart attacks along the lines of the figures from Edinburgh (Fig. 3.2).[23]

Mounting Need and Demand

During the 1960's there was a consumer boom in medical care: home-helps, clin-path, prescriptions in general practice, hospital admissions (Table 3.4). There are few numbers like the admissions for tuberculosis, or the falling length of stay in mental hospitals, to place alongside the increases. How to find the resources?

The *over 75s* are the fastest growing section of the population. With high living standards there are more *diseases of affluence* such as diabetes and coronary thrombosis and these are even more difficult to cope with than the (abundant) residue of the diseases of poverty. Treatment of *chronic relapsing disorders,* metabolic, mental, malignant, in an *ageing population* alleviates more often than it cures, so the prevalence of chronic disability in middle and old age is increasing: the "model" of the future is likelier to be diabetes and, even more depressing, the arthritides, requiring care over rest of the lifetime, than tuberculosis responding so well to direct attack or, a fortiori, pneumonia. *Extended survival:* there must be several thousands with severe brain damage from congenital malformation, motor-vehicle accidents, stroke and senile dementia, salvaged each year and added to the most needy in the population. *Public expectations* are rising in the field of mental health; there is little basis for this in any growing capacity to help, but we have to try harder. *Present standards of provision* in several parts of the NHS, in long-stay wards for example, are no longer acceptable to public opinion. *Technology* increasingly is presenting fresh options; shortages prevent runaway expansion, but it will be important to identify which prostheses and transplants should be carried out, and when; or, and these may be easier to assess for cost-benefit, what new preventions to adopt? As said, moreover, *provision of a service* generates and critically determines demand —

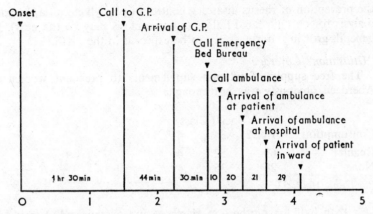

Fig. 3.2 Median time intervals between events for episodes of acute heart attack referred to hospital by general practitioners.

The Edinburgh Community Study. Armstrong, A., Duncan, B., Oliver, M. F., Julian, D. G., Donald, K. W., Fulton, M., Lutz, W. & Morrison, S. L. (1972) *Brit. Ht J.* **34**, 67; and personal communications.

TABLE 3.4
"ADMISSIONS" TO HOSPITALS

National Health Service
England and Wales

Condition/Main Diagnosis	1961	1971
	(thousands)	
Tuberculosis	45	21
Other infections	59	46
Bronchitis	68	58
Lung cancer	35	43
Other malignant disease	169	215
Cerebrovascular disease	69	95
Acute myocardial infarction	53*	87
Gynaecological conditions	166	248
Cataract	26	36
Hyperplasia of prostate	26	31
Poisoning	28	100
Head injuries	89	140
Schizophrenia†	26	36
Depressive psychosis†	41	66

Hospital In-Patient Enquiry (HIPE). OPCS.

Annually. c.10 per cent sample. Totals, excluding maternity, were 3,217,000 in 1961 and 4,179,000 in 1971.

*1962. †Mental hospitals, 1960, 1969, 100 per cent count. DHSS.

the prevention of rhesus disasters, control of phenylketonuria, haemo-dialysis for chronic renal failure (amniocentesis may be the next). In general, growing shortages are to be expected in the NHS.[24, 25]

"Utilisation"/Coverage

The free supply of vitamin supplements to pregnant women in Aberdeen obviously was not enough:

		Social Class	
Consumption	1 & 2	3	4 & 5
Regular	69	52	41
None	28	35	49

Per Cent, 1948–53

Less than half the mothers in classes 4 and 5 (expectedly) regularly availed themselves. As the authors said, "Ignorance and apathy seemed to play a great part. Many women believed that the vitamin A and D tablets were laxatives. The orange-juice concentrate was often disliked or thought to cause heartburn." (Often even less is still known of consumer attitudes, even today.) In this favourable ante-natal situation, those most in need "took-up" the service least,[46] the classic failure in "compliance" now being repeated in cervical cytology. How to get the community's social welfare services utilised is a recurrent problem among the aged. A campaign to inform them of their entitlement and a more dignified procedure sharply increased the number of old-age pensioners receiving supplementary benefit (no longer "national assistance"). Doctors make little use of available welfare services that could be of relief to *them* as well as their patients. Of course, many services would be overwhelmed if all who could benefit suddenly applied.* Which only goes to show what comprehensive models are required. "Means tests" are a remarkably powerful disincentive to the use of services. In general, only about half are taken up.

The functioning of health services might be described as a dynamic "system" that is changing rapidly, each element affecting the others and none to be understood on its own: "no one of them can be taken as the causal determinant, each being emergent . . . from the interplay of all of them."[26] In Britain today, in the extreme case — with a per-forated ulcer, say, or smallpox or childhood cancer or gross delusions

---

*"The review of the welfare arrangements to ascertain the extent of the success of the services already in existence and to discover the need for additional services was undertaken in the form of a house survey. Very soon it became apparent that the existing services in relation to meals-on-wheels, chiropody and bathing assistance were insufficient. Unfortunately at the same time it also became clear that the Council would have to impose severe restrictions on the budgets of all departments. To continue the survey therefore appeared pointless as we should quite certainly discover a need, and equally certain be unable to meet it." From an annual report in the mid-1960's.

— what very likely will happen is that *need=demand=supply=utili-sation*. In most questions of admission to hospital, however, need is not absolute and there are multiple influences at work, social and cultural as well as medical, involving personal factors and familial support and not merely the availability of services. This has already been illustrated by the conflicting pressures over maternity beds; it is evident in the "disposal" of old people with serious disabilities in general hospitals, mental hospitals, communal homes, sheltered housing, and (mostly) their own bedroom. To sort out such situations should often be the first line of enquiry. Data on the provision and utilisation of services ("delivery") for defined "need", "client" – groups are the easiest to obtain and at present the best way into study.

GEOGRAPHY OF HEALTH SERVICES[27-30]

Other countries with different histories, economies, ideologies, have other systems of medical care. Our own universal commitment discourages deliberate experiment (though there is plenty unintended) so study of others' successes is especially worthwhile. Consider these token figures for comparable *community general hospitals* in a recent year:

	New England	Uppsala	Liverpool
Operation Rate per 1,000 male population Tonsillectomy & Adenoidectomy	6·8	1·5	2·9
Hernia repair	4·9	3·5	2·6
Prostatectomy	1·8	1·4	0·7
Average Stay days/males "Ts and As" (5–14 yrs.)	1·6	4·5	4·4
Hernia repair (45–64)	7·3	9·9	14
Prostatectomy (65+)	15	30	31

From Pearson, R. J. C., Smedby, B., Berfenstam, R., Logan, R. F. L., Burgess, A. M. & Peterson, O. L. (1968). *Lancet*, 2, 559.

Average length of stay in the three countries is falling steadily. However, the capability of our hospitals would be transformed if we could emulate this aspect of the American scene — though our domiciliary medical and social services might not cope (do the American?). We ought to find out more about needs/demands, about patients (how sick, for example) and families; doctors and nurses; to evaluate outcomes in health and comfort; money costs and payments in the three health-care systems and, especially, about what in fact is done inside hospital.

And has to be done inside: the statistics have to be translated from "beds" and "days" and throughput into diagnosis of the actual needs of the people for medical, nursing, and other services — and the specific skills and tasks entailed in meeting them.

QUALITY OF MEDICAL CARE [31-38]

Because of popular expectation — it is now assumed to be individual right and public good — and because of the resources involved, medical care has become a leading concern of social policy. But it is proving hard to appraise how well the services are doing their job, and so to render account to the public. Objective standards of performance are likely increasingly to be demanded of medicine and the other helping professions. They are increasingly interested, but poorly prepared for it.

Questions range all the way from ethics through education to economics, and they can be considered under three heads:

What services are actually delivered—the supply and the use
The effects of services on health, the wanted and the adverse
    reactions
The costs

I can describe only a few sorties . . . If there is little service, little application of new knowledge, there can't be high quality. Disparities of delivery, of provision and take-up, have already been cited, though of course we have none on the scale that is commonplace in developing countries. The National Health Service by increasing and distributing geographically specialist skills — to help mothers at high risk, for example — improved quality. The fewer the dentists, the less the "conservative" dentistry. Table 3.5 is an example of those bleak

TABLE 3.5
DISTRIBUTION OF DENTAL SERVICES IN ENGLAND AND WALES
1970

Region	Population per dentist	Courses of treatment per 1,000 population	Ratio filled: extracted permanent teeth	Proportion of courses that included full dentures
Wales	6,434	193	1·3	9·4
Midlands	6,331	264	1·7	6·6
Northern	6,028	239	1·3	8·5
E. & W. Ridings	5,737	277	1·7	7·4
N. Western	5,576	262	1·6	7·3
Eastern	4,913	284	2·8	3·8
S. West	4,248	335	2·7	4·3
Southern	3,862	486	3·5	3·4
S. East	3,063	457	4·5	3·6

Department of Health and Social Security.

"two-nations" divides, distributive injustice. Knowledge of regional needs, e.g. rates of caries, would probably only aggravate the disparities, a picture by social class would be even worse.[24]

Diphtheria immunisation provides a textbook case. Research in North America in the 1920's and early 1930's established its preventive value: yet in England, as late as in 1941 — but the figures have already been given (p. 4). The Ministry of Health reported shortly before that:

"Continuous if slow progress is being made, particularly in some of the larger provincial cities, although none of them has yet succeeded in immunizing the 50 to 60 per cent of the child population which is necessary before the incidence of the disease is affected. Chester, with an estimated number of 45 per cent, is probably the best immunized town in the country. London (inner) appears very low in the list with an estimated number of 5·3 per cent of her child population immunized."

Observer Variation

What is to be made of the difference in these two estimates of prevalence of *otitis media*?

As a defect found at school health inspection (1951),
7·6 per 1,000 examined
As a cause of rejection for National Service (1954–55),
32·0 per 1,000 examined

Such a finding is unlikely to be unique and, in fact, my colleague identified a long list of physical defects that apparently were missed at the "school medical".[39] What is happening at school inspections may be surmised from reports like these:

Prevalence of Cardiac Defects Requiring Treatment or Observation per 1,000
Children Inspected
County Boroughs of England
1965

Barnsley 1, Barrow in Furness 15, Bath 13, Birkenhead 8, Birmingham 13, Blackburn 3, Blackpool 6, Bolton 10, Bootle 13, Bournemouth 9, Bradford 23, Brighton 33, Bristol 20, Burnley 21, Burton-upon-Trent 4, Bury 21.
The Health of the School Child (1966). HMSO, London.

Only a gross example, very likely, of what in some degree is inevitable in routine clinical data-collection. Because of observer-variation the material is not valid enough to identify groups or individuals at special risk. Agreed definitions could help, systematic training, the use of "reference" case-material, routine duplication and spot checks; all ought to be built into the system. With computers and record-linkage the result of later examinations might be fed back. Are there adequate incentives to be careful in local schools? Are the doctors under pressure — and if so can it be relieved? (There is no reason to suppose that top consultants — or public health nurses — not specially trained for the job, and monitored on it, would show less observer-variation.)

Glover Phenomenon

To proceed. The next Table is from a pioneer study of over thirty years ago:[40]

Tonsillectomy Rates per 1,000 School Pupils, 1936-8

Manchester	11	Leeds	38
Bradford	12	Leicester	36
Gloucester	12	Exeter	40
Birkenhead	3	West Hartlepool	39
Isle of Ely	4	Soke of Peterborough	55
Cambridge	13	Oxford	40

Annual Averages

The quality of treatment received by the children in these towns surely varied enormously; not to mention the man-hours and money that might be spent otherwise. Don't such (random) figures raise the question what are the valid clinical indications for tonsillectomy, the most popular operation in the book, falling but still well over 100,000 a year, and the biggest element in hospital "waiting lists"? In how many other examples would such comparative studies, such *community* perspective, stimulate fresh *clinical* thinking?[41] [42] The same kind of distribution is evident in many fields, for example in the mean length of stay in hospital [43] (for tonsillectomy, 3·0 days in the fastest hospital region to 5·8; for varicose veins from 8·4 to 18·0 days). Table 3.6 is not merely a matter of outlying observations and, hopefully, 10 years old, the variation is chiefly of historical interest.

Case-Fatality in Teaching and Regional Board Hospitals

Figure 3.3 and Table 3.7 are challenging enough, though data are also needed on morbidity and disability. Routine national statistics analysed with a purpose can so "discover" problems.[44] Possible explanations for the different outcome in the two types of hospital, such as the greater staffing resources of the teaching hospital (TH) are obvious, but, plainly, much more information was needed. So we followed up the crude observation by survey, in a few representative teaching and regional board (RB) hospitals, of all the admissions for hyperplasia of the prostate.[45] Among other reasons this was chosen as probe and "tracer" because, on average, 1 man in 3 or 4 after 65 years of age may expect to need treatment, so first-class facilities should be widely available. The correct way to tackle such a many-sided problem is to *randomise* all patients in a big enough population between one kind of hospital and the other. Results of such an experiment, too, could have more impact. But this was out of the question; so in the search for "avoidable" factors, we had to make do with retrospective *standardisation* for as many relevant, favourable and unfavourable, features as we could — the age of the patients, social class, general

TABLE 3.6

RANGE OF PRACTICE OF THE 17 SINGLE-HANDED GP's IN AN ENGLISH INDUSTRIAL TOWN

Early 1960's

Rates per 1,000 local Residents on List

Service	By Lowest 3 GPs in Range	By Highest 3 GPs in Range
Total remedies prescribed	255	648
Antibiotics, etc.	7	68
Chloramphenicol	0	7·8
Patients referred to consultant physician	1·8	10
Utilisation of free-access		
X-Ray	1·9	64
Pathology	0·0	9·2
Home nursing	1·6	17·4
Attendance by patients on their "list" at hospital "Casualty" for minor conditions	7·6	35·5

Total list size varied from 1,400 to 3,600; aged over 65 from 7% to 13%.

The period observed was the same for all the doctors and varied from 1 to 12 months per "service".

Average results for doctors in partnership were similar to the average results for the single-handed G.P.s.

Draper, P., personal communication.

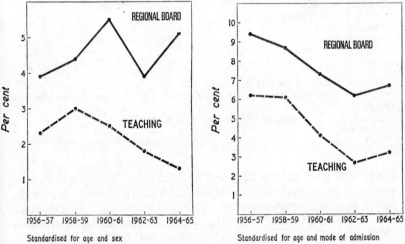

Fig. 3.3 Case-fatality in teaching and regional board hospitals of England and Wales. National Health Service.

Hospital In-Patient Enquiry. Personal communications.

TABLE 3.7
CASE-FATALITY IN TEACHING AND REGIONAL BOARD HOSPITALS

1967–70
England and Wales
National Health Service

Condition/ (Type of Admission)/ Sex and Age	No. of "Admissions"		Case-Fatality (%)	
	T.H.	R.B.H.	T.H.	R.B.H.
Hyperplasia of prostate (All admissions) 65–74	554	3,841	*1·6*	*3·1*
Acute myocardial infarction (Immediate admissions) 45–64				
M	816	7,286	*13·5*	*17·3*
F	199	1,861	*16·1*	*20·4*
Chronic bronchitis (Immediate) M 55–74	587	5,687	*9·9*	*14·7*
Appendicitis (Immediate) M and F 0–14	718	9,161	—*	*0·08*
Peptic ulcer (All) M 45–64	992	5,704	*1·7*	*2·5*
Diabetes (All) F 45–64	309	1,967	*2·6*	*5·2*
Head injuries, skull, face and bone fractures (Immediate)				
M 0–14	871	7,035	—**	*0·4*
M 15–24	742	5,020	—**	*1·4*

Ten per cent national samples.

Hospital In-patient Enquiry. *Annual Reports;* and personal communications, OPCS.

Ashley, J. S. A. & McLaughlin, C., personal communications.

* 0 deaths.

** 3 deaths.

state, local medical condition and so forth — to achieve fairer comparisons; it is some consolation that such an approach will provoke less change in the customary behaviour of the hospitals. The care given was observed, and the immediate results, the disability and mortality till the end of one year (there is a more detailed discussion on p. 271). This kind of audit, of "process" *and* outcome, might regularly be made within the new health regions and areas. "Accountability", indeed, a vogue word of the early 1970's, might well be adopted.

Meanwhile, Table 3.7 (a sample Table) represents the kind of unpleasant social fact that too readily is swept under the carpet. It indicates
how the quality of services is a major element today in preventive
medicine, another illustration how *health services affect the people's
health.*

Is Community Health Benefited?

Quality of medical care thus can have several meanings: the provision
of service accepted as norm, hospital confinement or FRCS specialist
surgery, for example; and it should be "audited" systematically to
check whether stated standards are reached and the take-up is as
intended — in the chronic disabilities these are often very complex
processes. But the "norm" so often is empirical only, hallowed by
politics and tradition, and not optimal, as shown by observation, still
less by experiment. So we have often to go further and ask, "evaluate",
what good the service does, what are the results, not the intention?
Recognising straightaway that the health service contribution to health,
to disease prevalence and to mortality for example, may be quite small
compared with other factors, personal, environmental and unknown,
a situation that requires the perfect and often still unachieved clinical
trial for an answer. Such measurements — how many have benefited?
By how much? — go beyond audit whether the "right" thing is done.
Consumer satisfaction is also important, of course, but not enough;
nor, a fortiori, whether the staff are happy in their work, essential
though job-satisfaction and careers so plainly are. Social policy
requires advance to *supply* $\rightleftharpoons$ *utilisation* $\rightleftharpoons$ *outcomes* $\rightleftharpoons$: to search for
effects in the health of the community. And the outcomes, in turn,
help in restating meaningful "needs" for medical care, in deciding
where health services are in fact most useful: *outcomes* $\rightleftharpoons$ *needs* $\rightleftharpoons$ in
the continuing planning process.

And it is here that knowledge of the population, and not merely of
the effective demand is essential. There is some experience. Thus,
local perinatal mortality rates are an established measure of the outcome
of obstetric care in relation to definable needs; though, as seen, biological and other social factors obviously are also involved and not always
easy to "standardise".[46] The rates for classes 4 and 5 in the Table on
p. 53 are disconcerting . . . Effort must now be concentrated on defining community health-benefits in life-span, in rescue and first-aid,
rates of recovery, more sensible behaviour, complications avoided,
symptoms relieved, lives more liveable, families coping; in return to
work, social roles preserved, less invalidity, disability postponed, old
people independent, dignity at the end. The example from the teaching
and RB hospitals suggests a priority for services in simple terms of
lives that might be saved. At the other extreme, to comfort, provide
human contact and safe lodging, to support the family, to prevent
physical deprivations, preserve a degree of independence, may be the
realistic benefits to aim for, and equally to be assessed.[47-50]

TABLE 3.8   HOW GOOD ARE HEALTH SERVICES?

EXAMPLES

| EXAMPLES OF | | 1. STANDARDS OF PROVISION |
SERVICE	and OBJECTIVES	*How near the best? Everywhere? How match defined needs? How adaptable to demand of the population? How integrated with other services?*
Maternity beds	Booked confinement in consultant-staffed beds for defined high-risk groups	National norms of staff and facilities are reached; corrected to meet current ascertained local needs in and out of hospital
Prevention: screening: cervical cytology	Hypothesis: a preventable cancer	Diagnosis and treatment procedures available for target groups. Built-in quality control of cytology
Diagnosis: what school doctors do	E.g. to pick up all cardiac defects requiring observation/treatment	Validity of cases identified is confirmed by special studies of "positives" and samples of the remainder
Intensive coronary care	Enough staffed beds, in average circumstances, for all who are under 70 and survive $\frac{1}{2}$ hour after onset of heart attack to be admitted quickly and stay for 72 hours	Clinical needs derived from ongoing IHD Community Register: facilities match in access and in capability
Treatment of hyperplasia of prostate	Hospital service available in accordance with assessed need	Specialist urology units have little or no waiting lists. Necessary facilities in hospitals available for emergency as well as planned admissions
Information system: death certification	Valid, informative, timely statistics; which are used	Certificates reach acceptable standards when compared with clinical records and necropsy findings. Quality of certification rising
Theory. Methods		*Medical audit. Codes of Practice. "Confidential Enquiries" on representative samples. Ad hoc surveys of the population. O.R. Work study*

2. UTILISATION	3. OUTCOMES IN COMMUNITY HEALTH ·	4. ITS EFFICIENCY/ PRODUCTIVITY
How complete is the actual take-up by "target" populations?	*What are the wanted effects? And the adverse effects? In community rates?*	*How economically are objectives in 1., 2., and 3. being achieved?*
High-risk pregnancies completely registered and admitted in good time	Reduction in complicated cases; in emergencies; and in perinatal mortality rates	
All in target groups are reached	Mortality of cancer of cervix falls more than expected on previous and others' experience; no serious harm from the screening and subsequent procedures	
	Children are helped at the right time and without producing invalidism	*High quality services, 1., 2. and 3., achieved by most productive use of re- sources of manpower, materials, money; this being settled by evaluating the alternative methods of*
Data again from the Register: what fraction of designated patients so reach the I.C. Unit? (And how many who shouldn't, do so?)	Significant improvement in local population rates of early mortality, of later morbidity; acceptable adverse effects	*achieving high quality 1., 2., and 3.; the accounting to include also other possible ways of using the the resources to achieve other objectives*
Ad hoc survey through doctors confirms success. Population survey neces- sary to identify those who didn't get treatment, and what are the unavoidable needs for emergency presentation	Optimum survival; minimal side-effects of operation; relief of symptoms, and they don't recur; minimal residual disability; social roles preserved	
Convenient usage in medical care organisation and in research		
Study of population take-up through medical records: comparison with assessed needs-demand. O.R. Feed-back of infor- mation to providers	*Community Diagnosis; movement of local health indices. Statement of optimal outcomes. Systems analysis. Sample-studies with follow up. Estimates of further needs that are generated*	*Systems analysis; input- output analysis; cost- efficiency, and cost effective- ness, analysis on the popu- lation base. Impact on other services*

Hazards of Health Services

The damage that health services do is an urgent consideration in this kind of accounting. Table 2.16 on page 69 is one way of looking at it. The official notification scheme for toxic reactions to drugs should help to avoid the disasters; this is yielding one report per 50,000–60,000 prescriptions. In the years 1948–65, 403 children in England and Wales having tonsillectomy died of the operation; thankfully, the number of deaths, though not so much of operations, has fallen sharply in recent years. The children crippled by thalidomide are on their slow procession through the special schools for the handicapped, following those made deaf by streptomycin who succeeded the infants blinded by oxygen. How count the moribunds of extended survival? . . . The damage that "social care" may do by labelling people, overprotecting and making them *more* dependent, weakening the social network, is becoming recognised . . . (How cost such "soft" outcomes?)

A last word on "quality". This is a highly sensitive area that ideally should be part of ongoing management itself, and intrusion by an investigator may be unwelcome. The bureaucrat under the public gaze has his own troubles, the ENT surgeon with what is left of his charisma, his. No prescription can be offered on how to win their participation, but that the enquirer be modest, objective and have a patent concern with the improvement of services. Myself I have an old-fashioned faith in saturating the services with *facts*.

Table 3.8 is an attempt to summarise. It mentions also 'economy":[51-54] the *costs* at which the sundry *objectives* of community health services and their effects on health and welfare are achieved.

*　　*　　*

COMMUNITY CARE

One of the main reasons for the reorganisation of health services is an epochal reallocation of roles. The trend now is to admit the sick to hospital as briefly as required for active treatment, then to return them to the "community". (The wording is unfortunate but by now too late to mend; its "institutions" surely are resource and part of the "community", and "care" has to be seen as a whole.) The motive forces are the character and natural history of predominant health problems, the possibilities of treatment — and ideological. A variety of long-term out-patient and day facilities are involved; teamwork between GPs — hospitals — the greater medical profession — "social welfare" — industrial rehabilitation; the co-operation of relatives, friends, neighbours, workmates, voluntary service, police, landlords, the public. Community care is a matter for the whole community, and it involves numerous untested and even unrecognised assumptions about the rights of the sick, the purposes of the family, kinship networks, the capabilities of local government, popular attitudes to deviant behaviour, the degree of public concern, levels of employment, and social security — not to mention the benefit to the patient.[49] The ambulant "chronic sick" are not a new phenomenon, but their numbers certainly are.[55] To help them medicine wants better understanding of physical potential of patients, their psychological adjustment and social competence. When disease has to be lived with for a lifetime it is the degree of ability and disability that matter. We want an epidemiology of these in which the working of health services will be a major factor.

The *Mental Health Act* (1959) was a powerful catalyst. But the provision of new "community" services, the education of all concerned, even elementary surveys of the needs, have been sadly insufficient. What the law (and public relations) say is one thing. In the contemporary climate of opinion, however, it would have been folly not to seize the opportunity, not to push through legislation; in fact, and traditionally, the law mostly puts into practice what already is on the way. So the mentally ill, partially recovered, leave hospital quicker than formerly. How is it working out? How are the patients benefiting? How many are chronically sick, how many are working, how many down-and-out, how many just vanished? . . Is the overall burden, the cost, less, or more, or merely redistributed? How many families are thriving, coping, desperate? What kinds of family, of patients, of community service? . . The table overleaf outlines the situation. Note the readmission to hospital and rapid turnover (the "revolving door"), the multiplying social service facilities outside that, however, still don't cope even on paper with current clinically presenting needs—this is the "sad illusion" often of community care.

The epidemiological method, with its inescapable questions about populations, all its patients and ex-patients, about all the co-operating and conflicting services, should be able to help. The picture has to be "systems", or "ecological": the more (successful) care is outside them the more intractable will be the residue inside the institutions, whether old people's ward, or approved school however named. Discussion today is still mostly about mental disorder; but other chronic disabilities — from ischaemic heart disease, bronchitis, the infirmities of age — present as many unanswered questions.* The frequent absence of services offers unusual opportunity for experiment.

---

*"Too Much of a Heartbreak" (title of television programme on spina bifida in South Wales, 25/3/71).

TABLE 3.9
MENTAL ILLNESS, MENTAL HOSPITALS, AND "COMMUNITY CARE"
England and Wales
National Health Service

---

(1) General Practice – i.e. The Total Population
Estimated no. of patients with major mental disorder = 500,000–1,000,000
    approx.*
Estimated no. of patients with conspicuous psychiatric morbidity = 5,000,000
    approx.**
No. of prescriptions for antidepressants, hypnotics, tranquillisers = 46,000,000 in
    1972.

(2) Mental Illness Hospitals, 1959–71
    First admissions rose from   55,000 to 66,000
    Non-first admissions rose from   51,000 to 117,000
    Total admissions rose from   106,000 to 183,000
    Discharges rose from   95,000 to 172,000

Resident Population
1954   1959   1971
152,000   143,000   110,000
    Those aged 65+ remained the same, 50,000 in 1959 and in 1971.

(3) New Psychiatric Out-Patients Mental Illness (all NHS Hospitals)
    Rose from c. 160,000 to 223,000 between 1959–1971.

(4) Local Authority Services
    Psychiatric patients in "Community Care"
        1959: 81,000 ("mentally defective")
        1970: 196,000 (incl. 104,000 "mentally handicapped").

    Mental-health social workers
        1959: 891   1970: 1,938
    Expenditure
        1959–60: c. £4,000,000.   1970–1: c. £34,000,000 (£21M on Training Centres
        for the mentally handicapped).

Notes on Table 3·9
(1) *The higher figure, about 2% of the population, are in contact with a psychiatric service during a year.
   **Including children, say, 100–150,000, at 5–14 years. During the year a very few of the 250 with "conspicuous psychiatric morbidity" in the "average" general practice will be in general hospitals, prisons, Communal Homes; 5 or 6 will be in the Mental Hospitals (above); perhaps 15–20 under care also in out-patients and child guidance clinics; and 5 or so in "community care".

(2) The Mental Health Act (1959) came into force in November, 1960.
   Deaths are not included in "discharges"; these account for most of the differences between Admissions, Discharges and Resident Population.
   In 1959, 61 per cent of resident population in mental hospitals suffering from "mental illness" were "voluntary"; in 1970, 93 per cent of residents were "informal".
   Since 1960 psychiatric beds in *general* hospitals have doubled to 11,400.

(3) Figures are not available for *total* number of persons attending, but only for total attendances at out-patients. New out-patients in other consultative departments rose during the period by 12%.
   New "day-care" patients are growing in numbers, from 5,700 in 1961 to 26,600 in 1971.

(4) There also were c. 4,000 with psychiatric disability on the "general" register of substantially and permanently handicapped persons (most local authorities, 1970). Voluntary agencies help with some others.
   Because of the "generic" approach of the new Social Services Departments, special figures for mental-health social workers are no longer available.

Annually: Ministry of Health/DHSS *Reports; Statistics of Health and Personal Social Services; Psychiatric Hospitals and Units in England and Wales.* HMSO. London. DHSS, personal communications.

Population, E & W	*Total*	*65+*
1959	45·4	5·4
1971	48·8	6·4
Millions		

ACTION RESEARCH

Graylingwell Hospital serves a community of some 400,000 people. The object of the "Worthing Experiment", in the words of its pioneer, was "to discover whether the provision of large-scale psychiatric treatment on an out-patient basis could materially affect the great annual increase of admissions to the hospital", from 574 in 1947 to 1,345 in 1956; i.e. to study through changing.

Community Care with appropriate medical and social services was provided for the three districts in turn; in each instance there was an immediate drop in local admissions, Table 3.10. Before and after studies showed that all kinds of patients were affected by the new programme and not merely those with minor disorders who might previously have been admitted too readily.

Sainsbury and Grad are further "evaluating" by comparing Chichester with a similar population in Salisbury, served by a similar mental hospital but not supported with the other facilities. It was found that only 14 per cent of referrals from Chichester, compared with 52 per cent from Salisbury, were admitted to the mental hospital. They also compared the outcome in terms of the effect on patients' families, how they were coping, what were their limits of adaptation, and found that Salisbury's more traditional service tended in general to give greater relief; though the families whose burden was judged to be "severe" were in fact helped equally.

Table 3.10 shows also that after the initial sharp reductions, admissions rose until, in 1965, the total was higher than at the start. In this period the local populations grew by approximately a fifth and the number of old people by about 40 per cent (Worthing is a leading "retirement area"). In small measure the psychiatrists were also again admitting more readily. But, more striking, referrals from the community have been rising with the development of the community service (*supply* $\rightleftharpoons$ *utilisation*). Thus, admission rates have risen significantly in Chichester for vulnerable groups, the aged, the poor, those living alone. In Worthing there has been a shift towards admitting patients more readily for rehabilitation and, at the same time, in discharging long-stay patients to accommodation in which they largely look after themselves. In other words, the community services meet more *needs* than before, and this is contributing to the increase in admissions.

It remains to be seen how far the experimental community service is reducing the prevalence of mental illness by achieving earlier treatment. There is a suggestion that it is having an effect in preventing suicide in geriatric patients by earlier recognition of depressive illness. Such systematic experiment in health services is only beginning.

TABLE 3.10
HOSPITAL AND COMMUNITY
Admissions to Graylingwell Mental Hospital in Relation to the Provision of
"Community Care"

Year	From Worthing	Admissions From Chichester	From Horsham	Total†
1956	645	444	219	1,345
1957	284	463	246	1,032
1958	247	228	256	759
1959	269	263	227	786
1960	295	293	239	853
1961	332	329	278	986
1962	325	389	311	1,086
1963	408	464	394	1,310
1964	427	493	334	1,305
1965	428	546	366	1,390
1966	426	560	309	1,346
1967	533	592	325	1,512
1968	504	604	177*	1,359*
1969	573	489	—	1,168
1970	642	637	—	1,404‡

Domiciliary social-medical facilities and day-hospitals were specially provided for Worthing and district in 1957, for Chichester and district in 1958, and for Horsham and district in 1964.

Carse, J., Panton, N. and Watt, A. (1958) *Lancet 1*, 39; and continuing personal communications from Sainsbury, P. & Grad, J. (1973).

*Horsham was removed from the catchment area in 1968.
†Includes a small number of "out-county" patients.
‡Geriatric assessment unit opened.

MORALITY OF MEDICAL CARE

How fair are the shares? Whose rights are respected? Whose business is it to assure that those at highest risk receive priority? There never will be enough medical care; the modern mood insists on exposing the shortages. Clinical freedom also implies a kind of rationing — so the professions must be accountable for that too. Resources are entrusted to us and it is wrong not to use them providently. Moreover, as if waiting-lists were not enough, epidemiology has uncovered a world of non-patients. Getting the facts can help to restate values and build a better system. One of the main uses of epidemiology is that it can so help social institutions to apply the scientific method to their own workings, professions to be professional; each physician to learn about his practice and himself.[24] [34] [54] [58-65]

4. Individual Chances and Risks

The chances and risks of having an accident for a schoolboy cyclist, young man on a motor-bike, or an elderly pedestrian; of developing leukaemia after X-rays for therapy or diagnosis; of rheumatic fever following a haemolytic streptococcal infection; of contracting poliomyelitis when protected by one "shot", two or three; of a 17-, 27-, or 37-year female becoming pregnant; of perinatal death to an elderly primip or worn-out multip; of future heart-attack from various levels of blood pressure or cholesterol; of an operative suffering byssinosis after exposure to this or that amount of cotton dust: these risks, chances, probabilities for the individual can be predicted, on average, from analysis of the collective experience of large numbers of representative individuals with the characteristics in question. For comparison, the experience of the general population, or of the rest of the population, will often also be required.

In practice, the incidence measures the *rate* at which new disease develops in the *group*, and the average *risk* of developing it for the *individual* member of the group. The simple arithmetic of individual risk is by addition of the successive incidence rates of the condition for the period required.

These rates, in the appropriate "population", are calculated for each year in the span of age for which knowledge of the risk is sought, and over the period being studied, and the rates are then added together. If the sum of the incidence rates per 1,000 equals 200, the individual risk is 1 in 5. If incidence rates are available only in bands of ages (decades, for example), such age-specific rates must be multiplied by the number of years in each band (10 in this example) before being added together, so that specific allowance is made for each year of age.

For greater accuracy the actuary's Life Table methods can be used, and these are essential if the incidence of the condition being studied is high at young ages, or there is considerable mortality from other conditions. The Life Table is also necessary in complex problems, like the chance of an individual having *repeated* accidents ("accident proneness") or spells of sickness; and in studies of *prognosis* — of renal transplant vs. haemodialysis, say, or to predict the chances of surviving a disease, or of relapse after recovery from it, and so on.

Figure 4.1 illustrates probably the best known fact of this kind. The average overall risk at live-birth of Down's syndrome (trisomy 21, nearly always) is about 1 in 600–700. The probability for mothers under 30 years of age is less than 1 in 1,000. The risk rises steeply thereafter to about 1 in 45 for mothers over 45 (i.e. also 44 in 45 chances that it won't happen). These data are Australian and the figures are typical of "Caucasian" populations.[1][2]

References on page 291.

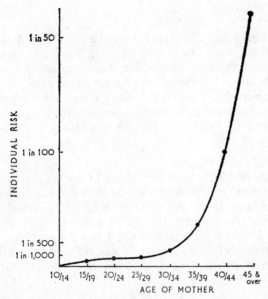

Fig. 4.1 Individual risk of bearing a 'mongol' child, according to age of mother. Collman, R. D. & Stoller, A. (1962) *N.Z. med. J.* **61**, 24.

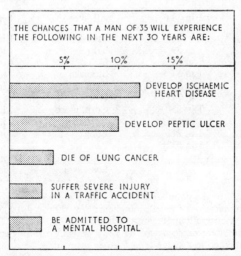

Fig. 4.2 Risks and chances of the average man from 35 years through middle age. Approximate figures, Britain. [3-8] 5% = 1 in 20, etc.

"Modern Epidemics"

Figure 4.2 gives a rough idea of the "risks" of the average man in Britain during his middle age; it complements Figs. 1 and 2 at the opening of the book and such data. In light of something like a one-in-eight chance of developing clinical coronary heart disease, as the Figure suggests, or one-in-ten for peptic ulcer (mostly duodenal), the term "epidemic" is warranted. Since these sums were done 10–15 years ago probabilities have changed, and knowledge of them; today, the figure for IHD would be far higher (about 1 in 5), for peptic ulcer lower (p. 16).

Risks of Malignant Disease

A colleague (B.J.W.) calculated Table 4.1 from the best data available in England; death certificates as well as clinical presentations are used for completeness. It shows the overwhelming contribution of lung cancer to malignant disease in men. Without it, the average cancer risk overall is 1 in 6 for men and still 1 in 5 for women — higher in women, as it was before the first world war, before the modern epidemic of lung cancer struck. One point from any number that might be

TABLE 4.1
INDIVIDUAL RISK OF DEVELOPING CANCER
Calculated from the Clinical Experience in 1960–2 of the Cancer Registries of Three English Hospital Regions, other NHS and Death Certificate Data; and from the Life Table for England and Wales

Males		Females	
Site	Individual probability	Site	Individual probability
All Sites	1 in 4	All Sites	1 in 5
Lung	1 in 15	Breast	1 in 20
Skin	1 in 39	Skin	1 in 49
Stomach	1 in 43	Colon	1 in 56
Prostate	1 in 57	Stomach	1 in 67
Rectum	1 in 71	Cx. uteri	1 in 80*
Colon	1 in 74	Ovary	1 in 90
Bladder	1 in 83	Corp. uteri	1 in 98
Pancreas	1 in 155	Rectum	1 in 100
Leukaemia	1 in 211	Lung	1 in 102
Testis	1 in 632	Pancreas	1 in 196
		Bladder	1 in 250
		Leukaemia	1 in 255

Just over a third of the population of England is included.

Personal communications from Birmingham: Waterhouse, J.A.H.; S.W. Region: Leyland, L.; S. Metropolitan Region: Payne, P.M.; Womersley, B.J.

The calculations were made *up to 85 years of age,* so the figures in the Table slightly underestimate the average *total lifetime* expectancy.

*Excluding carcinoma *in situ,* the figure is 1 in 79: the national campaign for cervical-cytology screening began in 1964/5.

made about this Table: compared to the probability of about 1 in 45 of developing skin cancer, the risk of dying from it (and appearing in the Registrar General's Mortality Tables) is about 1 in 750, another order of magnitude.

Average *lifetime* probabilities are not enough. The administrator, planning a screening programme for cervical carcinoma in situ, must also know that the "need", the average risk of manifesting clinical invasive disease, is 1 in 2,053 by age 35 but three times greater, 1 in 677, by age 40. To have a chance of preventing invasive cancer, his programme should start by 30 or 35 years at latest. . . . Or, another aspect: in assessing, and explaining to all concerned, the hazards of *industrial* bladder cancer, it is necessary to establish also the relevant individual risk for the *general* population: 1 in 2,597 men by age 45 and 1 in 668 by age 55; or 1 in 83, "total", as shown — substantially less than in the dyestuffs workers (1 in 10, or even 5).

Risk to Individual Cigarette Smokers

"Statistics of excess deaths among cigarette smokers as a group may not give the individual smoker a clear idea of how much worse off he is than his non-smoking contemporaries. Table 4.2, derived from Doll and Hill's study of British doctors, shows the chances that an average cigarette smoker who consumes various numbers of cigarettes per day has of dying within the next ten years, calculated for four decades between the ages of 35 and 74. The significance of these figures may be illustrated in terms of a lottery by supposing that for each ten-year period a man draws a ticket from a box containing one ticket marked 'death' among a number of blanks. If he draws the marked ticket he dies within the next ten years. The ratios in Table 4.2 indicate the number of tickets among which the one marked ticket is placed. Thus, for a non-smoker aged 35, there is one marked ticket for the next ten years in a box of 75 tickets but for a heavy smoker of this age the marked ticket is one among 22." *Smoking and Health Now.*

The main measurements, or "instruments", of epidemiology are the *incidence* of new cases (particularly useful as already seen in historical study, Chapter 1), the *prevalence* of all cases (measuring the burden of chronic disease on the community, Chapter 2), and the *death rate*. The estimate of *individual risk* is simply derived, and it also has its uses; in particular, for expressing the *cumulative impact* of conditions with a long-term incidence (commonly also rising as age advances). Thus doctors were found to have an annual incidence of clinical ischaemic heart disease of 3·4 per thousand at 45–49 years of age, rising to 17 per thousand at 60–64 years; the corresponding prevalence rates were 17 and 90 per 1,000. It tells something more, that the chances of the individual doctor developing the disease during middle age, from 45 to

TABLE 4.2
INDIVIDUAL RISKS AND CHANCES IN RELATION TO SMOKING HABITS
Experience of British Doctors 1951-8
Men
(1)   Risks of Dying from All Causes Within the Next Ten Years

Decade	Non-Smokers	Ex-Smokers	Cigarette Smokers	Other Smokers	All Doctors
35–	1 in 90	1 in 49	1 in 46	1 in 62	1 in 54
45–	1 in 27	1 in 19	1 in 13	1 in 19	1 in 16
55–	1 in 8	1 in 7	1 in 5	1 in 12	1 in 7
65–74	1 in 3	1 in 3	1 in 2	1 in 3	1 in 3

Later data, up to 1965, shows that at age 35, the risk of the cigarette smoker dying within a decade ranged from 1 in 47 in light smokers (1–14 per day) to 1 in 22 in heavy (25 or more per day); etc. The figures for non-smokers, referred to in the text, were now 1 in 75 instead of 1 in 90, etc.

(2)   Chances in 100 (%) at Age 35 of Surviving to Age 65

Non-smokers	85
Ex-smokers	81
Cigarette smokers	73
Other smokers	86
All doctors	79

The later figure for non-smokers was 82%.
Doll, R. & Hill, A. B. (1962 & 1971). In *Smoking and Health* and *Smoking and Health Now*. London; [9] [10] and personal communications.

TABLE 4.3
RISK OF DEVELOPING ISCHAEMIC HEART DISEASE

Estimate of the number of male medical practitioners who, not having previously been clinically attacked by it, would get ischaemic heart disease before reaching certain ages

Age x (years)	Of 1000 men aged x, the number indicated below would get clinical ischaemic heart disease before age–					
	40	45	50	55	60	65
35	3	10	27	67	130	200
40		7	24	65	129	200
45			18	59	124	196
50				43	110	184
55					72	152
60						90

Ischaemic heart disease refers to the clinical manifestations: sudden death; other "coronary thrombosis" and myocardial infarction; angina pectoris; together with a small number of cases of "coronary insufficiency".[5] [6]

65, was about 1 in 5 (Table 4.3). Such analysis of the crude data of Table 2.11, (there are no figures on spontaneous abortion, for example, or on the number of girls appearing more than once), yields a quite unexpected proportion of teenagers bearing children. Sometimes, however, this method may be a quite *in*effective means of expression. There are nearly 400,000 casualties from road accidents every year in Britain;[7] but the individual risk is about one for every quarter-million motor-vehicle miles, a self-defeating kind of "fact". There may be only 1 chance in 7,000 or even 10,000 of dying from tonsillectomy — 9,999 didn't — but it has added up to over 400 disasters since 1948.[11]

EPIDEMIOLOGY AND CLINICAL MEDICINE

The calculation of average risks and chances is one of the ways that generalised experience can be related to the particular individual, facts about groups or populations applied in the clinical situation when decision by and about individuals is involved. What is the risk of vascular complications from the pill, relative to other relevant risks (next page)? Of malformation after rubella? The "empirical chances" of bearing another child with cleft palate (in comparison with the rest of the population)?[12] [14] What are the chances of the vigorously exercising, non-smoking Jack Spratt, converted to the Sanitary Idea of the Day, avoiding a heart-attack in his fifties, sixties? Relative to the chances in the mass of the population on quite other regimens? This kind of estimate is produced by forward-looking, "prospective", studies, and much that is being learned about the relations of health and disease to the mode of life is readily expressed in such probabilities; which is one advantage of having a population well trained in weighing the odds.

Prediction Research

"Prediction is essentially a best estimate of future probabilities in the light of our knowledge about past patterns"; it aims at "measurable uncertainty".[15] The term "prediction research" seems to have originated in criminology[16] and its need for tables of the likely results of "treating" such-and-such an offender this way and that. (The basic fact in that field, however, is that the individual chances — or risks — of being caught at all may be too small to be any deterrent in the first place.) In epidemiology and preventive medicine prediction research is coming to be used in the practical application of what we've been considering in this chapter: to identify *individuals* at such high risk of manifesting particular trouble that action should be taken; or, if it helps, to identify high-risk *groups* which are very specific. On present evidence, a middle-aged London busman who happens to be in the top quarter or fifth of the distribution of casual systolic blood pressure (at 170 mm Hg and above), has a 1 in 2 risk of developing cardiovascular disease within ten years — several times the risk of the

TABLE 4.4
RISK OF DYING IN WOMEN AGED 24-34

England and Wales
Estimates for One Year

	Risk of Death in a Million such Women
Healthy women taking oral contraceptives	
From childbearing	2
Venous thromboembolism and cerebral thrombosis *attributable* to oral contraceptives	13*
Women using the diaphragm	
From childbearing	23
Women using the safe period	
From childbearing	46
Pregnant women	
From childbearing (including 13 from puerperal venous thromboembolism)	228
Women having Therapeutic abortion	110
Total Population	
From childbearing	34
Road vehicle accidents	49
Cancer	137
Venous thromboembolism and cerebral thrombosis	11

*The figure is probably lower now it is appreciated that risk is related to oestrogen dosage, and this has been adjusted.
Inman, W. H. W. & Vessey, M. P. (1968) *Br. med. J.*, *2*, 193; Doll, R. & Vessey, M. P. (1970) *Brit. med. Bull.*, *26*, no. 1, 33; Vessey, M. P. (1970) *J. clin. Path. 23*, Suppl. 3, 62; and personal communications; Vessey, M. P. & Doll, R. (1974) *Brit. med. J.*, *1*, 158; Beral, V. (1974) *Lancet*, *1*, 1280; Potts, D. M., personal communication. Mortality data from Registrar General, 1966.

Failure rates for different methods of contraception are estimated to be as follows, though the orders of magnitude are more valid than the actual numbers:

Oral contraceptive	1% per annum
Diaphragm	10% per annum
Safe Period	20% per annum

men in the lowest ranges, Table 4.5. Giving points to the busmen for plasma cholesterol concentration, etc., as well as blood pressure, improves the individual prediction.

TABLE 4.5

INDIVIDUAL RISKS OF DEVELOPING CLINICAL CARDIOVASCULAR DISEASE IN TEN YEARS

By Level of Initial Blood Pressure.[7]
Middle-aged London Busmen

Casual Systolic Pressure (mm Hg)	Nos. of Men	%Men Having First Attack			Men Dying All causes (%)
		Coronary Heart Disease* (%)	Cerebrovascular disease (%)	Other vascular disease (%)	
-129	118	9	2	2	17
130–	216	10	3	4	17
150–	171	17	5	4	26
170–	103	25	9	6	49
190+	39	33	21	10	54
Total Risks	647	1 in 6·3	1 in 20	1 in 25	1 in 3·7

Gardner, M. J., Kagan, A., Meade, T. W. & Morris, J. N. In preparation. [17-19]
* All clinical manifestations.

Multiple Factors

Various techniques are used to combine several risk factors more efficiently for prediction of individual risk; and *multiple logistic analysis* is one method that is often used for estimating the probability, *P*, of developing a disease over the period of time being studied.[17-24]

TABLE 4.6
INDIVIDUAL RISK OF HEART-ATTACK IN TEN YEARS

Prediction Based on Nine Factors
Middle-aged London Busmen

593 men were scored for nine risk-factors as determined at their initial examination: Systolic blood pressure; plasma cholesterol concentration; smoking-habits; whether they were drivers or conductors; skinfold-thickness; history of parental mortality etc.[17 19]

Fifths of Men by Scores	*n*	No. of Heart-Attacks when Men were Scored for the 9 Risk-Factors
1 Lowest score	120 ⎤	1 ⎤
2	119 ⎦	5 ⎦
3	118	16
4	118	13
5 Highest score	118	28

"Heart-attack" = acute myocardial infarction and sudden death ascribed to coronary heart disease.

Epidemiology of Health. — Using this method, Table 4.6 shows that the 40 per cent of the busmen scoring lowest on the nine risk factors were approaching immunity to heart-attack during middle age: 6 in 239; i.e., c. 1 in 400 men, per year.

"At-Risk Registers"

To assess and *register* infants born apparently healthy who are at high risk of later manifesting a serious handicap, deafness, for example, or cerebral palsy, so that health and social services can be mobilised in the hope of reducing disability, makes good sense. The probabilities predicted should be materially greater than for other infants, and the chances of benefits worthwhile. But there is no short cut to such information: a large cohort of "representative" mothers and children, with their ranges of social and biological characteristics, of pregnancy and obstetric experience, has to be followed up and suitable treatments then evaluated. In this way, groups of the newly-born may be defined that are specific enough to warrant bothersome and time-consuming screening and surveillance and sensitive enough not to bring the exercise into disrepute — and whose improved welfare justifies the diversion of scarce resources. (This is the kind of enterprise that requires close collaboration of different parts of the Health Service, plus basic epidemiology, plus clinical trials of methods of helping; then the relevant information system — modern Community Medicine.) Meanwhile, inherited deafness in the family, a history of maternal rubella, very low birthweight, haemolytic disease of the newborn, these surely indicate vulnerability and entry on a register. One such initiative in Reading,[29] using such simple criteria, has identified a minority of 30 per cent of newborn infants among whom 50 per cent of particular defects developed subsequently.[24-30]

An individual approach is likely to be one of the preventive strategies against several chronic conditions and it is beginning to be practical for clinical medicine and health-services administration. So this use of epidemiology to estimate individual risks and chances will be coming into its own.

5. Identification of Syndromes

One of the paths of progress in medicine has been to define "syndromes": by clustering of symptoms and signs, regularities of natural history and outcome; in common morbid anatomy and, later, biochemical disturbances; by discovering that apparently unrelated phenomena have the same causes. Hippocrates describing consumption may be cited; or, crossing the centuries, Sydenham's "uniform and consistent" distinction of measles from other specific fevers, gout from other rheumatism. The separation of gonorrhoea and syphilis, Kraepelin's classification of the psychoses, Bright's disease, acute myocardial infarction are classical examples. A great many syndromes have been delineated in modern times, by clinical and a variety of laboratory methods: Sheehan's, Conn's, echo virus, for example; Burkitt's lymphoma; carotid obstruction; kwashiorkor (unbelievably late); analgesic and Balkan nephropathies; phenylpyruvic oligophrenia; the affectionless thief; the illness that occasions admission to the mental hospital and the "social breakdown syndrome" produced by the treatment. Now there are new possibilities of pattern-recognition by computer-analysis, and another chapter may be opening with chromosome typing, the tall-subnormal-delinquent-XYY male, for example.

"Syndrome", thus, is used here very widely for the definition of entities, e.g. single gene-molecular disorders like the haemoglobinopathies at one extreme, and description of "reaction types", such as the collagenoses or the autoimmune, with shared characteristics at the other. Each generation will "split" and "lump" to suit its own purposes.[1-5]

Epidemiology has characteristic "use" here. Analysis may show that what has been commonly lumped together wants taking apart because its components are differently distributed in the population; conversely, the apparently unrelated may be linked because they are similarly distributed. In short, the epidemiological behaviour of phenomena is helping to identify "syndromes". In the 1920's there was less appreciation than today of the two main types of peptic ulcer, of the differences in natural history, gastric mucosa and in the role of hypersecretion, etc. Clearly (Fig. 5.1) these two ulcerations had to be distinguished. The poverty gradient in the certifications of gastric ulcer (GU), and the absence of anything like it in the "new" duodenal ulcer (DU), suggested that these are different diseases (with some

References on page 292.

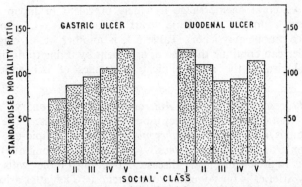

Fig. 5.1 Peptic ulcer: distinction of duodenal from gastric ulcer in 1921–3 by the social-class distribution of their mortality. Males, aged 20–64. England and Wales.[7] [32]

necessarily different causes). A later morbidity study found the same. There is gross international variation in the ratio of gastric to duodenal ulcer. Family studies indicate specific inheritance of one or other. The recent decline in DU mortality (p. 17) followed 10 or more years after that of GU (supporting a standard of living hypothesis for the latter).[6-11]

Syndromes of Atherosclerosis

Simply to label *ischaemic heart disease* (IHD) and *cerebrovascular disease* (CVD) as complications of "atherosclerosis" is little justified by clinical experience, in light of the anatomy or pathology of the affected vessels, or in the relation of the two conditions to hypertension. Viewed epidemiologically, again they are different. Ischaemic heart disease was known last century but seemingly uncommon, cerebrovascular disease as now was common. IHD apparently is increasing, CVD (congenital aneurysms doubtfully excepted) shows no such trend. There is a gross excess of IHD but not CVD among middle-aged men compared with

TABLE 5.1

TWO SYNDROMES OF "ARTHEROSCLEROSIS": ISCHAEMIC HEART DISEASE AND CEREBRO-VASCULAR DISEASE AMONG MEDICAL PRACTITIONERS[12]

Number of "First Attacks"
Males aged 40-64 years
1947-50

"Atherosclerotic" Condition	General Practitioners	Other Doctors
Ischaemic Heart Disease	82	33
Cerebrovascular Disease	14	13

Insured population of Medical Sickness Annuity and Life Assurance Society Limited.

women. Cerebral haemorrhage is widely prevalent in Japan and in developing countries, ischaemic heart disease not yet. The small experience among physicians, Table 5.1, is another bit of evidence*. The reader can continue this line of argument by trying to distinguish, epidemiologically, the main clinical syndromes of ischaemic heart disease.

Two Processes in Coronary Atherosclerosis. — Coronary "athero-sclerosis" is a complex of distinct though related processes. The salient distinction is into (1) *mural atheroma* (? essentially lipid-cholesterol deposition); and (2) *lumen stenosis* (? essentially thrombotic) which may lead to ischaemic heart disease. Atheroma of the walls of the coronary arteries is far commoner than stenosis. The latter arises only on the basis of the former, but many with much atheroma at necropsy show no particular narrowing while some with little atheroma show a great deal, even amounting to complete occlusion. Historically, the Table on page 15, there is evidence that acute coronary thrombosis and chronic coronary occlusion, and ischaemic myocardial disease, have increased but not that mural atheroma has.[13] The occupational distribution of the two processes again is different. Judging by the frequency of acute infarction in population studies, physically active and heavy workers less often have fatal acute massive thromboses than do sedentary and light workers. Similarly with complete or near-complete occlusions of coronary arteries found at necropsy. There are no major differences, however, in the amount or severity of mural atheroma:

Coronary Atherosclerosis and Physical Activity of Occupation
Deaths from Causes Other than Ischaemic Heart Disease
Males, Aged 45–70[14]

	Occupation		
Coronary Arteries	Light	Active	Heavy
	(1392)	(1377)	(836)
	%	%	%
Much mural atheroma	21	17	18
Calcification reported present	23	20	21
Lumen occlusion of a main artery	5·9	4	3·1*

National Necropsy Survey.
(Number of cases in brackets.)
*0·01 > P > 0·001.

*Table 5.I also shows how an epidemiological observation can be made in the absence of denominator numbers: these two disorders were occurring in the *same* population-at-risk.

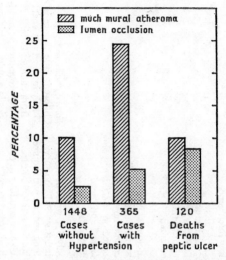

Fig. 5.2   Coronary atheroma and coronary occlusion, National Necropsy Survey, deaths from causes other than ischaemic heart disease. Males aged 45–59.[15]

Figure 5.2 is another illustration; I hope it speaks for itself and can only speculate about rich cream diets, Sippy *et al*. Finally, setting up a "model" of coronary atheroma and coronary stenosis from all the data available to us of the contemporary *prevalence in the middle-aged male population,* there seems again to be a difference. Thus, close on 100 per cent of men show mural disease at necropsy, most of them having a little or moderate amount. But only a minority have naked-eye stenosis of a main coronary artery, and in most of them it is severe/occlusive. Speculating, the occlusive phase once started tends to build up by positive feedback.[15]

Such identification of "syndromes" may also be of immediate practical interest. Thus, if the modern epidemic of IHD is due to an increase of coronary thrombosis, a new frequency of the occlusive phase and/or of related myocardial pathology, two models of defence are opened up: against the ancient and underlying atheroma, or against the occlusion and myocardial disease which are more likely to be associated with "modern" social changes. Once the latter phase is in the ascendant, moreover, there may not be much point to attempting to control the lipid-cholesterol-atheroma phase.

Identification of syndromes by their *causes* is the ideal method, e.g. tabes and GPI as syphilitic, or the manifold tuberculous diseases. But failing this, useful progress may still be possible.

Severe Subnormality and Slight

Table 5.2 sets out these two classical syndromes and follows through with other uses of epidemiology as in Chapters 2 and 3.

TABLE 5.2 TWO GRADES OF MENTAL HANDICAP [16-20]

THE GRADES ARBITRARILY DEFINED	CAUSES	COMMUNITY DIAGNOSIS	DISABILITIES/NEEDS/SERVICES	COMMUNITY PROGNOSIS
SEVERE – Intelligence quotient more than 3 s.d. below mean, i.e. IQ score is under 50: *Imbeciles* (severe and moderate retardation, WHO) IQ 20–49 *Idiots* (profound retardation, WHO) IQ under 20	Whole brain pathology, e.g. Chromosomal abnormality Single gene-molecular abnormality Congenital malformation Brain damage due to bio-chemical lesion, injury, or infection. Unknown; a few presumably the tail-end of the normal distribution First-degree relatives are rarely affected	Minimum incidence per year = 3.7/1,000 live births; i.e., 6-7 now in average town of 100,000 Prevalence at ages 0-19 there-fore=a little less than 3.7/1,000. Nos. about 120 in town of 100,000 Prevalence in adults=mini-mum of 1.8/1,000, i.e., about 130 in town of 100,000 All affected subjects in England now known to educational or medical services by 5-7 years of age Found throughout the *social classes*–but more than expected in lower	These vary widely Large proportion have medical problems as well low intelligence Special educational facilities needed. Their right to this is now accepted Lifelong support of individual and family by community is needed, based on *clinical, psychological* and *social* diagnosis Only 5% work in open industry. All who survive long enough will require special residential care Unable as adults to esta-blish independent households Genetic counselling. Diagnosis of PKU, etc. Challenge to joint effort by health and social-services administrations	*Future prevalence rates* Children: little change is likely in short run apart from changes in birth rate New preventive possibili-ties in amniocentesis, etc. Adults: rising by about 1% per year because of increased longevity

MILD— IQ between 2and 3 s.d. below mean, i.e. IQ score is 50-69 Other terms: *Feeble-minded, Morons*			
Majority show no brain, chromosomal or single gene pathology, i.e. no *qualitative* abnormality. Difference from those with normal IQs is *quantitative*	Incidence of children with IQ 50-69 is about 15-20 per 1,000 live births, i.e. 30-40 born per year into town of 100,000	Small proportion have additional clinical lesions
Evidence of multiple genetic factors; and unfavourable social environment, including? infantile malnutrition (sub-culture)	Majority in *classes 4 and 5*. Virtually none without evident brain pathology in *higher* social classes	Minority have other problems than low IQ: e.g. come from broken homes, and may need residential care (e.g. in hostels) and social casework. Special problems with large families
First-degree relatives are similarly affected more than expected from frequency in general population	True prevalence of children with IQ 50-69=15-20/1,000 depending on social class distribution of population: say 400-600 in the town of 100,000	Majority find employment in open industry and manage to set up independent family units
	Prevalence of such children receiving special education =10/1,000 (these "mildly subnormal" are the majority of "Educationally Sub-Normal" children)	*Future incidence and prevalence rates* should decline with spread of family planning and environmental improvement
	Prevalence of adults *known* to social agencies as mildly subnormal falls steeply with age and overall=1·8/1,000 adults 30 in the town). They are in fact absorbed into the general population	

High Blood Pressure Without Evident Cause —
Is There a Specific Disease?

In the general population, up until old age, blood pressure is fairly "normally" distributed with a tail to the right. Most of those at the positive end of this distribution constitute a group having high blood pressure without evident special cause (such as renal disease): do they represent a specific syndrome of essential hypertension? Or are these individuals merely different in degree from the remainder, one extreme of the continuous distribution of blood pressure in the population? Pickering has proposed the latter explanation; he believes that age, and environmental causes as yet undetermined, are of major importance in determining blood pressure at all including high levels. The contribution of heredity, as in other such continuous distributions, is polygenic, it is suggested, and small. Contrariwise, Platt emphasises that only in some persons does pressure increase materially in middle age. In the majority of those having high blood pressure without evident cause, he postulates, this is determined by a small number of genes, environment being of less importance; the majority of hypertensives it is thus claimed are qualitatively distinct from those who merely happen to be at the high end of the "normal" distribution. (Compare "severe subnormality", with its excess of special groups at the very low end of the IQ distribution.) Meanwhile, there is no clinical or laboratory biochemical method of further distinguishing individuals supposed to be afflicted with this specific disorder of essential hypertension, and the epidemiological evidence is inconclusive, but mostly pointing Pickering's way which is inherently the more likely explanation in so common a condition. These questions have been more clearly — and con brio — argued elsewhere.[21-23]

Our own contribution, analysing busmen's blood pressures — this segregated a group of hypertensive drivers on the basis of a family history of hypertension inferred from premature parental death — received no support in larger studies of miscellaneous industrial workers.[24 25] The evidence however is not consistent: thus, systolic blood pressures did not increase in all individuals of a cohort of aviators followed for 24 years. The increase of mean blood pressure with age in the group as a whole reflected the consistent rise in pressure experienced by a small number of these men as they grew older. These men also showed greater gains in weight and their parents were shorter-lived.[26]

In Miall's cohort study, by no means all showed a marked rise of pressure with advancing years. He suggests that when the blood pressure does so increase, this is dependent not merely upon age, but on the height of the pressure already reached: in those individuals whose blood pressure rises, the level of pressure itself has initiated a vicious circle with movement upwards (a qualitative factor). And the actual rise of pressure, he further postulates, is proportional to the pressure already attained. A possible reconciliation between "Pickering" and

"Platt" is thus offered.[27] [28] Analysis of the Framingham data, however, does not show any general tendency for an individual's future blood pressure to be correlated with his initial level.[29]

Meanwhile, it is immensely worthwhile to discover symptomless hypertension (p. 105), because life expectancy is directly associated with the level and, often, something can be done about high levels. A fortiori, will this be so if Miall is right and catching higher pressures early will prevent subsequent rise to even more dangerous levels.

Quantity and Quality

Definition of "disease" syndromes by degree not absolutes, in shades of grey not black or white, in terms of those at a tail-end of a continuous distribution and *quantitatively* different from the majority — this provides an explanation for most of neurosis, personality disorders, delinquent behaviour, alcoholism, "slight" mental subnormality, senile dementia; in glaucoma, hyper- and hypothyroid disease, diabetes (for a start, the positive end of the glucose-tolerance curve), hypercholesterolaemia. The object of arbitrarily so defining a "syndrome" is usually clinical and practical. These situations may be contrasted meanwhile with *qualitative* distinctions and syndromes: most of severe subnormality, for example; the chromosome defects, polymorphism. specific gene-enzyme disorders, autoimmune reactions; being pregnant and not; the critical periods of the life-cycle; passing an exam and failing; having faith or no; self and not-self.

The situation is complicated by the transformation of quantity into quality: through entry into a vicious circle, or through critical-mass, break-point, saturation, or threshold effects. The intensity of exercise adequate to stimulate cardiovascular health; benign vs. malignant hypertension; the degree of coronary stenosis that does and doesn't disable; the level of intelligence below which it isn't possible to function independently in a particular culture; the prognosis of very small as distinct from merely small babies; plasma concentration of cholesterol over 400 mg. may be enough by itself to cause major trouble: these are the kind of situations in mind.

Summary

Table 5.3, overleaf, is a model of what has been said. In the first column several problems are stated, about the nature of the apparent excess of "appendicitis" in young women, for example, or the course of coalworkers' pneumoconiosis. The second column lists the data that were analysed, e.g. large representative series of cases, or vital-statistical records. Column 3 shows the criteria on which these data were classified: by clinical condition; by host factors, or behaviour and environment; and by making "secular" comparisons of the site of perforated ulcer last century and this, or of the cell-type of bronchogenic carcinoma during the modern epidemic. In the last column the results are given in terms of *syndromes* that were identified from the mass-data of col. 2

Thus "appendicitis" in young women divides into two, and the surplus of the disease in them beyond what is expected on overall sex and age trends (in any one year it is enough to occupy 100 surgical beds) is probably not true appendicitis. The common squamous and oat-cell cancer of the lung is related to cigarette smoking — as might be anticipated from the histology — adenocarcinoma has not been so related. In the last illustration, a vulnerable group for stillbirth is identified;

TABLE 5.3

IDENTIFICATION OF SYNDROMES BY EPIDEMIOLOGICAL METHODS: SOME EXAMPLES

Problem	Medical Data Available	Epidemiological Analysis	Result
Homogeneity of "Peptic" Ulcer[31-32]	National death certificates, 1921-3 Surgical records, late 19th and early 20th century (large series)	By site and— social class secular trend sex	*Duodenal* ulcer distinguished from *gastric*
"Appendicitis" in Young Women [33-35]	Hospital admissions (national sample) Death certificates	By age By sex By clinical severity By civil state	Large group (3,000-4,000 per year in England and Wales) which is probably *not* appendicitis distinguished by its peak at 17 years of age, and its occurrence only in females. There is no corresponding excess of peritonitis or fatal cases. Frequency declines with age in both married and unmarried women
Natural History of Pneumoconiosis [36]	Radiological follow-up of populations of coalminers and ex-miners	By exposure to coal dust	*Progressive massive fibrosis* (which can and does develop without further exposure to dust) distinguished from *simple pneumoconiosis* (which doesn't)
Histology of Bronchial Carcinoma[37 38]	Large (national) series of cases	By smoking habits By historical trends By sex	*Squamous* and undifferentiated, characteristically "exogenous" carcinoma are related to smoking; unlike *adenocarcinoma*
Unexplained Stillbirth[39]	Clinical records of total "population" Stillbirth certificates	By age and parity of mother By period of gestation	A group of "unexplained" still-births distinguished by their *post-maturity* and occurrence especially in *elderly primiparae*

Action Research—or "experimental epidemiology". In Aberdeen they began earlier induction of labour in the vulnerable group thus defined, and caesarean section is done more often. The statistics show a substantial fall of stillbirths and first-week deaths among these women (the lines for Parity 1 at ages over 30 in the first two sections of Fig. 5.4 indicate the scope for reduction).

this discovery led to successful clinical-preventive action and it has been rewarding, moreover, to study the group in the laboratory — anoxia was found to accompany the postmaturity and cause the foetal deaths.

Clinical phenomena awaiting such ventures in clustering by epidemiological methods are easily listed: the assorted social and biological phenomena of ageing; cardiomyopathies; toxaemia of pregnancy; vast areas in psychiatry (the schizophrenias for a start), cerebral palsy. And, though progress is disappointingly slow, ischaemic heart disease.

IDENTIFICATION OF NON-SYNDROMES

"Physicians appear to have a special love for syndromes. The idea connects two medical phenomena and the hypothesis in these cases is simply that the two phenomena occur more frequently together than can be accounted for by chance association. An example is the Paterson-Kelly (Plummer-Vinson) syndrome, in which the dysphagia is associated with iron-deficiency anaemia. The hypothesis of association can, of course, only be adequately tested by comparing an unselected group of people with this particular type of dysphagia with a group of the same age and sex, chosen at random from people without dysphagia living in the same area as the former. This feat has finally been carried out by Elwood and his colleagues,[40] using a part of the population of the Rhondda Fach, and to everyone's surprise no difference as regards anaemia was found between the two groups."[41]

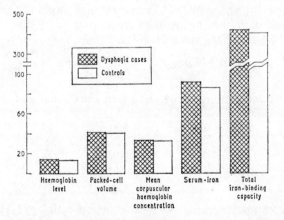

Fig. 5.3 Mean levels of haematological variables in women with dysphagia and in their controls.[40]

ASSOCIATION OF DISEASES —

A step further.

Examples abound of syndromes or diseases being connected — with varying justification. The difficulty, apart from coincidence, is that a patient with more than one disorder is more likely to be admitted to hospital. Coronary and other thrombosis, diabetes with IHD are cited; peptic ulcer and coronary occlusion (Fig. 5.2); pernicious anaemia and cancer of the stomach; ulcerative colitis and cancer of the colon; uveitis and spondylitis; social and mental health with physical health in the aged; infection and malnutrition in developing countries; the diseases of civilisation from constipation to hypercholesterolaemia and heart-attack. The association of acute leukaemia with mongolism was shown epidemiologically before the common chromosomal abnormality was discovered.[42] As the death certificate is modernised, and computer-tabulations made of the multiple pathologies that so often are present in the aged, we should learn more about connections between them.

"The question of *associations between diseases,*" wrote J. V. Neel, "has long intrigued medical investigators. So long as the predominant diseases were caused by single agents which, with appropriate techniques, could be isolated, relatively little was done to exploit the potential value to the epidemiologist of disease associations. Now, however, that our attention is more and more occupied by diseases caused by genetic susceptibilities or environmental insults with long lag periods, the question of associations assumes new importance, since a single gene or a constellation of genes may predispose to several apparently distinct diseases, and a single newly introduced environmental insult, such as radiation, may result in abnormal cell proliferations recognisable both as leukaemia and as one or more other types of malignancy." In *The Use of Vital and Health Statistics for Genetic and Radiation Studies.* (1962). WHO, Geneva.

I wonder if a relevant experience is to be found in the health of the wartime British Army.[43] [44] Time after time morbidity among men from *peptic ulcer* was higher than in women of similar rank. For example, the discharge rates in 1945:

(BOR) Males	(ATS) Females
216	46

In the same data, and typically, these were the discharges for psychoneurosis:

737	900
Total 953	946

(Rates per 100,000)

Does this complementarity point to common aetiology? The figures illustrate the need to consider epidemiological problems in terms of all relevant events in the population. This has to be done at the simple verbal level, and at biological and social levels. In some of the communist countries, mental and nervous disorders "appear" less frequently than in the West. But hypertension with nervous manifestations apparently is widespread. What would be the result there of this kind of simple arithmetic? And how does the common alcoholism fit into the picture (ecology)?

—AND THEIR DISSOCIATION

This is a fertile field for clinical speculation and inspiration: rheumatoid arthritis/jaundice, bronchitis/emphysema, ulcer/ pregnancy, disease from ageing. Epidemiologically, the chapter opened with an account of GU/DU. The grandest dissociation of all was Jenner's. Discovery of the protection of mottled enamel against dental caries was the beginning of fluoridation.

Figure 5.4, overleaf, a massive record-linkage job, illustrates from elementary human biology. The notion of *perinatal mortality* has many origins in clinical obstetrics, pathology, the difficulties of vital statistics, in administration and in forensic medicine; it has many advantages for international comparison. The differences in the Figure are a warning on its limitations in drawing lessons on aetiology. Thus, *mortality in the first week of life* — indeed in the very first hours — includes patterns both of *stillbirth* with high rates in elderly primiparae (and an association with post-maturity), and of *post-neonatal mortality* with high rates in multiparae, young and grand (and an association with prematurity). The causes of death are also different: for example, anencephaly in stillbirth; and hyaline-membrane disease in the premature liveborn.

*   *   *

Several "uses" of epidemiology are being proposed, but variations on a theme may be a better description. Thus, data from historical study, and community diagnosis, have been exploited to identify syndromes. Equally, defined syndromes have helped to clarify some issues of previous chapters. The same epidemiologic data in fact are being organised to ask a variety of questions, serve several purposes.

Fig. 5.4 overleaf:

Numbers: Live births, 1,322,150
Stillbirths, 28,956
Deaths in first week, 17,359
Deaths between 1 and 4 weeks, 4095
Deaths between 4 weeks and 6 months, 10,270
Deaths between 6 months and 1 year, 3952
Deaths in the second year, 1566

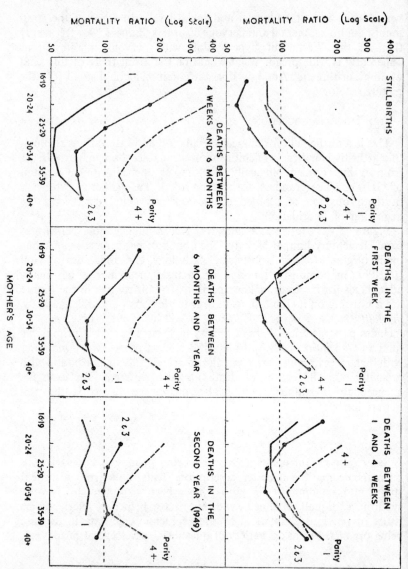

Fig. 5.4   Stillbirths and deaths in the first week (perinatal mortality); deaths in the remainder of the first year; and in the second year. The pattern of mortality, at various stages, on analysis by mother's age and parity (number of children she has borne). Stillbirth rates are calculated per 1000 total births (live and still), the other death rates per 1000 live births. In the figure, the various rates have been expressed as mortality ratios (log scale), the experience of all mothers being regarded as 100. Single, legitimate births, 1949/50. England and Wales.

Morrison, S. L., Heady, J. A. & Morris, J. N. (1959) *Arch. Dis. Childh.*, **34**, 101. Heady, J. A. & Morris, J. N. (1959) *J. Obstet. Gynaec. Brit. Emp.*, **66**, 577.

6. Completing the Clinical Picture

The clinician's experience of the chronic diseases is likely to be incomplete. In the less common conditions numbers may be too few, with attendant troubles of chance variation. But even when numbers are large his experience may be peculiar and his patients unrepresentative, i.e. the picture may be biased. The reasons for this are manifold — in personal specialism and reputation, for example, or in geographic, social or administrative situations. Such limitations apply also to the work of a hospital or any other clinical facility. Selective processes affecting admission to hospital may be explicit and obvious, by severity for example; but they can also be subtle, complicated, unrecognised and unsuspected. All this is to refer only to patients who present to medical attention. But advanced disease may be symptomless till the end, and even those suffering severe disability may not seek help. At the other extreme, much minor illness is ignored. In short, a clinician's picture of chronic disease is likely to be incomplete, all clinical experience is liable to be so. The epidemiologist, concerned with the total of defined cases in a defined population, and not merely with patients who present in particular hospitals, clinics or practices, can help to provide a fuller picture than is obtainable in any or all of these. This fuller picture may prove to be a different one. The epidemiological method thus is helping to *complete the clinical picture* and "natural history of disease".

1. COMPLETING THE PICTURE IN BREADTH

An Illustration from Ischaemic Heart Disease
Soon after beginning to work on the epidemiology of coronary disease I came across this example of how unrepresentative is the picture of it in hospital. Searching the pathological archives of a great teaching and by tradition "district" hospital, I was puzzled at the rarity of spontaneous *ruptured ventricle* despite the numerous examples of other manifestations of ischaemic heart disease,[1] and the hospital's cardiologists agreed that they scarcely ever saw a case. The answer eventually dawned on me, and it was confirmed by the pathologist responsible for the medico-legal necropsies in that part of London. "Oh yes," he told me on the telephone, "I get two a week." The coroner's pathologist (the Medical Examiner) dealt with almost all these cases.

References on page 293.

TABLE 6.1
HOSPITAL AND COMMUNITY: RUPTURED HEARTS[2]

1957–8

| Age (Years) | HOSPITALS | | | | | | | | |
| | 13 Main Teaching* | | Other Hospitals | | Coroners' Mortuaries | | Estimated Total in London | | |
	M	F	M	F	M	F	M	F	M+F
–69	15	4	13	4	86	60	114	68	182
70+	4	13	11	19	145	240	160	272	432
Total	36		47						
	83				531		274	340	614

*12 Undergraduate TH + Hammersmith Hospital.
  "Inner" London.

Some years later we returned to this question, and the detailed results are illuminating.[2] During the two years 1957–58, in all of London's hospitals, 83 ruptured hearts, presumptively due to ischaemic disease, were found at necropsy. However, in a two in three sample of coroners' pathology, drawn from the same population over the same time, there were 345 such ruptured hearts. Scaling-up the coroners' figures to give an estimate for the people of London, it was obvious that the condition is quite common (Table 6.1). On these figures, about 300 cases each year were being recognised in London, or 100 per million of the population. About one in 100 deaths in old people seem to be due to ruptured heart.

Why were so few (less than 15 per cent) dealt with in hospitals? I can only speculate. Ruptured heart is one of the forms of "sudden death" from IHD, and all of these are under-represented in hospital. Ruptured heart affects mainly the aged, and there are special difficulties in their admission to hospital. Moreover, myocardial infarction in old people often is painless — not Harvey's "mighty seizure" — producing perhaps yet another episode of confusion; often, too, the victims were living alone. In consequence, even if they were "admitted" to hospital it would often be as the "D(ead) O(n) A(rrival)". For such cases, special arrangements are made in London through the system of coroners.

Overall, the largest group, it will be noticed, were old ladies. But this does not imply a higher frequency in them: as will be expected there were, then, in London nearly twice as many females over 70 as males. The number in old ladies, more likely reflects the trend to a similar rate in the two sexes among the aged. There is a widespread clinical impression, epidemiologically so far unconfirmed, that the relative female immunity to ischaemic heart disease, which diminishes after the menopause, disappears altogether in old age. Certified national coronary death rates in old age do converge, for what specific cause- of-death data after 65 or 70 years of age are worth (which is not very much); but apart from these figures on ruptured heart there is little information on the incidence or prevalence of IHD in old people.

To sum up: the clinical picture in London's hospitals of ruptured ventricle was incomplete, indeed it was wrong: wrong, grossly, on size, wrong about age, wrong even on sex. And wrong, it may be added, on the possible contribution of anticoagulants: these were being taken by 16 per cent of the hospital patients but only by 2 per cent of all the cases.

Clinical Medicine and Epidemiology

The first point to make then is this: clinicians deal with patients, epidemiologists with populations. In studying the natural history of disease, the epidemiologist, for the numerator of the "rates" he is always seeking to produce, must as a first step and at the very least find all the patients in the population (the denominator), *wherever* they happen to present. Surveys usually are needed for this, and it is to surveys of one kind and another that the epidemiologist devotes most of his time. In the present instance, to estimate the number of ruptured hearts in the population of London was relatively simple, because of the practice whereby nearly every unexplained death in London is investigated by necropsy. Mere addition of hospital numbers and those from the coroners' mortuaries gives a useful picture, though it will be an underestimate because of cases wrongly diagnosed before death and not reported to the coroner. (Ruptured ventricle from IHD is virtually unmistakeable — but only if the heart is examined.) The position will be quite different in other places where there is routine post-mortem examination in only a small fraction of "sudden" unexpected deaths that evidently are due to natural causes. (What is the position in the reader's community? What is the validity of local statistics on mortality from IHD?)

To generalise, ischaemic heart disease "presents" in many places; general practice, consulting practice, the works' clinic, a variety of hospitals, diverse medical wards, surgical wards, general and special out-patients, general necropsy rooms, as medically unattended sudden death, the coroner's mortuary. It also presents in many ways: as sudden death in the apparently healthy, classical cardiac infarction, an atypical chronic and serious illness, angina of varying severity, "confusion" in the elderly, congestive failure, with dysrhythmias, these ruptured hearts. Since it presents in different ways in different places, more of one type here, of another there, information from any physician or any particular facility is liable to be incomplete — and may be misleading. Only an inclusive study in a big enough community, using a Register for example, can provide a picture, even of clinically presenting IHD, in proportion and as a whole.

Working of Health Services. — Today, the clinical picture less and less can be taken for granted. *Community care* is dispersing patients, with serious mental disorder for example, so that the most determined efforts are needed to keep systematic track of them. And *treatment* is drastically altering the outcome: in spina bifida, for example; patients with ventricular fibrillation are snatched from the brink; chronic bronchitics rescued winter after winter. In such situations, long-term follow-up of all diagnosed patients in an appropriate population is the least on which a modern "clinical" picture of *the unnatural history of disease*[3] can be based.

"District" and "Teaching" Hospitals. — The figures on ruptured heart show the incompleteness of hospital data for a grave illness. Even in this instance, however, the picture in many teaching hospitals, which are the source of most statements on pathology (and where students learn most of their medicine), is particularly unrepresentative. Buerger's disease, if there is such an entity, is not restricted to Russian Jews: "It was Mount Sinai Hospital in New York City which at that time was largely limited to Russian Jews".[4] More subtly, there may be hundreds or thousands of patients on the "books" of a university diabetic clinic, but numbers alone will not ensure that they reflect the occurrence of renal or retinal or ischaemic disorder in *diabetes* and not merely in a particular and probably quite indefinable group of *diabetics*. Patients from a wide region suspected of such "complications" will often be selected for referral to university clinics, etc. For a start, it would be better to assure that all patients with definable diabetes in a large population, in general practices for example, are studied; this is an epidemiological question and that is the right way of asking it.*

Irregular Epidemiology. — This happy phrase was coined at a WHO meeting in a plea for the amateur, for the encouragement of the clinician as "naturalist" to extend his interest to the population from which his patients are drawn. No one with the sketchiest history of epidemiology (of Pott, Gregg, Burkitt et al) can be unenthusiastic about such a plea. These pages, however, may be read as a caution (gentle) to the clinician tempted to translate hospital numbers and ratios — numerator data — into statements about the frequency of disease at various times or in particular race, sex, age or other — denominator — groups. In each specific question it is wise to ask who the patients represent, what the selective processes are likely to be, and how such bias might limit the inferences that can be drawn.[5-9]

---

*Grouped hospitals, and even a single district hospital, may be adequate in contemporary Britain to give a balanced picture in some conditions: cancer in the young and some cancers, including bronchogenic probably, in middle age, perforated peptic ulcer, schizophrenia with gross disturbance and frank delusions, smallpox, haemophilia with bleeding, serious accidents. Out-patient and Casualty records must also be examined, of course. The situation is changing as the teaching hospitals progressively assume "district" or "area" responsibilities.

TABLE 6.2
NATURAL HISTORY OF ADDISON'S DISEASE
1960–64 incl.
North-East Metropolitan Region, National Health Service
Both Sexes   Ages 25–69

	Numbers
Cases known to clinicians at 1 Jan. 1960	74
Deaths from 1 Jan. 1960 to 31 Dec. 1964:	
In above cases	1
In cases newly recognised by clinicians	1
In cases unknown to clinicians and recognised only terminally or at necropsy	10
Total Deaths	12

Six of the 12 fatal cases were tuberculous, compared with 23 of the 74 living "prevalence" cases.

Mason, A. S., Meade, T. W., Lee, J. A. H. & Morris, J. N. (1968) *Lancet*, **2**, 744.

Clinical Disease, But Not "Presenting"

To continue. Clinicians deal with their own patients, and I have considered the limitations this imposes. But some individuals with manifest, even advanced disease, and symptoms enough, do not complain, are not patients. They learn to put up with their trouble (headaches, for example, "rheumatism", or urinary difficulties); they may be afraid; but in most instances little is yet known why they do not adopt the "sick role" (in the jargon), why even gross disabilities are not felt as "needs" for medical care, then translated into "demand". This is a serious obstacle in cancer control, a recurring tragedy in glaucoma though less so now in cataract, an everyday problem with old people. In Addison's disease (Table 6.2) "completing the clinical picture" seems to have identified two syndromes: the "chronic" cases, under medical care, with excellent prognosis; and another group, presenting clinically only at the end — if at all — and responsible for most of the deaths. It is common for diabetics to give a history extending over several months when they are first detected, it may be with a "complication". Many people with severe emotional and social troubles deny them altogether: the depressed, of course, alcoholics, the family failures. And there is the "dark figure" of crime that never reaches the public view (blackmail, domestic cruelty, sexual assault, petty stealing). For a more complete picture of any of these, ad hoc community survey will be required, not merely the assembly of what is known to community services.[10][11]

Advanced Disease Which Is Not Manifest

Just before the second world war, in my first exercise in epidemiology, I made a systematic physical examination of the 1,350 men employed in certain grades by a Midlands municipality and found eight with textbook neurosyphilis.[9] None had any symptoms that bothered him; none any idea he had syphilis; none was under observation or treatment. Such cases, often burnt out, with nothing to bring them to the physician, must somehow also be included in the "natural history". Twenty per cent of first episodes of transmural infarction in Framingham were silent, diagnosed only on the electrocardiogram.[12] Routine physical examination by doctor or subject may disclose a symptomless invasive cancer. Even severe anaemia or hypothyroidism may not be "manifest" clinically, the women having vague if any symptoms, adapting at that level of efficiency. Kidneys can contract silently until acute failure precipitates a crisis.

The discussion has now shifted to disease that does not turn up of its own but may be found on ad hoc search, to all the "cases" as defined in a population, not merely the patients.

2. ICEBERG PHENOMENON

The main interest in extending beyond the clinical presentation lies in the deeper ranges, in *early* stages of chronic diseases which may be revealed.

Early, Presymptomatic, Diagnosis

I intend "early" to refer to stage and degree of development. Such early disease often is slight, "presymptomatic"; because of the reserves of organs and systems it does not reach the clinical threshold. At this stage, it is postulated, tissue and functional disorders may be reversible or, at the least, halted. This is therefore the most important group of cases to be sought.

The notion derives from nutrition, from the subclinical "malnutrition" or "hidden hunger" which is so much more common, in vitamin or protein/calorie deficiency for example, than florid deficiency states — these form the tip of the iceberg. Recognition of subclinical infection in meningococcal disease, diphtheria, poliomyelitis clarified, indeed transformed, our picture of their natural history. Mild beginning signs have long been familiar in tuberculosis, toxaemia of pregnancy, lead poisoning, children's deafness, dental caries, and they are now being described in many chronic diseases: in airways obstruction, byssinosis, cancer of skin, lip and tongue, congenital dislocation of hip, renal tract infection, prostatic hyperplasia, depression, senile dementia. Such early stages may be impossible to distinguish at present from healthy variation, from values and changes that do not matter in themselves or appear to precede trouble often enough to be worth noticing. This attempt to complete the clinical picture of chronic diseases again promises to yield not merely more information but greater understanding. Thus, population surveys of blood pressure and blood sugar levels have transformed our picture of hypertension and diabetes, disposing of any simple notions of "cut-off points" between health and disease.

PATIENTS AND POPULATIONS

The survey of *diabetes* carried out in Birmingham by the Royal College of General Practitioners and the Medical School, using the glucose-oxidase paper strip for urine examination together with the oral glucose tolerance test (GTT), provides figures that can be referred to the "levels" that have been proposed:[13]

Prevalence of Diabetes per 1,000 Aged 50+
        Both Sexes

1.	Clinical	(a) Patients presenting	16
	Detected on survey		
		(b) "Florid", with symptoms or complication	4·7 ⎫
	Sub-clinical	(c) "Florid", without symptoms	3·2 ⎬ 17
2.	Mostly sub-clinical	(d) "Early" diabetes	8·6 ⎭
		Total	32 per 1,000

The first line (a) gives the frequency of patients in this population, in each thousand at these ages. Included in line (b) are cases as in (a) who surely should have complained, but did not; many of them as already noted would later have "presented" to their GPs, with a history. Line (c) gives the proportion found in the survey to have a diabetic response to the glucose load but no symptoms; and the last line (d) represents lesser, "GTT", or "borderline" disease, corresponding to "early" in the present account, and with trivial if any symptoms. Diabetes was defined on the presence of glycosuria, plus the results of the test, so division into "florid" disease, "early" (and of course "healthy") is quantitative — and operational; there is no break in the continuous distribution of the blood sugar levels. In this study the GTT was administered only to those having postprandial glycosuria at the first screening, and, conventionally, the response regarded as "diabetic" if the capillary blood sugar level exceeded 180 mg per 100 ml at one hour and 120 mg/100 ml at two; the diabetes, further-more, was regarded as "early" when the fasting value was below 130 mg per 100 ml, "florid" if above that. This screening procedure is highly specific, but not sufficiently sensitive — there are numerous false negatives — and additional cases that fulfil the criteria are readily detected when the glucose load is given to everyone. Questions arise at once about the relationships between these several "constructs".

Thus, how many in lines (c), (b), (a) pass through a recognisable stage of early, subclinical but detectable abnormality (d)? And over what span of time? Such progression seems to occur fairly commonly. However, follow-up study has shown that in practical terms most new subjects/patients with *clinical diabetes* are recruited from the great majority who did not show glycosuria on the initial test (and administration of the GTT to all does not alter this).

Latent Disease. — The study was continued in depth. A random sample of subjects over 50 years of age who did not have glycosuria were given 50 g of glucose and their blood-sugar levels measured. Thirteen *per cent* of them now produced a diabetic-type curve, and a sizeable minority also had glycosuria. This large group may be regarded as having "latent" diabetes. But such labelling begs a lot of questions, if only because these findings may not matter so much after 60 years of age (when they are particularly common). Consideration has scarcely begun of the volume of disease which can be detected by such special challenge and that may correspond to cases that become clinical, are activated or, just as mysteriously, decompensate under stresses of infection, pregnancy, social or emotional crisis.

Figure 6.1 is a theoretical summary; Table 6.3 represents another practical approach to these questions.[14] It gives the number of patients "presenting" clinically with various conditions in an average general practice in this country, then estimates what may readily be found on ad hoc search — some of it advanced, and some of it early and subclinical disease . . . *Lung cancer* often grows rapidly and early detection by screening with mass miniature radiography seems unlikely to be rewarding. The *breast* lesions are the numbers to be expected on routine clinical examination plus mammography. "Non-presenting" *obesity* is estimated from the proportion of London busmen with trouser-waistbands of 42 inches and over; alternatively, 1 or 2 s.d. above the mean waistband could be used as a practical definition. . . Detection of significant *hypertension* is by a "cut-off" point at which most clinicians would seriously consider treatment. And so on.

Problems abound that might be illuminated by assembling complete pictures of early together with advanced disease. What is the association of *early warning signals* — transient ischaemic attacks, morning joint stiffness, suicidal threats, truanting — with the established pictures? How do major *accidents* differ from minor and from near-misses? The protean manifestations of *alcoholism* have to be categorised, from the incipient drinking problems presenting to (or being concealed from) GP to the varieties of disabled. Nothing is known, in an affected population, about the majority of those having *haemoglobin SS*. Do they in fact manage on their own? "The total picture of *schizophrenia* is not conveyed by hospital data. Such figures do not take into account the schizophrenic private patients of psychiatrists, or the undefinable

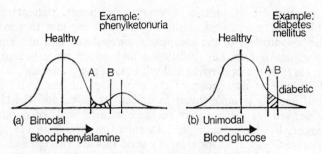

Fig. 6.1 Bimodal and unimodel distribution of attributes.
A–B = "early", "borderline" disease.

Wilson, J. M. G. (1974) In *A Companion to Medical Studies* (ed. Passmore, R. & Robson, J. S.), Vol. 3, Part 2, p.76.1. Blackwell, Oxford.

TABLE 6.3

PATIENTS AND POPULATIONS

Estimates Adjusted to an Average General Practice of 2,500 Persons Britain[14]

Condition	Approx. Average No. of Patients During a Year	Approx. Additional Cases which may be Detected on Survey
Cancer: New cases[15]		
Lung[16]		
(M, all ages)	1–2	1 in 2 years on MMR
Breast[17]		
(F, 40–65)	1	5 with suspect lesion, 4 of them benign, on biopsy
Diabetes[13]	10	10–20
Obesity[18]		
(M, 45–64)	2	25
Anaemia[19]		
(F, 15–44)	12	40–80 with Hb < 12 gm./100 ml.
Deafness[20]		
(65+)	20	40
Ischaemic heart disease[21]		6 with angina pectoris
(M, 45–64)	5	2–3 with silent "Q" waves
Hypertension[22]		Diastolic BP, 105 mm Hg +
(45–64)	M 5	M 16–27
	F 12	F 13–34
Alcoholism[23]	5	15
Depression[24]		
(F, 45–64)	10	8
Children with special handicap[25]		
(5–14)	15–20	15–20

(Sex, and/or age, in brackets)

group on the list of practically every practitioner, patients whose schizophrenic-like reactions continually impair response to treatment for other conditions; or the completely unregistered and undiagnosed schizophrenics not in any institution and under no psychiatric or medical care; or the borderline and mild cases, the 'schizoids', more or less identifiable in any group of the population at any level" . . .[15] *Industrial hazards* is understated in official statistics, and the clinical picture derived from these may be inaccurate as well: of dermatitis, skin cancer, byssinosis, accidents. In each instance there are special circumstances, and it is prudent to seek out all the clinical cases, however disguised or "selected out" of the industrial population, and to survey ad hoc for the subclinical.

3. PRECURSORS

The next dimension to be considered in the natural history of the chronic diseases is that of *precursors*. The term is used to distinguish breakdown in the body's regulatory mechanisms, in defences and adaptation; identifiable abnormalities which, on experience, are liable to lead up to recognisable disease.[26] [27] The analogy with the study of acute infections and infectious epidemics is now more remote.

The main finding of the Framingham and similar prospective studies is that men who have a high concentration of plasma cholesterol are at greater risk of developing ischaemic heart disease than comparable men with lower levels; and so on, down the scale. (One per cent difference in the blood level $\equiv 2 \cdot 7$ per cent difference in the individual risk.[28]) Hypercholesterolaemia thus is an abnormality systematically preceding the onset of ischaemic heart disease, a "precursor" in the present sense. The point of it may be illustrated by the contrast between the futility of lowering high cholesterol concentrations *after* ischaemic heart disease is manifest — the prognosis is not improved — and the abiding hope that to reduce them *before* will reduce the risks of heart-attack occurring at all.

Functional and structural precursors, as diverse as the chronic diseases themselves, are now actively being sought, "qualitative" yes/no signs, and "quantitative" that will be more difficult to define usefully. The proposition is that causes in inheritance, experience and mode of life may be translated into disease via such identifiable precursors and, among other uses, these enable the identification of individuals at particular risk. Carriage of inborn errors of metabolism; endocrine abnormalities preceding the onset of breast cancers; immunologic reactions (e.g. the presence of antinuclear substance); "precancerous" lesions like carcinoma-in-situ; pre-psychotic "character disorders"; fatty liver (for cirrhosis); or gastric ulcer (for carcinoma); evidence of sensitisation to the rhesus factor; bacteriuria in pregnancy for pyelonephritis and renal failure: these exemplify disorders that at present, if sometimes diffidently, can be postulated as precursors. "The high incidence of foetal complications of pregnancy in women destined to become diabetic many years later supports the existence of an active metabolic aberration long before the insulinogenic mechanism becomes overwhelmed (and hyperglycaemia appears). This is to speak of a diabetic trait which precedes the beta cell decompensation, the deficient insulin activity; it is prior to diabetes, prediabetes, not mild diabetes."[29] There is prospect at the molecular level of new understanding of precursor disorders and their transition into disease, as in gout or Parkinson's disease.

There is no formula for identifying precursor stages, though it is worth considering if established associations of the chronic diseases *could* be precursors, then testing by prospective study. In disease of later life that has important genetic causes, is laid down in childhood or merely is long to incubate (all three apply to atherosclerosis), it is reasonable to hope that precursor derangements will progressively be discovered. How to define "precursor" levels among graded relationships, like that of serum cholesterol apparently to coronary heart disease, will have to depend on the purpose. For example, among such a population of men, above what level is there, say, twice the average incidence of IHD, or twice that in the rest of the men; or, above what level would it be justifiable to intervene with currently available remedies?

TABLE 6.4

POSSIBLE PRECURSORS OF CHRONIC DISEASE

Estimates Adjusted to an Average General Practice of 2,500 Persons
Britain

Disease	Approx. Nos. with possibly Precursor Abnormalities who may be Discovered on Survey
Cancer of cervix[30]	5 (F, 30+) with carcinoma in situ
Gout[32]	20 (M, 30–59) with blood uric acid level of 7 mg. per 100 ml. and over
Glaucoma[33]	75 (M & F, 40–74) with ocular hypertension
Ischaemic heart[21][34] disease	20–25 (M, 40–49) with casual SBP of 160 mm Hg and over 25–30 (M, 40–49) with casual plasma cholesterol level 250 mg per 100 ml and over
Chronic bronchitis[35]	40–50 (M, 35–44) with smoker's cough
Chronic pyelonephritis–renal failure[36]	10 (F, 5–14) with persistent significant bacilluria

(Sex, and age, in brackets)

How hypercholesterolaemia "works" is not clear. If it is directly involved in the pathogenesis of IHD, as is commonly postulated, lowering the level would reduce the incidence; controlled trials alone can give the answer and they are proving exceedingly difficult to carry through. Possibly, cholesterol level is merely an association of the operative disorder of metabolism and lowering it, by itself, could be pointless. Discovery of such an "indicator", however, would still be worthwhile by helping to identify a high-risk group deserving of special attention in the detection of early disease.

Table 6.4 (previous) has a few numbers, guesses of what again may one day become essential measurements for community health and their movement, over time, important health indicators. It illustrates the present (very imperfect) capacity to postulate "healthy" groups among whom risk is substantially higher than in the remainder of the population. In glaucoma, the conventional cut-off point of 21 mm Hg in pressure screened out too many false positives to be useful. About 2 per cent of those examined, two standard deviations upward from the mean, had pressures of 25 mm and over, a far more practical figure. "Completing" the clinical picture in this way again looks like changing it: the great majority with high intraocular pressures don't have glaucoma, a few with low pressures do . . . In the blood pressure and plasma cholesterol, the upper 16 per cent of individuals are identified, those more than 1 s.d. above the age-specific means; so yielding manageable numbers at far higher risk for future IHD than the remainder . . . A fifth of the 5 per cent of the men with such uric acid levels developed gout, far more than at levels of 6–7 mg and about seven times the incidence in the remainder; the combination of positive family history and such biochemistry may indicate preventive intervention to reduce individual risk.

Normal, Normality: The Average and The Healthy

The question of what is to be regarded as "normal" arises many times in the book and it is very practical. The word has two meanings. First, (a) the *average,* or *typical,* or *mode,* as 98·4°F (37°C), seeing the GP four times a year, drinking some alcohol. The other meaning, of normal, (b), is the *healthy,* the *right,* the optimum: for example, ideal weight, the normal intestinal flora, BBC English, 80 mg alcohol/100 ml of blood, a model child, the norm of 2 "acute" beds/1,000 people. The two usages often coincide, as in the notion of the "normal range"; but they are liable to be very different. Eating a lot of saturated fat, coronary atheroma, being physically unfit, dental caries, disc degeneration, intestinal parasitism in the tropics, the consumption of sundry medicines and other typical ways of living in other cultures all are normal (a) but abnormal (b) — "we are all ill". Taking vigorous exercise, having a plasma cholesterol level under 200, loving your neighbour as yourself, are abnormal (a) but normal (b). An outlying, "abnormal" observation (a), of IgG immunoglobulins for example or of blood sugar, may immediately indicate trouble, significant clinical disease. But the better understanding of (b) is our main concern.

Among Englishmen, casual systolic blood pressure in early middle age varies with numerically few exceptions from 85–135 mm Hg; this is the normal range (a). Subsequently, however, even within that range more coronary heart disease is liable to develop on a basis of 130–135 mm Hg than from 85–90, and quite small variation seems to matter. Strictly, "normal" or healthy blood pressure in the sense of (b) should refer to levels not associated with above average or, it may be insisted, any morbidity, now or in the future; which becomes a very academic notion. "Ideal weight" in life insurance has such connotations, is supposedly associated with maximum longevity (very low weights are associated with their own troubles, and this may be true also of blood pressure).

In questions of behaviour, a major factor in redefining normal or normative (b) is the appreciation of what (a), the average or typical, actually is, in fact as distinct from fantasy or theory: viz. the debunking of the public Victorian attitudes, conventions and taboos on sexual behaviour, or the Kinsey Report in our own times.

The practical importance of understanding the normal is evident in such questions as the early diagnosis of chronic disease and the definition of precursors. The statistical average or the typical (a) is most useful in epidemiology, as in clinical medicine, to illuminate (b), what things are "right", and what is "wrong" or liable to become so. Ranges and levels, and "qualitative" states, of biological and social variables which carry few symptoms or signs of pathology, and predict trouble-free futures, again are likely to be important new measurements of community health.

We have moved on from *facts* of advanced or early disease to *probabilities*. What these precursors identify are groups vulnerable for a high incidence and individuals at high risk, whether high enough to warrant interference will depend on the magnitude of the danger, the chances of reducing it, and the implications of doing that.

4. DISPOSITIONS

Precursors merge into the earlier stage of *personal dispositions* to disease: by which is intended the operation of adverse causes in individuals and groups who thus have a greater chance of being affected by disease and, in theory if not yet often in practice, by precursor disorder beforehand. Intense research is yielding patchy knowledge of such causes in inheritance, experience, and the current mode of life, and their consideration belongs to the next chapter. Anticipating: middle-aged men who have an unfortunate family history are fat, smoke cigarettes, eat a "Western" diet, take inadequate exercise, are "disposed" to ischaemic heart disease; cigarette smokers also to chronic bronchitis and, of course, lung cancer; men who are blood-group O and non-secretors to duodenal ulcer; emotionally deprived young children are candidates for a multitude of behavioural disorders. Together with the precursor states, such personal dispositions have come to be known as "risk factors".

Information for Research and for Service

Several *communication systems* are needed to provide a more complete clinical picture of the chronic diseases and describe their natural history, and to provide intelligence for community health services. We must seek precursor states and relate them to subsequent pathology; elucidate the beginning, often undifferentiated, stages of disease and the events in progression; unravel the causes of remission, recurrence and disability; measure the effects of treatment at the several stages.

The first of these instruments is the *Chronic Disease Register*. The clinical picture "in breadth" of some major chronic non-communicable diseases could well be transformed if all the patients in specified health areas, districts or regions — depending on the scale of the problem, the NHS offers several possibilities — were notified to ongoing registers, then chronicled in their courses; as is routine in tuberculosis and some other handicaps, and during the 1930's was being established for rheumatic heart disease. The Table on page 48 is the beginning of such a register for IHD. These data were used to study the natural history — the modes of presentation, and, by follow-up, the average chances of survival, of further heart-attack, of return to work and of total disablement. As said, such population registers are more than ever necessary because the "community" at large, rather than its "hospitals", progressively is carrying the main burden of the chronic sick. Such registers could be invaluable in the search for new syndromes and other new associations — including hopefully the causal. By classification also in terms of disabilities and not merely diagnoses, they would simplify the study of *need⇌delivery* of local health and other social services and make it easier to audit and evaluate them. In common clinical situations requiring long-term surveillance, "dispensarisation", in hypertension or diabetes, for example, such registers could serve both individual management and community planning. Numerous practical problems straightaway arise, from that of the confidentiality of health (and social service) information to the "compatibility" of sundry records for computer-processing.[38]

Secondly: the *linkage of records,* medical and social, so that the relevant experience of individuals can be pieced together. This is implicit in the Register, but extends wider. At present, clinical and official health records are dispersed in "births and deaths", general practice and miscellaneous hospitals, sickness-absence, a variety of welfare agencies, criminal statistics, special registers like cancer: hundreds of millions of relevant entries are made each year. For study of the major chronic conditions, that may develop over half a lifetime and last the remainder, it could help enormously if there were a system of *individual identification,* so that extracts of various documents could be brought together automatically as needed — for a local IHD register or a national research project. This sort of machinery is particularly necessary to serve the shifting population of a mobile society — such as the advanced industrial society in which the chronic non-communicable diseases are likely to predominate. The continuing growth of clinical specialism, fragmentation often, is another impetus.

Cohort studies, the follow-up, over many years if necessary, of whole "populations" of representative individuals are a third requirement; I have already mentioned this approach in Chapter 4.[40] [41] "Many years" may be the operative words. Blood lipid patterns of the sexes diverge in the 'teens, though ischaemic heart disease is uncommon even in men before the forties. Such cohort studies offer probably the only hope of distinguishing early and maybe fleeting pathology from healthy variation; what quantitative and qualitative deviations matter in the outcome? What are the mechanisms of progression of smoker's cough into chronic bronchitis, and under what conditions is there regression? Particular infections in childhood may be crucial in chronic bronchitis of middle age. The possible metabolic and vascular hazards of the Pill are so being studied. The evolution of subclinical urinary infections into pyelonephritis (and chronic renal failure?) might be described. A systematic beginning has to be made in the long-term study of the immunologic group of disorders. Of course such studies would be enormously easier with readily available record-linkage. Follow-up of cohorts could give the answer to many puzzles in the *natural history of old age.* For example, simple questions like: does disability precede or follow retirement? Do the levels of plasma cholesterol (or of diastolic pressure, or body weight) fall in the aged, or does the reduction of average levels that is commonly found with age in population samples merely reflect the death and exit of persons with high levels? What is superimposed disease, and what the physical, mental and social processes of ageing? To understand any observation among the old (including the question why they have survived), it is of little help to make comparisons with the contemporary middle-aged who may have led quite different lives.

The natural history of health and disease is one thing. The other dividend of the follow-up of representative populations is likely to be in the *search for causes* — the subject of the next chapter. In many of the chronic diseases of middle and old age clinically presenting states often are advanced, complicated, of multiple pathology. To search for original and preventible causes in the presence of cor pulmonale, "cardiomegaly", senile dementia, end-stage kidney, hobnail cirrhosis, a blood pressure already set high and producing complications, among hooked addicts or in skid row, is to choose the worst time for answering the most difficult — and important — questions.

Finally in this collation: *family studies*. Plainly, many of the chronic disorders run in families, and there is now a great range of conditions — diabetes, pernicious anaemia, hypertension, various cancers, the connective-tissue disorders, auto-immune disease, inborn errors of metabolism, delinquency and other deviance, the inter-generational "transmitted cycle of deprivation", etc, — in which family clustering is being studied for overt disorder and covert, for relevant precursors, and for dispositions in common experience as well as heredity. Whole families are studied as they occur in a general population sample, or against appropriate "controls" selected to represent the population. With computers, it is not SF to think of *family-linked* records.[42-48]

NATURAL HISTORY OF CHRONIC DISEASES —

Table 6.5 now abstracts the main features of this account of the natural history of the "chronic diseases", the term which has come to be used for these long-developing and usually long-lasting metabolic, malignant and mental disorders. Presenting mostly in the second half of life, the chronic diseases increasingly dominate the practice of medicine in advanced societies, where most dangerous infections and undernutrition are under control, standards of maternal and child health are high, medical care is abundant and the population commonly has many old people. By the time they are *clinical* (section 1 of this chapter), cancer, ischaemic heart disease, diabetes, only too often are established and severe, the chances of cure small, and a remitting downhill course only too likely. Of greatest interest in *sub clinical* disease, section 2, are the reversible lesions which may be detected. (There is no reason to suppose that all chronic diseases progress through such an early stage; moreover, the Table presents only an "ideal type" in progression, and there are easily recognisable variants and gradations, galloping highly malignant cancer, for example). Earlier still come the prodromal, *precursor* disorders discovered before what is currently recognised as disease develops (section 3.). Finally, the *dispositions*-causes. Logically, it would be preferable to turn the Table on its side so that the traffic of events could be emphasised, traffic that often can move in either direction, halted in mid-course at the least. But I wanted to attach the scheme to the clinical picture, to look at these notions from the clinician's point of view.

— AND THEIR CONTROL

This model of the chronic diseases is abstracted so that, in turn, a useful model can be outlined of the possibilities, of control and prevention.[49 51] At each stage action may be possible, and it is worth identifying groups among whom it is particularly necessary or likely to be of benefit; each "stage", moreover, is vulnerable to the next. The unity of therapeutic and preventive practice is illustrated, and the need, I hope,

TABLE 6.5

ABSTRACT OF A MODEL OF THE NATURAL HISTORY AND CONTROL OE
"CHRONIC" DISEASES

POSSIBLE "STAGES" IN DISEASE	THEORY OF CONTROL
Advanced Disease	*"Tertiary" Prevention*

Irreversible changes present
Mostly *clinical*, and (in Britain)
   having medical care
Often incurable
May remit and relapse
Psychosocial repercussions often are
   serious
	of *deterioration*
	of *relapse*
	of *complication*
	of *disability*
	of *dependency*
	
	By finding cases not under care
	By (anticipatory) medical and social care
	By rehabilitation

Early Disease	*"Secondary" Prevention*

Pathology can be reversed
Mostly *subclinical*, with minor or no
   symptoms, detected on search, or
   becoming manifest only on
   challenge
	of *continuation* of disease (so reducing
	   the prevalence)
	of *progression*
	of *severity*
	of *illness*
	
	By detecting disease early and curing or
	   at least halting it

	"Primary" Prevention of *occurrence of disease* (its incidence)
Precursor Disorders	

of function and structure occurring
   during the pathogenesis
Silent, discovered only on search
	By discovering and controlling precursor
	   disorders

Dispositions	

I.e. the presence of identified causes of
   disease in heredity and previous
   experience; in environment and
   personal behaviour; in other
   diseases
	By measures directed to individuals
	   and groups so vulnerable
	
	By general measures in the population-
	   at-large to promote health and prevent
	   disease

for new unions between clinical and community medicine, between medical education and medical care. Today, the practical questions are very topical. What is and is not worth including in the examination of the well? Who is to be responsible for screening, surveillance, preventive treatment of the apparently healthy? How are these to be related to ongoing health services? And what is entailed for health-service administration? What is the scope for social action; when can it be mass, and when must it be individual medicine? How much priority to the enterprise?

At the *clinical stage* of declared, even advanced disease, foresight is needed and a policy for looking ahead and trying to avoid "complications", decompensation and deterioration: stroke in hypertensives, suicide among the depressed, blindness from cataract, detached retina in severe myopia, mutism from deafness, fixation of abnormal posture and movements in cerebral palsy, contractures after stroke, bedsores in the aged, kyphosis in spondylitis, somatisation of neurosis, the family disorganisation so often threatened by chronic disease. Monitoring should be mentioned, of post-thyroidectomy and gastrectomy, of hydatidiform mole. And penicillin and surveillance of those who have had rheumatic fever, for example. This is good clinical practice, requiring often a high degree of community organisation. (I suppose I should mention here the new clinical-preventive responsibility in monitoring powerful medicines taken over a long period — e.g. the Pill.)

Prevention of Disability

A more general question arises — one of the grand questions, and today's severest test of the quality of medical care. Why is it that with equal pathology and physiological disorder, some victims lead independent lives with real satisfactions, while others are personally *handicapped* and socially incompetent? We are very ignorant. Often, the most useful thing that can now be done in the manifold chronic diseases, and throughout old-age, is to seek to prevent common disabilities and social breakdown, to sustain independence (physical, emotional, economic). The medical and social care received; personality resources, attitudes to the illness and family relationships; occupation record; external stresses — whole-man medicine, again. . . But such issues will surely be more easily resolved if those who do cope — healthily — are studied as much as those who cannot, i.e. if the "careers" of all or representative cases in a population having particular basic pathology are studied.[52]

The other issue at the clinical stage is represented by the old people, depressed or failing, who do not themselves seek help despite multiple pathologies, so that only too often they "present" in a crisis of the kind that might be avoidable, when neither their families — nor society nor medicine — can readily cope. Or by the florid diabetes with symptoms and often "complications" that commonly remains undiagnosed, three or four cases on the figures already given in the average general practice. Or by the fact that the slowly developing malignancies with long clinical histories offer the best prospects: How not to miss them? There is no argument on the need for action in such instances only the question of how to take it, another aspect of the epidemiology of the non-patient. To many practical people these are the "preventive" priority today.

Secondary Prevention

Causes of the chronic diseases are only slowly being found (e.g. most cancers), knowledge is often difficult to apply (e.g. on cigarette smoking), and even when applied it could be the next generation mainly who will benefit (in any lesser incidence of mental disorder, very likely). But because often their incubation is long and they present insidiously, the chronic diseases offer special opportunities. There is now a hope, a *hope* rather than a *promise,* that it may be possible to catch some chronic diseases early and to knock them out or, at the least, to halt progression. In such ways prevalence might be reduced, much misery avoided and the burden on the community lightened. The long build-up of coronary atherosclerosis, the slow progressive destruction of kidneys or liver, the downhill career before schizophrenia is recognised, these illustrate the theoretical and unrealised potential for helping. Pulmonary tuberculosis and toxaemia of pregnancy are the classic examples.[53-57]

Detection of early and slight cases is now a basis for much routine preventive activity in the personal health services and in industry. The search is eminently worthwhile for reproducible and valid methods of such screening for early disease, yielding few false negatives (diseased individuals who are not detected by the test), and not too many false positives (individuals without the disease who are positive to the screening test) — provided something acceptable, useful and reasonably harmless can be done about what is found, and the cost in health-service resources is realistic. In breast cancer, seeking hopefully for stage 1 grade I disease,[58] the combination of clinical examination and mammography looks promising; though meanwhile there are many false negatives.[17] In phenylketonuria there is hope of preventing intellectual deterioration.[59] In acute schizophrenia, prompt diagnosis and treatment often give remarkable results. When borderline, subclinical diabetes is detected in middle age infection can be controlled, and such acute complications as coma; but it is doubtful whether the main process itself can be arrested and florid diabetes — or its chronic cardiovascular complications reduced.[60] Stopping smoking in those with "simple bronchitis" (smoker's cough), in the hope of halting progression to serious trouble, makes sense, though results meanwhile are disappointing. Whether infirmity and tissue degeneration in an ageing population will be prevented if disorder is treated earlier in middle age remains a key — and open — question.[61-63]

Primary Prevention

Earlier detection and treatment, even when feasible, often cannot be the answer. Much metabolic disease is florid from the start, cancer anaplastic, dementia progressive; renal and retinal manifestations of diabetes may present quite early; about a quarter of first heart-attacks in middle-aged men fulminate clinically as "sudden death". At the stage of precursor disorder (section 3), the occurrence of disease in those at special risk may still be averted — that is the hypothesis — by modifying the environment and mode of life, and by specific treatment. The search for such precursors — and for early presymptomatic disease — in the ostensibly healthy non-complaining population, in the hope of helping them, is now called "prescriptive screening". Such an approach to primary prevention is already standard in industry (poisoning can seldom be completely eliminated), in seeking punctate basophilia for example, or determining blood cholinesterase levels to anticipate organo-phosphorus poisoning.[64] It is clear that control of moderate and severe hypertension — half of it is symptomless — will reduce the incidence of stroke:[65] the issue is now one of education of all concerned, of long-term public compliance in a twilight role neither sick nor well, and the organisation of services. Hypercholesterolaemia today presents the hardest clinical and community issue. A level of 300+mg per 100 ml places middle-aged men at three times greater risk of heart-attack than their fellows whose plasma level is under 250 mg. Yes; but there is no convincing evidence yet that lowering the high level will in fact reduce risk. And there may be a million middle-aged people at such risk in this country.[66]

By now there is much information about mass-screening by exfoliative cytology for discovery of intraepithelial, non-invasive, in situ changes in the cervix (and, in early surveys particularly, a bonus of invasive cervical cancer, and of endometrial cancer of the body of the uterus, may also be anticipated). Analysis of the later results of the famous experiment to eradicate the disease in British Columbia shows overall reduction of incidence, and mortality is now falling more than elsewhere in Canada. The reader should study the exceedingly complex issues involved in achieving retrospective clarity when public — and professional — opinion forced the development of screening ahead of the evidence that it was effective.[67]

The practical problems in cervical cytology, since it is national policy in this country, are those of "compliance", and to reduce observer-error and false-negatives by training the readers (and not overloading them). The "positive" yield on average is only about 1 per cent, of whom rather less than half will be confirmed as carcinoma in situ, the rest being still earlier dysplastic lesions of even greater obscurity. Limited resources should therefore be concentrated where they are most likely to be rewarding, and epidemiological studies have given strong indications: parous women of the lower social classes from the age of 35 should be given priority. Among them, as seen, the lifetime probability in this country of developing invasive cancer may be 2 per cent, 1 in 50, or even higher. But these are the very women who, expectedly on public health experience, are most reluctant to participate in the screening programme.[68-70] The problem is serious because mortality in middle-aged women is stationary, and the current increase of sexual activity and of venereal disease may presage a rising incidence of carcinoma in the years ahead . . . The discovery of atypical cells in the bronchi of smokers suggests that it may eventually be possible to identify such changes also by cytological study of sputum: which personal information, together perhaps with blood levels of relevant enzymes,[72] might concentrate the minds of some at least of our 2½ million heavy smokers more effectively than health education on general statistics of probability seems able to achieve.

The radical approach to primary prevention by improving healthy growth and development, strengthening population defences, the reduction of evident causes of disease, is the other half of the next chapter.

*　　*　　*

The facts dictate a piecemeal and opportunist strategy for *control of the main chronic diseases:* by applying what is known about causes; by attempts at removal of pathogenetic precursors, however little is understood of the mechanisms involved; by earlier detection to give treatment a better chance; by bringing advanced disease into treatment before breakdown. The future of medicine, clinical medicine and all of it, will be in pushing practice back from section 1. of this chapter to 2., 2. to 3., 3. to 4. At each stage, a controlled trial is indicated before new practices are introduced. But this in real life will often be to ask too much of the public and of medical science which, between them, and often, have been unable to carry out the necessary studies: for example, the blind randomised trial of modified diets in thousands of representative men with hypercholesterolaemia, from youth or early middle-age onwards, to discover whether the incidence of IHD can thereby be lowered. Here is one of the awesome dilemmas of modern medicine. . . Another will arise from the creation of a new role in society, the "at risk" role,[73] and asking huge numbers of people who are coping tolerably well, to alter their self-image, accept labelling as not quite normal – and to behave accordingly. With what consequences? Not disregarding the indirect and remote? How strike an (ecological) balance-sheet? . . . Anyhow, where are the health-service resources for the mass screening? For the subsequent load of treatment? What that is less useful could be diverted? How state acceptable priorities?

7. In Search of Causes

The main use of epidemiology is to discover causes of health and disease so as to increase understanding, and hopefully also help improve the condition of the people.

Examples can readily be drawn from the classical epidemiology of *airs, waters, places*. Over the centuries, knowledge grew about the influence of climate and season (malaria, rickets), of geography (cholera following the trade routes) and of geology (the role of iodine and later of fluoride were so discovered). Pioneers described the "unhealthiness of towns" (bowel infections, bronchitis) and of country (pellagra, mental deficiency). They identified "dangerous trades" (the calamity of sailors or miners' sickness). When affected populations are so characterised by their environment and ways of living, epidemiology is in fact beginning to discover "causes" of health and disease, knowledge which it may be possible to apply in prevention. Commonly, this has happened before particular diseases were at all fully understood, as in the achievements of Lind and the scurvy, Pott and chimney sweeps' cancer, Snow and the cholera.

"Ways of living" have often been described only very generally and causes, therefore, postulated only in broad terms of the satisfaction of elementary human needs: *general, non-specific conditions of health, and of the production of disease* have been postulated. Such are the relationships between income levels, and family limitation, and maternal and infant welfare, and child growth; of the purity and abundance of water-supply to alimentary infections; of living space and population density to respiratory infection. However "general", such principles must not be underrated. They include much folk wisdom about healthy living acquired over the centuries, and the history of the search for means to avoid epidemics, to survive at all, shows how elementary observation and the courage to draw the lesson can transform the quantity and quality of life. Each level of understanding has its own value and, like the notion that "filth" is dangerous, to identify such ways of living may be the start of effective action to alter them. Thus, the epidemiological researches on the *Sanitary Condition of the Labouring Population* were a landmark in social history. In the middle of the Industrial Revolution the findings of bacteriology were anticipated and public opinion aroused; Chadwick and the other social reformers and doctors showing how people might better live and work together

References on page 295.

in the towns of the new Britain. They campaigned effectively for sanitary improvement, a cleaner water supply, sewage disposal, ventilation, "hygiene". And they spelled out in crude detail how the spread of disease, the chances of living and risks of dying, varied with the social environment. Of course mistakes were made, as about the dangers of the "miasma" that emanated from faecal pollution, though it was the stench as much as anything that got the drains laid.

VICTORIAN THUNDER

TABLE 7.1

(1) SANITARY RAMBLINGS IN THE STREETS OF BETHNAL GREEN[1]
1846–7

Dis-trict	Total No. of Streets	Clean	Very dirty	Sew-ered	Privies full	Nuis-ances	ZYMOTIC DISEASE Cases attended			DEATHS
							All	Diarr-hoea Etc.	"Typhus"	
no. 4	133	19	61	5	35	2,303	422	157	138	27
no. 5	66	22	13	6	10	552	66	12	23	6

Populations were c. 16,000 in each district.

District No. 4: "Characterised by Grossest Foulness"
"This district exceeds all in filth, disease, mortality, poverty, and wretchedness; it abounds with the most foul courts and is characterised by the prevalence of the greatest nuisances, and perennial foulness, everything degrading to our civilisation. Notorious as the hot-bed of epidemics, the drainage is characteristic of primitive barbarism. Ventilation is in the most defective state; the atmosphere is most oppressive, and loaded with unhealthy emanations; it is a common practice to retain the faecal remains in the rooms in order to avoid exposure and the perfect nastiness of the common privies. The tenements are unfit for human habitation; they are much under the level of the neighbouring road, and are very damp; they smell most offensively. The third walk is still more filthy than the rest; excrements are scattered about, all the privies are full and over-flowing, and the soil desiccating in the sun. One stand-pipe, beside a dung-heap, is the only means by which 30 houses are supplied with water; of course, quarrels for precedence and to ensure a supply are common. The whole of these gardens are in a condition alike disgusting and disgraceful. Being private property, they are never cleansed by the parish, but are left in a perpetual state of dirt and nastiness; they are excessively damp, and most noisome. Disease is always common here; some of the worst cases of 'typhus' fever were removed from this locality to the workhouse."

District No. 5: "A Healthy District"
"This district is by far the most respectable of the five medical parochial districts. The remarkable exception of the chief parts from fever and the other epidemic diseases is no doubt to be attributed to the comparative cleanliness and good drainage. . . Great complaints, however. No one could possibly doubt that such enormous heaps of decaying animal and vegetable remains must prove injurious to health. The senses revolt, the feelings are roused with indignation and depressed by despair, when such atrocities are seen perpetrated in the very face of society. The laws which

imprison and transport for petty theft, view with calm indifference this wholesale, barefaced and violent robbery of the health of communities. People, helpless and impotent, cry out in puerile indignation against such abominable and pestilential conservations of refuse; but, the sordid gainers, firm and entrenched in the stronghold of legal quirks, and laxity, and the astounding indifference of governmental and local authorities, set their feeble cries of suffering and despair at defiance . . . "
Gavin, H. (1848). (A not unworthy footnote to *annus mirabilis*.)

(2) Life Chances in the 1840's, Preston, Lancs.

	Gentry	Trades	Operatives
Born	1,000	1,000	1,000
Remaining alive at end of:			
1st year	908	796	682
5th year	824	618	446
20th year	763	516	315
40th year	634	375	204
60th year	451	205	112

Clay, The Rev. J. (1844).[2]

(3) An Experiment on the Grandest Scale

Mortality from Cholera in the Four Weeks Ending 5 August 1854

Water Company	No of Houses Supplied	No of Deaths	Death Rate per 10,000 Houses
Southwark and Vauxhall*	40,046	286	71
Lambeth**	26,107	14	5
Rest of London	287,345	277	9

Snow, J. (1855–6).[3]

* Supplying down river water "containing the sewage of London".

** Upriver water "quite free from such impurity".

During the whole 14 weeks of the epidemic the mortality rate from cholera was 153 per 10,000 of population supplied by the S. & V. Co.; 26 per 10,000 supplied by the Lambeth Co.; and 30 per 10,000 in the rest of London.

(4) IN A 300 YEAR TRADITION

(*Miners' Sickness*)

Mortality of Men in Cornwall
Rates per 1,000 per Year
1860–2

| Ages | All Causes | | Pulmonary Diseases | |
	Metal Miners	Males exclusive of metal miners	Metal Miners	Males exclusive of metal miners
15–24	9·44	7·50	3·77	3·30
25–34	9·57	8·32	4·15	3·83
35–44	15·12	10·08	7·89	4·24
45–54	29·74	12·50	19·75	4·34
55–64	63·21	19·96	43·29	5·19
65–74	110·51	53·31	45·04	10·48

Farr, W. (1864) *Evidence to Royal Commission on Condition of Mines*. London.

A MODERN HYGIENE?[4]

Sex and Age

General causes of contemporary health, disease? . . . I won't attempt a systematic account of the satisfaction in society today of human needs, physiological needs, needs for human relationships and social networks, through a hierarchy of needs for medical care and social security and family planning, all the way to personal autonomy and something to live for . . . Table 7.2 (on the risks of being mortal) deals with the basics, recalling much that has already been mentioned in the book, especially in Chapter 2, and starts by bringing Graunt up-to-date on *age*, page 146. High in utero and infancy, the force of mortality rises steeply again from early adult life. At the turn of the century, about 25 per cent of deaths occurred in infancy and 25 per cent after 65; now the corresponding figures are about 2·5 per cent and 70 per cent. Two general points. As the organism ages, it becomes progressively more vulnerable, is in general less able to withstand physical, mental and social stresses. Many conditions are "age-bound", start and stop, occur only or mainly or importantly at particular "epochs", "critical periods", "milestones", phases of biologic and social development and particular needs.[5][49][50] For example, hyaline membrane syndrome (neonates), cot-deaths (at about 10 weeks), kwashiorkor (after weaning), leukaemia (5–9 years), stealing (the secondary school), motorbike accidents (late teens), hard-drug addiction (early 20's). The old are subject to falls, become hard of hearing, they forget.

TABLE 7.2
THE DEATH RATE – ALL CAUSES

England and Wales

(1) Influence of Age

	IMR	1–	5–	15–	25–	45–	55–	65–	75–	85 + Years
Male	20	0·78	0·39	0·93	1·6	7·1	20·6	52·6	118·6	248·3
Female	15	0·64	0·26	0·40	1·1	4·3	10·2	27·1	76·9	198·0

(2) Sex

	IMR	1–	5–	15–	25–	45–	55–	65–	75–	85 + Years
Male	133	122	150	233	145	165	202	194	154	125
Female	100	100	100	100	100	100	100	100	100	100

(3) "Civil State"

	All in Group	Married	Single	Widowed	Divorced
Male	100	94	128	158	138
Female	100	92	118	122	103

(4) Living Conditions

	All in Group	Good ——————→ Bad			
Male	100	98	110	115	123
Female	100	97	104	109	116

(5) Residence: Unhealthiness of Towns

	All in Group	Rural Districts	–50,000	Urban Areas: Population 50–100,000	100,000+	Conurbations

Male	*100*	88	99	97	107	107
Female	*100*	93	99	98	104	104

(6) ARTS, TRADES, PROFESSIONS
Men Aged 20–64

All Occupations = *100*		Medical Practitioners	90	Tailors	126	Publicans	150
Teachers (not music)	66	Clerks	101	Ticket Collectors	135	Watchmen	163
Farmers	70	Barbers	113	Shoe Repairers	140	Sandblasters	173
Drillers	85						

(7) CIGARETTE SMOKING

	All in Group	Non-Smokers	Ex-Smokers	Cigarette smokers No. per day		
				1–14	15–24	25+
Ages 45–54	*100*	60	84	90	117	166
Ages 55–64	*100*	79	94	116	134	168

(8) WEIGHT
Mortality Relative to "Under" and "Over" Weight when Taking out Insurance: Policies Issued at Ages 40–49

	Underweight			Ave. Weights	Overweight				
	−30 lb	−20 lb	−10 lb		+10 lb	+20 lb	+30 lb	+40 lb	+50 lb
Male	100	95	100	*100*	100	120	125	135	145
Female	85	90	90	*100*	100	110	120	130	140

Notes

(1) Infant Mortality (IMR) = deaths in the first year of life per 1,000 live births.
    Other death rates are per 1,000 persons living in the specific sex and age groups.
    1970–1. From Registrar General.

(2) Male death rates as percentage of female death rates.
    Ages as in (1) above.
    1970–1. From Registrar General.

(3) In this and tables (4)–(8), the death rates and ratios for the sub-groups are expressed as percentages of the death rate in the whole age group being studied.
    Ages 55–64.
    1970–1. From Registrar General.

(4) Mortality in relation to a composite index of adverse local social conditions – unemployment, house-crowding, etc. County boroughs, i.e. large towns, of England and Wales, grouped into four by size of index.
    Ages 45–64.
    1958–64. Gardner, M. J., Crawford, M. D. & Morris, J. N. (1969) *Brit. J. prev. soc. Med.*, **23**, 133.[17]

(5) Ages 45–64.
    1970–1. From Registrar General.

(6) Standardised Mortality Ratios (SMR) of particular occupations; i.e. death rates, from all causes, of the men in these occupation-groups, adjusted for differences in age composition. The ratios are expressed as a percentage of the death rate for all the men in the country aged 20–64.
    England and Wales
    1949–53: R.G. *Occupational Mortality Supplement.* HMSO. London.

(7) Male Medical Practitioners, United Kingdom.
    1951–8. Doll, R. and Hill, A. B. In *Smoking and Health Now*. (1971). London; personal communications.

(8) Men: height = 5 ft. 7 in. – 5 ft. 10 in.   Ave. weight = 167 lbs.   370,000 policies.
    Women : height = 5 ft. 3 in. – 5 ft. 6 in.   Ave. weight = 141 lbs.   90,000 policies.
    Policies were issued during 1935–53; "lives" were traced to the end of 1954.
    The women weighing 30 lbs. less than average experienced a death rate, from all causes, 85% of that for all these women; i.e. a mortality ratio of 85, etc.
    U.S.A. *Build and Blood Pressure* (1959), Society of Actuaries. Chicago, Illinois; personal communications.

Part (2) of the Table summarises the *sex* difference in mortality. Higher death rates in males are universal now in advanced industrial countries; when maternal mortality in England was common, the overall rate at relevant ages often was higher in women, as it still may be in low-income countries. Prenatally and during infancy major biological causes are postulated for feminine superiority. Thereafter, ways of living may be very different — in occupation, for example, or (still) cigarette smoking, in the behaviour that the culture expects. How much is biological, what social, is a continuing debate on the sex ratio in ischaemic heart disease, psychoneurosis, porphyria, hypertension (its incidence and disability), fractured neck of femur, crime; in everything to do with sexual behaviour.[6-8]

Civil State[9-13]
I leave it to the reader to sort the variation in part (3) of the Table: that due to personal selection, as of the sick in not getting married, and that to protection of health by matrimony (despite its fatigues), the medical causes of divorce, the psychological expressed in the physical, chance effects, etc. "Standardised mortality ratios" (SMR, all = 100) for different causes are given by the Registrar General in his *Commentary* for 1967. Here are some of the most interesting:

	Married	Single	Widowed	Divorced
Male				
Resp. tuberculosis	79	203	147	212
Cirrhosis of liver	88	142	138	220
Accidental poisoning	64	157	225	346
Suicide	68	152	125	184
Female				
Ca cervix	98	47	243	295
Ca breast	96	124	98	87
Suicide	76	122	154	233

Ages 15–84. 1965–7.

Hospital "utilisation" shows similar variation.
These figures of the "broken-hearts" syndrome are remarkable:

Mortality and Bereavement

	Ratios
Married Men at Ages 55–89	100
Widowers within 6 months of loss of wife	139
Widowers at 6 months to 1 year after loss	106

England and Wales, 1957.
Young M., Benjamin B., Wallis, L. (1963). *Lancet* 2, 454.

(A pointer also to surveillance by medical and social services, to "crisis-intervention"?[14] [36])

Social Conditions

Returning to the theme of the poor and the well-to-do, an over-abundance of preventable squalor and ignorance still disfigure our society, physical and economic deprivation if not Victorian destitution still contribute only too much in avoidable misery. But (4) the range of mortality in middle age with living conditions, shown in the Table, is even greater than expected. Standardising further, were it possible, for cohort of birth, and for early life-experience, would probably explain much.

Politically, and in social policy, there is continuing concern with —

The Regions[15] [16]

These mortality ratios are the simplest *community diagnosis* of quality of life, and the most elementary data for resource-allocation by social and health services, for priorities and efforts at "positive discrimination" in favour of the greatest needs:

Age/ Sex		E & W	Mersey-side	Tyne-side	SE except London	East England
55–59	M	100	122	125	88	83
60–64		100	122	118	89	86
55–59	F	100	119	113	90	92
60–64		100	116	110	88	89

1960–2.
Registrar General. *Area Mortality*. HMSO, London.

Gross differences persist (1971) and, of course, "depressed" Regions are now an EEC not just a British issue. Complementary data on morbidity are available in the *General Household Survey* and for sickness-absence; and the record is overflowing with figures on low wages and unemployment, inferior educational opportunities, urban squalor: well over 100 years of figures of disadvantage, deprivation, words that are in danger of the banal.

Population Density

The trend of mortality in Table 7.2 (5), illustrates what is left of the pastoral dream — quite a lot! — though a North/South differential (it is decidedly colder in the northern towns) also is supposed to be involved. Whatever the differences in smoking and other behaviour between town-dwellers and country people, a large part of the variation probably is or was soot and dirt, evident when these same *total death rates* for 1958–64 (a) are recalculated in terms of the degree of local air pollution:[17][18]

	All England & Wales	Rural Districts		County Boroughs		
		Agric.	Indust.	Clean	Intermed.	Dirty
M	100	73	94	97	112	124
F	100	89	104	94	108	114

And these are the ratios for *mortality from respiratory disease* (b) which really determine the general picture:

	England & Wales				
M	3·7 per 1,000 =100	62	93	116	153
F	0·82 per 1,000 =100	76	84	118	141

Ages 45–64

This is *air pollution* from domestic coal-fires, mostly. (Of course the healthier may abandon less pleasant — less healthy — districts, whose statistics thus are aggravated.) Such disadvantages in death rates are relics of bygone days, that have not passed. Nevertheless, contemporary discussion of *crowd diseases* and the "urban factor" in health is more likely to be concerned with the psychological and social, with mindless planners and soulless developers, inner-city blight, with teenage misbehaviour, racial friction, population pressure on amenities (England is the most crowded country in Europe), the "turmoil of pedestrains and vehicles, the noise, the stench and the general misery when it is raining, bus queues waiting in patient wretchedness";[19] I've already touched on this.

Occupation

Table 7.2 (5) also involves local employment, "of what trade is he?" Byssinosis is common among both men and women of some of the "dirty" Northern towns, whereas the overall SMR in agriculture, concentrated of course in the "rural districts", was about 70. The figures on occupation (6) illustrate selections "in" and "out", and the environmental causes and effects that produce the range of occupational mortality. Many watchmen have taken the job because they are disabled; because of the risk of silicosis, the sandblaster is in truly a "dangerous trade" (with $\frac{3}{4}$ more than the national average death rate). So are the steeplejack, window-cleaner, bullfighter, fisherman, anyone working in asbestos.[20-22]

These figures from two physically active occupations (Table 7.3) make a good text on occupation as a factor in health and ill-health, physical, mental and social: on choice of job, the impact of work, how and where people have to live, attitudes to illness, thresholds of need and demand for services.

TABLE 7.3

SICKNESS–ABSENCE OF MEN IN TWO PHYSICALLY ACTIVE OCCUPATIONS
Britain 1961–2
Rates for All Men = 100

Agricultural Workers	Diagnosis	Coal Miners – Face Workers
67	All Causes	188
40	Acute upper respiratory infections	234
60	Influenza	234
47	Bronchitis	205
55	Chronic sinusitis	300
33	Coronary heart disease, etc.	61
45	Psychosis and psychoneurosis	196
60	Arthritis and rheumatism	338

Proportions of insured men in these occupations with a spell of incapacity for work certified to causes stated.
Ages 15–63; standardised.
Incidence of Incapacity for Work in Different Areas and Occupations.
Ministry of Pensions and National Insurance (1965) HMSO, London.[23]

EPIDEMIC CONSTITUTION

Parts (5), (6) and (7) of Table 7.2 represent progressive directness of personal responsibility. *Cigarette smoking,* (7) gives further detail, is a cause of premature death from several conditions and not merely from lung-cancer, though its relationship to that is of course strongest. The cigarette is a tragic accident of human history; less dangerous solace, even in the quantities required, might have done as well. On the present rate of progress it may be the end of the century before we are freed of it. At the prices charged it is of course also the indulgence of a high standard of living.

Eating too much and taking too little exercise are involved in a multitude of modern pathologies. The figures in part (8) of the Table are of under- and overweight, not strictly of leanness-obesity. Water, muscle and bone masses make a large contribution, but there is little doubt about the significance of the extremes, at least, of such ranges.* Because of selection of applicants for insurance, and the likely exclusion of the most obese as well as those who already are ill, the figures must underestimate how overweight shortens life, in particular by cardio-vascular disease. These figures, being related to the 40's, include *middle-age spread,* though there is little direct evidence from cohort study that many individuals do in fact put on fat after 40, despite the all too solid incidence in my (non-medical) friends; muscle flabbiness may be responsible for some of the extending waistlines. British data[24] (unfortunately they include a small number of women among the large numbers of men) also give the record at specific ages. This was the subsequent *mortality at 50–59 years of age, of these selected people, relative to weight when taking out insurance:*

Underweight on acceptance	80 % of Standard Mortality (at 50–59)
Average weight	100 %
20–30 per cent overweight	123 %
30 per cent and more overweight	165 %

Extrapolating from the little available insurance data, some of the excess mortality might be avoided by reducing to the normal average. (This may itself be high, though in men, if *lower* weights are accepted as the healthy norm, the risks are little different.)

How many of the population are considered "fat", must depend on the cut-off point, a useful notion only if related to data as in (8). "A quarter of the women in Britain are fat", laments my morning paper, "their hips range from 42 inches to 5 feet" ($1\frac{1}{2}$ metres): unaccept-able to modern sensibilities. About 10 per cent of London busmen aged 40–64 (6 per cent of the conductors and 13 per cent of the drivers) had a waist measurement of 100 cm plus; in 16 per cent of the drivers and 6 per cent of the conductors [18 25 26] the suprailiac skinfold was 25 mm plus — a simple measurement. These mortality data do not deal with lowering of resistance and morbidity: with excess diabetes and hypertension that are not lethal, gall-bladder and other gastroin-testinal disorders, skin sepsis, emotional embarrassment, inefficient respiration, osteoarthrosis, immobility in old age; nor with the proven syndromes, associations, if still difficult to interpret, of obesity with high — undesirable — levels of so many physiological functions. Nor with the added misery of the obese when ill or having an operation. De-finition of a graded character like leanness–fatness in terms of *health-disease,* and thereby of the indication for action, makes good sense. But it is not yet possible to produce much data to compare with the death rates. Table 7.4 is a sample.

*Typically, the correlation between weight, and the sum of the three standard skinfolds' thickness, in bus drivers is $+0.76$ and in conductors (men) $+ 0.78$.[18]

TABLE 7.4
LEANNESS-OBESITY AND BLOOD LIPID LEVELS[18] [28]
London Busmen
Ages 40–64

Blood Lipid	Skinfold Thickness mm			
	–21	22–32	33–51	52+
	mg/100 ml			
α-Lipoprotein cholesterol[1]	52	48	45	49
β-Lipoprotein cholesterol[1]	173	192	203	209
Serum triglyceride[2]	83	92	119	158

Sum of triceps, subscapular and suprailiac skinfolds.
503 men. Age-standardisation makes little difference.
[1]Courtauld Institute of Biochemistry. [2]Department of Biochemistry, St. George's Hospital.
Non-fasting.

Exercise of Mind and Body

Mass overnutrition and underexercise are products of modern technology and a *high standard of living.* Overeating still is part of the approved life style and we are under strong pressures to live it, overeating in general and of particular nutrients. Physical inactivity reflects social-economic progress and is inherent in it: expending too few calories for energy balance, and exercise inadequate for cardiovascular health. Physical activity-inactivity in turn represents an even more general cause, particularly relevant to an ageing population. The exercise of functions is necessary for their health, "that which is used develops, and that which is not used wastes away" (Hippocrates). The need also for sensory input, for human contact, affection and emotional response, for mutual aid and social ties, is crucial to healthy functioning throughout life, in childhood, on the factory-floor, in retirement perhaps above all.[29]

Too Little and Too Much —

of a good thing: the satisfaction of human needs, any needs, has to be seen also in terms of excess inputs as well as deprivation, whether of calories or exercise, oxygen, vitamin D, saturated fat, mother-love, acceptance/rejection, social bonds.

The Figure on page 120 is a classic model of such U effects, of too little, optimum, too much.

"Stress"[30-37]

Social and psychological changes in the life-situation which are perceived by the individual as threatening, or are greater stimuli than needed for health — "it is changes, of all things, that rouse the temper of man and prevent its stagnation" (Hippocrates) — these represent another "general cause". They contribute to uncountable unhappiness, sundry functional disorders, accidents, mental breakdown, deviant behaviour; delayed recovery and disability from injuries; decompensation and disability in the chronic diseases, in peptic ulcer, diabetes, heart-failure even.[37-38] The role of psycho-social stresses in the incidence of organic disease, through physiological disturbance and visceral reaction, is less clear, though this is a promising field in ischaemic heart disease[39][40] (and was in duodenal ulcer), and there are classic examples in phthisis, thyrotoxicosis. Even in the most stable situations there is the possibility of trouble, a fortiori in times of flux and social dislocation. The obligation on epidemiology is to seek common patterns of stresses, and supports, in relation to definable human potentials and limits. Particular stresses of the times we live in (and not of the human condition) have been illustrated before, and there are only too obvious possibilities in the pace of contemporary change, the sensory over-stimulation, conflict from the multiplication of roles, isolation and estrangement in large organisations, the wear and tear of metropolitan living. The word "stress" is coming to be used for any stimulus to the organism, but more usefully refers to stimuli imposing detectable strain that cannot readily be accommodated.

INDIVIDUAL VARIATION, DISPOSITIONS[41-50]

What we are mainly considering in heart-attack, for example, is the ordinary business of daily life as the average man has to live it in western societies: some or many cannot take it and develop major chronic diseases. Further causes in the immediate "life-space" of human relationships and social networks, of marital, other family and work situations remain to be explored, to mention only some obvious gaps. Equally, host differences in vulnerability, in defences and the resources that can be mustered, will have to be clarified if more useful probabilities are to be attached to many of the non-specific causes being described, if the distribution within social systems is to be better understood, chance effects reduced to what is truly random — and the knowledge more readily applied for health. "Every individual has his breaking point".

"Thus, then, on the night of the tenth of May, at the outset of this mighty battle, I acquired the chief power in the State, which henceforth I wielded in ever-growing measure for five years and three months of world war. During these last crowded days of the political crisis my pulse had not quickened at any moment. I took it all as it came. But I cannot conceal from the reader of this truthful account that as I went to bed at about 3 a.m. I was conscious of a profound sense of relief. At last I had the authority to give directions over the whole scene. I felt as if I were walking with destiny, and that all my past life had been but a preparation for this hour and for this trial. I thought I knew a good deal about it all, and I was sure I should not fail. Therefore, although impatient for the morning, I slept soundly and had no need for cheering dreams. Facts are better than dreams"[51]

The study of *individual susceptibility* involves enzyme profiles;[52] the range of physiological response to eating the normal quantity of carboydrate or saturated fat; the variety or responses to medicines. The inborn, and learned, adaptive and maladaptive responses to psychosocial stress are a major field for investigation; the roots of personality in childhood experience, how ghosts of the past wreak havoc in the present. The epidemiologist must be on the look-out for new methods and ideas from the consulting room and the laboratory.

Genetic differences relevant to the major chronic diseases, and accounting presumably for some of individual susceptibility, are beginning to be identified. Thus the blood groups and secretor status in cancer of the stomach and peptic ulcer may be mentioned;[41] α-antitrypsin deficiency, pulmonary hypertension and emphysema;[46][47] a new era may be opening with the possibilities of HLA tissue typing of genotypes for major disorders — multiple sclerosis for example.[53]

Such *general causes* of health and disease in human needs, potential and limits, in biology and conditions of living, in the way we lead our lives; in prevalent hazards, and defences, in organism, family, community; the definition of vulnerable groups and susceptible individuals — on such knowledge and understanding the community physician will base his strategy for promoting the people's health through social policy and health services.

*   *

*

This chapter provides examples of the "uses" of epidemiology in the *search for causes* of the chronic non-communicable diseases. Studies of varying sophistication are reported, from first turning of the ground to planned experiments. By way of recollection and prospectus, Table 7.5 ranges from founding fathers to some of the growing points. Often, in these examples, epidemiological observation provides the critical evidence: there is nothing as convincing from clinical experience nor yet any human or animal-experimental model.

TABLE 7.5

IN SEARCH OF CAUSES OF THE CHRONIC DISEASES

SOME CONTRIBUTIONS FROM EPIDEMIOLOGY

In 1662 *Graunt* the London haberdasher "buzzling and groping" in The Bills of Mortality, related sex, age, seasons of the year and the environment (London vs. Country people) to mortality. Statistics, the numerical study of matters of concern to the state, developed in Germany and France. During the Industrial Revolution, *Chadwick* related health to the standard of living: health could be improved by environmental hygiene, the "sanitary idea". At the General Register Office, *Farr* (1839–80) founded modern vital statistics, using general and specific mortality rates to measure the healthiness of populations – of the whole country, of districts and of particular occupations.

* * *

Three Classics from Nutrition
Lind and the calamity of sailors, Takaki and beri beri, Goldberger and pellagra; in the search for causes they made experiments as well as describing and analysing.

Congenital Malformations
Rubella virus is the proven cause of a small fraction of congenital defect. . . Thalidomide calamity led to intensive and continuing search for teratogenic agents, to a new appreciation of iatrogenic disease, and to national and international systems of monitoring the adverse effects of medicines . . . The unequal ethnic incidence of anencephaly persisting in disparate environments, and the clustering among maternal relatives and among children of first-cousin marriages, point to multiple genetic and environmental causes.

Mental Subnormality
Multiple genes and social and cultural deprivations are involved in the production of "slight subnormality", the greater part of the negative tail of the distribution of intelligence in the population. Trouble from this – and so of claims on services – diminishes as children leave school and change their social roles; i.e. it depends on the way they adapt and how society now perceives the "subnormality".

Disease and Ageing
Cohort and prevalence studies in relation to personal and environmental factors of the variation with advancing years in physiological functions – e.g., hearing or respiration – distinguish ageing from the "degeneration" of diseases and the effects of external poisons such as the cigarette. Atherosclerosis, hypertension, osteoporosis, chronic bronchitis, emphysema, nerve deafness, senile psychosis . . . have been shown not to be mere or inevitable processes of ageing; so there is more hope of preventing them.

Malignant Diseases and the Mode of Life
Percivall Pott described soot-cancer of scrotum, so starting experimental carcinogenesis.
A clustering of occupational bladder cancer has been demonstrated, and its causes, e.g. β-naphthylamine. Much direct preventive action has now been taken – however little is understood of the carcinogenesis.
Sexual behaviour, the age at first coitus, its frequency, the number of partners, is postulated as principal cause of the common squamous (environmental) cervical cancer; personal penile hygiene, circumcision possibly, as a primary protection: in

turn, these factors are expressions of the society and culture. There are some indications that a venereal virus infection is involved in the carcinogenesis. Epidemiology of precursor carcinoma in situ is beginning to be analysed.

Gross geographical differences in incidence are yielding clues to environmental causes at present for example in cancer of oesophagus. Clinical observation – laboratory research – "shoe-leather" and statistical epidemiology, collaborating on a grand scale have identified and plotted Burkitt's lymphoma; a viral cause (Epstein-Barr) now looks likely.

Dangerous Trades

Old specific industrial hazards (e.g. byssinosis) as well as new (e.g. hepatic angiosarcoma from working in plastics, PVC) are being intensively investigated . . . The role of work in general health, and among the multiple causes of major chronic diseases, is still often neglected; (the study of leisure is only beginning).

Social Sciences

Collaboration is promising for framing hypotheses on aetiology of health and disease arising from people's behaviour; though social scientists are as helpless as the rest of us in knowing how to change behaviour.

Multiple Causes

These evidently are involved in the common chronic non-communicable diseases, and in kindred problems like accidents or drug-addiction. Different combinations may be operative in different situations, as seen in dental caries and gout; they may add together as in cigarettes and air-pollution, or multiply – cigarettes and asbestos. Different causes may be involved in the same disorder, for example congenital malformation; and the same cause in several recognisable disorders, as in the London smog. General non-specific causes of health and disease in the mode of life are evident throughout.

Cigarettes are the specific agent of modern-epidemic lung cancer. But the notion that they have no indispensable causes is beginning to be postulated for some of the more important chronic diseases, in particular coronary heart disease.

Disease; its Course and Outcome; Illness; Disability; Invalidism

Causes of the incidence of chronic diseases and of their prevalence are being distinguished. Because of the ubiquity of the chronic diseases, and their association with age, and because services rarely cure but often at great and growing cost keep alive (as exemplified in diabetes, say), disability is a central problem in modern society. Its causes may be very different from those of the incidence of disease – e.g. in the contributions of psychosocial factors and of the quality of medical care.

Experimental Epidemiology

Field trials can test hypotheses about causes by removing them under control; at the same time, such trials are trailers of what the unintended consequences of such action might be; planned experiments can illumine how multiple causes are connected and reveal their relative importance. Unfortunately, strict experiments (randomised, double-blind and long-term) which involve changes in everyday behaviour are proving impractical, though limited attempts are being made in direct search for regimens of prevention.

Health and Prevention

Epidemiology at present is mainly concerned with disease and the absence of defined disease. But a more positive approach to *health* beyond the traditional areas of childhood and maternity is emerging, e.g. in study of the use of mind and body, and the avoidance of multiple deprivations, in promoting physical, mental and social health in the elderly.

MODERN EPIDEMIC

Plainly, many causes are involved in *Coronary* or *Ischaemic Heart Disease,* personal and environmental causes, biologic and cultural. None so far proposed, saturated fat, cigarette-smoking, physical inactivity, or the pressures of running the System provides simple answers. Their unravelling has proved difficult, if only because the ways of living evidently concerned are so ordinary, everyday and widespread in modern industrial high-consumption societies; those with the disease, it is postulated, are unable to adapt to the normal (approved as well as typical) mode of life. Characteristically, taking the common diet of England some men have high blood lipid levels, others, for no reason that meanwhile is apparent, low. Surveys confirm clinical experience of the importance of the family history,[2][8] which is partly explained in resemblance of blood pressure levels, blood lipids and glucose. The ubiquity of coronary atheroma, the underlying pathology, makes it improbable that heredity is decisive in this, though conceivably it could be in massive thrombosis, in the conversion of omnipresent harmless mural into the dangerous lumen-occlusive disease. A suggestion has also been made in terms of balanced polymorphism: that such conditions as obesity, diabetes, hypercholesterolaemia, atherosclerosis and IHD are so frequent, and so often associated, because they represent the survival of genes for withstanding undernutrition, from times when such genes were advantageous to an age of plenty when manifestly they are not.[9-11]

Table 7.6 overleaf provides estimates, some rough but hopefully the right order of magnitude, of the extent of the "epidemic". It can also be regarded as a revision in *Uses*: on community diagnosis, the individual risk, in completing the clinical picture, the iceberg phenomenon, definitions of health, the natural history of disease, new measurements, the actual and potential needs for health services, etc., etc. IHD is the leading cause of untimely death in the western world, but it is the morbidity figures that make the point: such a mass disease cannot be due to way-out behaviour or exceptional stresses.

If ischaemic heart disease were not so clearly the product of many causes, we would have to invent them: so the natural history requires. The basic local pathology is coronary-*lumen occlusion,* which develops on coronary-*mural-atheroma.* These two processes — syndromes — are related but not the same, nor is the former any simple function of the amount or severity of the latter. They must therefore have different causes; and since both pathologies are necessary for ischaemic heart disease this must have multiple causes.

A step back. *Hypercholesterolaemia and hypertension* are important precursor mechanisms of ischaemic heart disease; they can be related to many of the levels in the Table. This is the main finding of the Framingham and similar studies in USA and in London.[2-4][20] Now these two processes are largely independent: those with one are not particularly likely to have the other, the correlation between them is small ($+0.23$ in our data). Though hypercholesterolaemia and hypertension may well

TABLE 7.6
EPIDEMICS OF CORONARY DISEASE[12-19]

Estimates of Average Rates in Men Aged 55–64
Britain 1950's–1960's

Between 0·5% and 1% in a year die of ischaemic heart disease (*mortality*)

About 1% per year manifest clinical IHD for first time (*incidence*)

About 2% per year suffer a first or later clinical attack of IHD (*attack rate*)

About 3% have recognisable clinical IHD (*point prevalence*)

  About 5% in addition give a history of IHD

  Some 5%–10%, not complaining, answer positively standard questions on angina of effort

  About 10% show minor subclinical ischaemic changes on the resting electro-cardiogram (and greater numbers on exercise)

About 25% have clinical disease, or subclinical often transient ischaemia, during a single year (*annual prevalence*)

Some 10%–20% have recognisable ischaemic myocardial changes at necropsy

Some 10–15% have occlusion of a main coronary artery at necropsy

  Some 20–25% have obvious narrowing of the lumen of a main coronary artery

About 25% have extensive confluent atheroma of the walls of the coronary arteries

  About 50% have moderately extensive coronary atheroma

  About 95% have naked-eye coronary atheroma

---

have common causes, such as obesity, they must also therefore have more important different causes: and since one or the other is so often involved in IHD — again this must have many causes.

Next, a look forward. *Cardiac infarction* occurs only in the presence of *coronary occlusion,* but is not the inevitable consequence of it. In death from IHD one or both of these may be prominent. So it is evident again that IHD must have multiple causes.

Clinically, the conclusion is the same. Death "out of the blue" in the young man, post-operatively in the middle-aged, in the old man excited by the television, shovelling snow or during a smog; infarction in the ovariectomised young woman, in the fat middle-aged diabetic, or the old lady with ruptured heart; the dissimilar syndromes of angina pectoris and classical infarction; necropsy revealing atheroma smothering the intima or but a solitary plaque, massive fresh thrombosis or none, minimal and maximal necrosis: its manifold presentations, variety of associations, and unpredictable outcome have accustomed the physician to think of ischaemic heart disease in "multifactorial" terms, of multiple events in individuals and their mode of life.

Ischaemic heart disease then is the product of many causes, and we have to try and identify their patterns. One day conceivably specific agents of IHD will be identified, but without other effective causes as well, these are unlikely to be any more "sufficient" causes of IHD than the bacillus is of tuberculosis. Meanwhile, the closest approximation achieved to necessary causes is the plane of nutrition of a population — high in saturated fat — and a high average cholesterol concentration.[21-23] This is fundamental, but so general a notion, the whole of the "western" world?, that it is of little practical help.

HYPOTHESIS ON EXERCISE

Figure 7.1 takes one postulated cause of ischaemic heart disease, inadequate exercise, and illustrates our attempts inch by inch to establish its reality, its contribution, and how it works.[14 24-27] When male government clerks, executive-officers and post-office telephonists, on prospective study, were all found to have the same kind of excess IHD over postmen that the bus drivers had over conductors, i. e. more of all first presentations of disease throughout middle age, Row 1 (a), and far more of the most serious form, the deaths in early middle age from acute dysrythmias that are the hallmark of the modern epidemic, (b), we "plumped" for the possibility that differences in the habitual physical activity involved in these jobs might be responsible for the differences in IHD. The conductors walk along the decks and engage in much stair-climbing in these double-decker buses; the postmen walked, cycled and often climbed stairs, carrying and delivering the mail, for about 70 per cent of the working-day. Bus drivers, and the government clerks, etc., are sedentary, or in quite light occupations. . . This seemed a more plausible proposition than one relating to "stress" arising from the emotional demands of the jobs, plausible enough for bus driving or operating a switchboard (at night often), but not for clerical work in the bureaucracy. We formulated a hypothesis to guide further investigation that —

Physical activity of work is a protection against ischaemic heart disease. Men in physically active jobs have less ischaemic heart disease during middle age, what disease they have is less severe, and they develop it later than similar men in physically inactive jobs.

Follow-up of the busmen[25] showed that the conductors throughout middle age recorded half the coronary death rate of the drivers — in sudden death, 3 - month and 3 - year mortality.

Several tests of the hypothesis have been made and two are illustrated. The second row of the Figure gives the main results from a *national necropsy survey* in which the jobs of the deceased were classified and agreed "blind" by experts as typically "light", "active", or "heavy" (giving a gradient and not merely a contrasting pair). Because of their many biases, necropsy data are usually unsuitable for epidemiological analysis. We thought it warranted here: an important and simple question was asked which could not be answered in any other way; particular efforts were made to obtain a representative sample; large

Light Workers · Active · Heavy

1. Incidence (First Clinical Presentation) of Ischaemic Heart Disease [24-26]

In London Busmen
(drivers & conductors)

(a) All forms, ages 35–64
(b) Sudden death, 35–49

In Government Employees
(male clerks & postmen)

(a) All forms, ages 35–59
(b) Rapidly fatal infarction 35–49

2. Prevalence of Ischaemic Myocardial Fibrosis [14]   National Necropsy Survey

3800 Deaths from other than Ischaemic Heart Disease, men aged 45–70

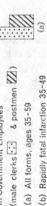

(a) All forms of ischaemic myocardial fibrosis   (b) Large healed infarcts
(c) Focal myocardial fibrosis in cases with hypertension and
(d) Focal myocardial fibrosis in cases without hypertension

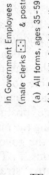

(a)   (b)   (c) and (d)

3. Ischaemic Heart Disease: Physical Activity of Work and Social Class

(a) Mortality, England & Wales 1949–53 [17,24,27]

Men aged 45–54

Social Class	Light	Active	Heavy
	Rates per 100,000 p.a.		
I	176	–	–
II	167	118	–
III	173	137	111
IV	153	121	116
V	175	145	91
All	173	135	102

Registrar General

(b) Prevalence of ischaemic myocardial fibrosis in deaths from other than Ischaemic Heart Disease [14,17]

Men aged 45–70

Social Class	Light	Active	Heavy
	Per cent		
I	13.7	–	–
II	13.4	9.2	–
III	13.8	8.0	8.2
IV	13.5	10.1	4.9
V	8.9	9.0	7.1
All	13.4	8.7	6.8

National Necropsy Survey

4. Coronary Artery Disease   National Necropsy Survey [14]

Deaths from other than Ischaemic Heart Disease, men aged 45–70

Main coronary arteries only:

(a) Extensive atheroma of walls   (b) Calcification present   (c) Slight narrowing
of a lumen   (d) Complete or near-complete occlusion of a lumen

5. Essential Hypertension

Evidence at necropsy, men aged 45-70 [14]

(a) E.H. present and related to death

(b) E.H. present and incidental to death

(c) No evidence E.H.

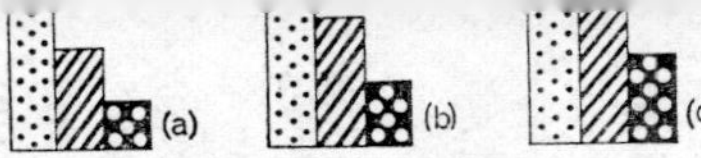

National Necropsy Survey

Casual diastiolic B.P. over 100 mm. Hg [17 26]

Age	Drivers	Conductors
	Per cent	
40–49	9.9	14
50–59	23.0	11
60–64	29.0	18

n = 852

6. Blood Lipid in London Busmen [17]

Ages 50-59

n = 272

Lipid	Drivers	Conductors
	mg %	
Plasma Cholesterol	249	235
β-lipoprotein	202	189
Sf 100–400	61	34

7. Physique and Obesity in London Busmen [17 26]

(a) % Uniform trouser waist 38″ and more

n = 958

Ht = 5′ 8″ – 5′ 9″

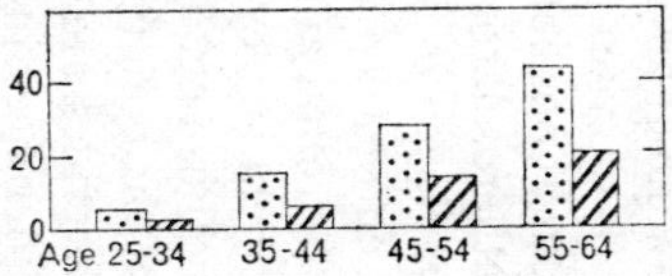

(b) Mean Skinfold Thickness

Triceps + subscapular + suprailiac

n = 550

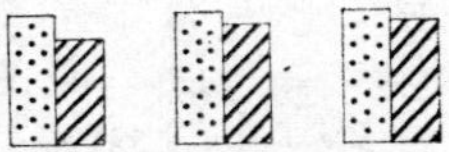

(c) "Sudden death" from Ischaemic Heart Disease Age 35-49

1949-1958 'Bus Fleet

n = 160,000 man-years

Trouser waist	Drivers	Conductors
	Rates per 1,000 p.a.	
32″ and less	0.8	0.2
34″– 37″	0.5	0.2
38″ and more	1.0	–

When necessary, rates were standardised for age.

Unless otherwise stated the "light" stippled columns = 100%, and the others are in proportion to this.

Fig. 7.1 Physical activity of work and coronary disease in men. Formulation and testing of an epidemiological hypothesis.[13 17]

numbers permitted a variety of built-in checks for internal consistency against the biases of disease-selection and of change of type of work because of illness; teamwork assured the reproducibility of the (blind) codings. The prevalence of ischaemic myocardial fibrosis in row 2 agreed with the hypothesis and amplified it in terms of the protection of heavy and active workers. Row 3 includes an analysis of Registrar General's data as well as these 3,800 necropsies. It seems to "explain" the well known social-class distribution of ischaemic heart disease by a rather obvious association: the higher the social class the less physically active on average the work.

The original observation, it may be said, still stands; the hypothesis has survived cumulative tests, independent, and different from the original. Most studies in other countries have been finding similar results.[2][28-34] But it still could be a hypothesis about something else. Despite what has been said, *psychosocial stresses* of occupation conceivably are the obverse of physical inactivity — in view of the generality of the findings in Rows 2 and 3, a hypothesis would have to be stated in such terms as the channelling of aggression and not confined to drivers vs. conductors. Meanwhile, no studies have been done on this. Some more likely alternatives can by now be dismissed. Differences in the *cigarette smoking* habits of drivers and conductors were negligible. Middle-aged conductors consume about 5 calories more per kilo of body-weight, a confirmation of their greater overall physical activity; but the *dietary studies*[35] show no interesting occupational differences in type or quantity of fat (or in sucrose) that are eaten.

Pathogenesis.[35-38] — We sought possible mechanisms, first comparing the prevalence of coronary atherosclerosis and its two main processes among men who had been employed in different kinds of work, row 4. There was substantially less chronic coronary occlusion, on the basis of not very different mural atheroma, among the more active workers, (d). We also made a clinical-field survey of blood pressure and blood lipid levels in a sample of the busmen. Judging by American and our own surveys the advantage of the conductors in levels of both, rows 5 and 6 — later data on triglycerides are similar — could account for much of the occupational differences in ischaemic heart disease. The means in row 6, without the scatter of observations, are of course of limited value as an index. In fact, conductors had very high blood lipid levels, cholesterol, e.g., of 300 mg per 100 ml, half as often as drivers. Drivers and conductors are a most cooperative and rewarding population for this kind of research, studying the whole fleet as in row 1, or samples as in rows 5-7. Until very recently remarkably alike in their social-economic circumstances, they do very different jobs, which are homogeneous and readily described.

Now for a fundamental question. It must be postulated that men who differ, in inheritance or experience, mind and body, will choose different kinds of jobs, for example jobs that are physically demanding or undemanding. We approached such personal "host" dispositions by study of *physique,* using data readily available for the busmen on uniform-size.[26] (The validity of the tailor's waist-band measurements has been confirmed, page 43.) The tailor's size, and the clinical measurement of skinfolds, row 7 (b), give similar results. The indication from our data and from an independent study of young recruits[39] is that liability to obesity, as well as to higher blood pressures and blood lipids, is brought by the men with them into their jobs, and in higher degree by drivers than conductors; these men don't differ only in their choice of job. Be this as it may, the differences in *obesity* do not help at all to explain the main differences found in ischaemic heart disease, rows 1 (b) and 7 (c). Measurements of weight, height (standing or sitting), breadth, sundry circumferences, and combinations of these, were no more rewarding than of obesity. . . This is a core issue for the understanding of the chronic diseases: to disentangle how much of an association found with mode of life is due in fact to initial dispositions, for example the selection of different jobs, and how much to the fact that 20, 30, 40 years are then spent living in different ways. The initial choice and the subsequent experience each may be related to the chances of avoiding disease and the risks of developing it.

All these observations are on *occupation,* and latterly we have switched to the study of exercise taken in *leisure-time:* not only because our busmen's population laboratory is dissolving before our eyes as more women are employed and many (if not enough) coloured immigrants, with all the new problems that this raises, but also because we are "health" people. Physical activity in work is dwindling and any future contribution of exercise to health must come from that taken outside of work, as even the conservative scenarios of occupations in the year 2000 predict. This is now our main interest.[40-42]

Vigorous Exercise in Leisure-time (VE)

Table 7.7 describes the findings to date. Estimates of aggregate physical activity during leisure among these sedentary and very light workers show little or no relationship to the incidence of ischaemic heart disease (A). But further scrutiny of the data showed that men who reported taking vigorous exercise, defined as activity likely to entail an energy expenditure of 7·5 kcal per minute (the standard definition of heavy industrial work), suffered less IHD in the next few years (B). This applied to total incidence as much as to sudden death, and there was no particular advantage to the younger men. A later electrocardiographic study found that men reporting vigorous exercise had substantially fewer ischaemic changes than their colleagues (C). The protection was as clear when all men with symptoms of effort pain or of dyspnoea were excluded from the analysis. "VE", it may be postulated, will be enough — above a threshold — to exercise the circulation, not merely the muscles, and as part of this to improve coronary blood -flow.

TABLE 7.7

PHYSICAL ACTIVITY IN LEISURE-TIME AND THE INCIDENCE (FIRST CLINICAL ATTACKS)
OF CORONARY HEART DISEASE[43]

British Civil Servants
Men Aged 40–45

(A)

Estimates of Physical Activity*	120 First Clinical Attacks**	240 Matched Controls
Mean total score	630	639
Mean score excl. sedentary and light activities	225	245
No. of men reaching "moderate activity"	70	147

*During two sample days in 1968–70. **First 120 cases, 1968–1971. $P > 0.05$.

(B)

Vigorous Exercise (VE)*	238 First Clinical Attacks**	476 Matched Controls
Active recreations	5	19
Keep-fit	3	16
Heavy work	19	78
Vigorous getting about	1	21
Climbing up 450+ stairs p.d.	0	8
Men reporting VE	25	120
Expected	60	

*During the two days in 1968–70. **First 238 cases, 1968–72. $P < 0.001$.

(C)

VIGOROUS EXERCISE IN LEISURE TIME AND THE PREVALENCE OF ELECTROCARDIOGRAPHIC
ABNORMALITIES

Sample of 509 Men	ECG Findings**				
	Myocardial infarction	Minor ischaemic changes	Ectopic beats	Sinus tachy-cardia	Men with any of these
Reporting VE* 125 men	0	6	3	7	14
Not Reporting VE* 384 men	11	42	27	34	83

*During the two days in 1968–70.
**In a clinical survey, 1971.
 Age distributions of the two groups of men were similar.
 Standard 12-lead resting electrocardiogram.

RISK FACTORS → PREVENTION → HEALTH[3] [44-46]

There are signs that three of the elements in the regimen of health postulated at the opening of the chapter, *weight control — no cigarettes — and adequate exercise,* are basics of healthy living in middle and old age, and, more specifically, that they give some protection against heart-attack. The first may be effective through its association with blood pressure, plasma cholesterol concentration and glucose tolerance. The evidence on the second is by now substantial, and interest has shifted to carbon monoxide blood levels as a mechanism.[47] Sample studies of the civil servants, according to vigorous-exercise habits, have found no significant differences between them in blood pressure and plasma cholesterol levels, in their smoking habits, in weight or in skinfolds-thickness; so a different dimension may be involved, as hinted also in the ectopic beats. Hopefully, the 50 per cent of the variance of coronary heart disease which is unexplained by standard risk factors will be breached . . . Primary prevention is the only strategy in sight; there is no indication that detecting early clinical C.H.D., in vulnerable groups for example, and seeking to arrest it, will give any measure of control. Meanwhile, this exploration of VE may also be regarded as a belated move to the study of *leisure and health,* of *re*creation in the coming age of leisure.

EXPLORING ARTERIAL BLOOD PRESSURE[1-4]

Next, Fig. 7.2 represents some attempts to clarify the mysteries of blood pressure levels in the population and of high blood pressure without evident cause, a disorder particularly of middle age. Such is the uncertainty on the natural history that even this apparently innocuous statement ought to be disputed. The search for causes is proving exceedingly hard.

Results of a survey in Scotland are given in part 1 of the Figure, which illustrates the rise with age of average systolic and diastolic pressures that are commonly found in *cross-sectional* population studies. The crossover is typical, and the greater number of hypertensive women during middle age has already been noted. Have many hypertensive men died? Unable to tolerate the high levels? The rise of systolic by comparison with diastolic pressure is familiar; a simple statistical expression, it is possible, of rigidity in large vessels and unrelated therefore to the central problem of essential hypertension. On the basis of *cohort* studies, the suggestion has been made that the effect of age in the rise of pressure is coincidental, and that the main

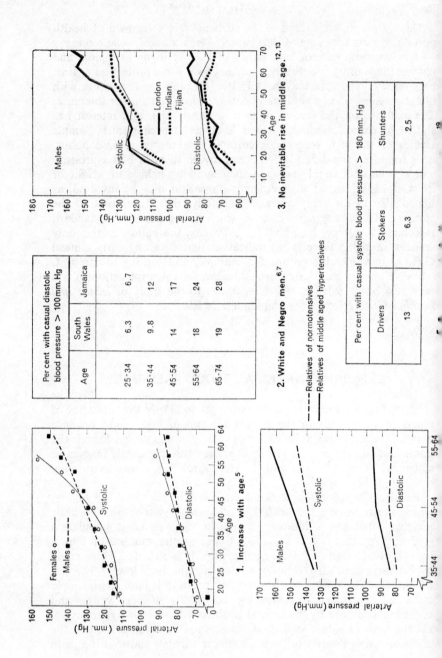

1. Increase with age.[5]

2. White and Negro men.[6,7]

- - - - Relatives of normotensives
———— Relatives of middle aged hypertensives

3. No inevitable rise in middle age.[12,13]

Per cent with casual diastolic blood pressure > 100 mm.Hg			
Age	South Wales	Jamaica	
25-34	6.3	6.7	
35-44	9.8	12	
45-54	14	17	
55-64	18	24	
65-74	19	28	

Per cent with casual systolic blood pressure > 180 mm. Hg		
Drivers	Stokers	Shunters
13	6.3	2.5

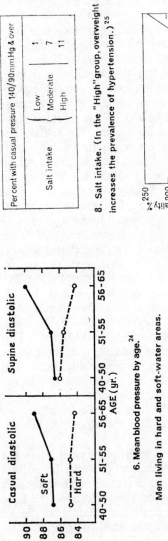

Per cent with casual pressure 140/90mm.Hg & over	
Salt intake { Low	1
Moderate	7
High	11

8. Salt intake. (In the "High" group, overweight increases the prevalence of hypertension.)[25]

9. Sex: actuarial experience.[29]

6. Mean blood pressure by age.[24]

Men living in hard and soft-water areas.

Obesity	Prevalence of hypertension	Incidence of hypertension	Incidence of hypertensive heart disease
None / slight	128	31	8
Moderate	229	38	13
Marked	368	54	16

7. Obesity : rates per 1,000 men, aged 50 – 59.[28]

Fig. 7.2 In search of causes of essential hypertension.

factor is the pressure already attained (p. 114).

Parts 2 and 3 of the Figure present contrasts from "geographical physiology", the former from random sample studies by Miall, who made the same observations among men in South Wales and in Jamaica. It has long been known that Negroes have higher blood pressure than whites, higher average pressure and more with high pressure;[8-10] hypertension and stroke, in fact, and unlike coronary disease present major problems across the world. But the acquired and inherited causes that are involved still are little understood; the epidemiological lead has been little taken up by clinicians, laboratory workers or social scientists.[11] Bacteriuria (and pyelonephritis) among the Jamaicans does not seem to be a major factor.[6] Note, also, in this Figure the disparity between high casual pressure found on population survey in South Wales and the morbidity from hypertension brought to general practitioners (p. 34), a difference of 16 per cent to 3 per cent. The accuracy of diagnosis is surely one factor and the lability of the casual consulting-room pressure another. But the complex of blood pressure/hypertension ± symptoms / atherosclerosis / cardiovascular hypertrophy / manifold morbidity/medical care (no chain of events implied) urgently wants disentangling in long-term follow-up studies. Part 3 shows that the rise of blood pressure in populations during middle age is not universal.[13-16] The thick line is from a London sample; the Indians and Fijians are described in a study, also cross-sectional, by Lovell and his colleagues. (A similar phenomenon has of course been observed among cohort studies of "western" populations, variable fortunate subsamples showing no increase in pressure over the years.[2]) Further genetic hypotheses (are they a peculiar isolate?) need examining, as well as host-factors and behaviour, e.g. in personality, salt-consumption; including the question of who survives to middle age. In one of the great experiments of opportunity,[16] they are now observing if such Polynesians being "westernised" through migration, or locally, develop changes in blood pressure and in the other risk factors for coronary heart disease.

Part 4 proceeds to family studies and compares the experience during middle age of relatives of normotensive, healthy — the lower lines — and of hypertensive subjects. The average increase among the former is less, scarcely any in diastolic pressure, the rise among the latter is "excessive", in Allbutt's phrase. Here again is an example of the wrong way of asking the right question: such cross-sectional group averages of blood pressure are a poor substitute for direct follow-up studies[18] of representative individuals with various family histories. The study of the disease in families, and the clustering of cases that will be found — positive correlations between the blood pressure of first-degree relatives are consistent but small — is another meeting ground for clinician and epidemiologist. Interpreting, how much is shared in the family must be kept in mind: living conditions, character development, human relationships, learning of behaviour patterns, including that under stress; genetic dispositions and their modification by environment and experience.

Part 5 is a collector's piece from an occupational study in Czechoslovakia. East European research in essential hypertension emphasises "psychosomatic" aspects, the nervous strain involved in the job (station-masters also had a high rate); although without knowing more about the particular situation it is difficult to dissociate this from the physical activity entailed. (Other sorties on the frequency of hypertensive disease in relation to *that* have already been mentioned.) The epidemiological method could be invaluable in testing the "neurogenic" hypothesis of essential hypertension;[11] [20-23] better measures of psychological factors for large-scale prospective studies are awaited.

Part 6 is drawn from a clinical sample survey in 12 towns, 6 with hard and 6 with soft water. Connection with blood pressure is a hopeful lead from our work on the "water story" and this behaviour of diastolic pressure a clue, possibly, to the protection given by hard water.

Dahl's figures (part 8) are token of the hypothesis that habitual sodium intake is related to blood-pressure levels; the epidemiological as well as experimental evidence at present is contradictory, but the hypothesis[25-27] has been gaining support, particularly in the East European countries. Again, it is suggested, chronic high salt ingestion leads to hypertension in the genetically disposed. Meanwhile, there is no link between the "salt" and the "water" stories, and since sodium is unusually high in hard waters this doesn't look promising.

Stamler's figures on obesity, judged by weight or skinfold thickness, give the prevalence rates in part 7, of defined hypertension at the start of his survey, and the annual incidence (first detection rates) for four years thereafter.

Part 9 is about "host" factors again, about sex, and it illustrates from actuarial data (using Life Table methods) the crux of the problem. Women, it is true, though they have more hypertension tolerate it better than men. But, more important, the Figure estimates for both sexes the individual risk of dying, on the average and in this kind of selected population, relative to blood-pressure levels at entry. Our own data, page 105, on the experience of the London busmen gives also some details foi vascular disease, responsible for the great majority of the excess risk in hypertensives. In general, blood pressure should be considered as part (9) for Table 7.2.

Action Research

The most famous attempt to deal with this situation, to detect hypertensives and to offer them preventive treatment gave satisfactory results:

Diastolic Blood Pressure	Number Randomised		Complications*			
			Numbers		Per cent	
mm Hg	C	T	C	T	C	T
115–129	70	73	27	1	38·6	1·4
105–114	110	100	35	8	31·8	8·0
90–104	84	86	21	14	25·0	16·3

Middle-aged men.
C = Control Group,   T = Treated Group.
*Principally cerebrovascular accident, coronary heart disease, congestive heart failure.
Fries, E. D. (1970). *Bull. Int. Soc. Cardiol.* no.II/4, p.6.

Study of the "mild", but common and important hypertensive group (d.b.p. 90–104) was incomplete, so that question remains open. Disappointingly, in the moderate and severe hypertensives, 105–129, no material reduction in coronary heart disease was achieved. Very likely, middle age is too late to start if that is the hope. . . Community control programmes of (often symptomless) high blood pressure is a hopeful "new momentum" in prevention to emerge from modern pharmacological, clinical and population research. It well illustrates many of the issues now facing health services and the community physician: to settle priorities; assess the cost-effectiveness of possible methods; public participation. The classical clinical trial has to be enlarged to long-term, maybe life-long, experiment on the problems of compliance, cumulative side-effects, the overall quality of life under various regimens – and to determine the critical ages for achieving the benefits at the lowest costs. Investigators in London have recently found that only about a quarter of the middle-aged severe hypertensives in a favourable situation were under care.[30] Which typical finding[31] makes it all the more difficult to understand the generally downward trend of mortality from hypertensive diseases observed in modern times in this and many countries.[32]

* * *

IMPROVEMENT OF CARDIOVASCULAR EPIDEMIOLOGY

In most field studies of blood pressure the first casual reading on a conventional instrument is the principal measurement used. This is subject to much observer-bias; that it may be the only practicable method is scarcely virtue enough. Here is a problem still requiring collaboration between clinicians, laboratory workers and epidemiologists: How should blood pressure be measured and recorded for population studies in this electronic age, which measurements are worth taking, and what other investigations can and must be made in large-scale surveys of arterial blood pressure? Meanwhile, sphygmomanometers such as the "random zero" apparatus that eliminate subconscious observer-preference, e.g. for terminal digits or for values below "cut-off" points, are increasingly popular. Other instruments are being developed for telemetry of pressure levels through the activities of the 24-hour day and — who knows? — they might be feasible even under free-living conditions on earth.

This questioning of the practice of most population studies of blood pressure is but one illustration. Needs can be cited throughout the C–V field. Here is a list that friends have helped me put together. Electrocardiograms (conventional or orthogonal) inexpensively recorded in the field on magnetic tape, or transmitted by land line, and read centrally by computers... Simpler renal function tests; biochemistry on a drop of blood; mass insulin estimations for relating to lipid-carbohydrate metabolism; trace-element measurement in tissues. . . Cheaper, and, more versatile autoanalysers. . . Easier, non-invasive, techniques for assessment of myocardial function; measurements of platelet and other mechanisms of thrombogenesis/lysis; usable enzymes as genetic markers. . . Methods of classifying individual diet on a mass scale; even crude measurement of exercise (continuous recording of pulse-rate which didn't cost a fortune would be an advance); a battery of hypothesis-based psychological tests that could also be related to physiology; field tests for rate of ageing... Further international standardisation like the Minnesota Code and the Atlanta cholesterol. . . Semi-quantitative assessment of arterial lesions. Simpler criteria and automated methods for progressive delegation of screening. . . Standardised community cardiovascular registers of incidence and prevalence, recurrence, disability; of medical-care provision and the results; and of social costs.

Work is needed in all of these areas. Some fresh ideas on the epidemiology of high blood pressure and of coronary disease would also be very welcome, there have scarcely been any since the 1950's. And a shift to study of cardiovascular *health* is long overdue ... On all counts, the notion of hypertension, atherosclerosis and coronary heart disease as "paediatric problems" represents a hopeful advance.[33]

MULTIPLE CAUSES[1-6]

For half a century, the triumphs of bacteriology and the liberation they brought from notions of "filth" and multiple vagueness led to "the germ theory" of disease. Today, there is no less interest in the *Treponema pallidum,* but we try to understand the occurrence of venereal disease among causes in *host* and *environment* also — physical, mental and social causes — in sex and age of course, and in the mores of the times, in the psychology of promiscuity, the means of contraception, the economics of prostitution, the horrors of war, a

References on page 299.

world on the move, the efficiency of health services — causes which in one combination or another help to explain the incidence of syphilis in the community (and illumine the individual case). However necessary they are, more than the spirochaete is involved in primary syphilis and a fortiori GPI, more than the haemolytic streptococcus in juvenile rheumatism, Koch's bacillus is only one of the causes of the manifold tuberculous syndromes.[7-11]

Sometimes of course one cause many predominate or even be sufficient. In malignant disease, retinoblastoma (heredity may be all), or cancer of the lip (the environment). Huntingdon's chorea, or the gene for achondroplasia. A plasma cholesterol concentration over 400 or 500 mg per 100 ml. Driving the car at 100 m.p.h. Or haemophilia; though the deficiency of Factor 8 seems to be insufficient itself to tip the balance into bleeding. Or a particularly traumatic emotional experience in childhood. Or an earthquake. But this kind of situation is uncommon. Coronary atheroma is necessary, but insufficient for coronary occlusion not to say heart-attack. ("General intelligence seems to bear about the same relationship to on-the-job creativity as weight does to ability in football. You have to have a lot of it to be in the game at all; but among those on the team — all of whom have a great deal of weight to begin with — differences in performance are only slightly, if at all, related to weight."[12]) Dispositions of inheritance or experience are plain in allergic asthma, but there are multiple environmental causes also, psychological and infective, which make for attack or no. Childhood poisoning is becoming commoner: because of the increasing number of drugs (cause), titivated often as coloured pills (cause), for which the popular appetite is voracious (cause), and readily indulged (causes in the grocer's shop as well as the National Health Service). The carelessness of parents and doctors, and the sex and stage of development of the child, exploring putting things into his mouth, provide the opportunity, are causes.[13 14]

A population incidence of disease, then, like any historical event or social fact, is the product of many causes. Various models, ways of organising them, are helpful. There is the *chain of events,* one thing leading to another:

> For want of a nail, the shoe was lost,
> For want of a shoe, the horse was lost.[15]

The child's poisoning; or the rationale of the death certificate. In juvenile epilepsy: a family history, brain damage at birth, fever in infancy, aggravating and perpetuating causes in a miserable home life and generally unsympathetic upbringing.[16] The "programming" of adult disease in childhood is seen in: inheritance → cystinuria → urinary calculi → pyelonephritis → hypertension and/or renal failure → death. The final link in the chain may be regarded as precipitating; as in the life crisis preceding a schizophrenic breakdown, or the smog that resulted in so many coronary deaths.

One scheme arranges causes into (i) *stressful experiences* and (ii) *deprivation,* affecting homeostasis, to which are added (iii) harmful *external causes* such as poisons and germs.[17] Kwashiorkor is thus interpreted by (i) the physiological and psychological strains of the weaning period, (ii) the deficiency of protein in the diet and excess of calories from carbohydrate, and (iii) the frequent coincident infections, combining to disrupt the metabolism and personality of the child.* "Deprivation", the denial of elementary needs, was dominant in disease-aetiology till recently in the West, abject poverty is still very much so in half the world, the most general and the most powerful of non-specific causes. The notion of deprivation can be elaborated in the social and cultural dimensions of protein–calorie malnutrition: poverty and ignorance; rapid industrialisation; the move to the (shanty) towns; the disruption of family life, and the employment of women away from home; breast-feeding stopped; local lack of protein-rich foods and the failure to make use of such as are available (including UNICEF milk) because of "tradition, taboo and magic".[19] My own interest in the epidemiological method was sparked by my first clinical teacher† and his description of the life of the underprivileged child as a cause of its juvenile rheumatism. Deprivation, extended to psychological needs and to social networks remains a dominant issue in the most affluent societies. Dwelling on "causes" we must not forget the great mass of trouble in malignancy for example, where very little is known, perhaps hints only of intrinsic, hormonal and immunologic processes. And we must always allow for chance, luck.

Patterns of Causes

For convenience, the pattern of multiple causes in the incidence of a chronic disease may be summed up like this. First to be distinguished, if it can, is the *necessary cause* or specific agent which has to be present before the disease can develop, and *other causes,* interacting together:

The salience of the necessary cause lies in the direct opportunity it opens for a "magic bullet" to disrupt the pattern and achieve prevention or cure, and in the relative ease of incontrovertible proof of its action

---

*Natura in reticulum sua genera connexit, non in catenam: homines non possunt nis catenam sequi, cum non plura simul sermone exponere.[18]

†iDr. F. J. Poynton, 1869–1943. Physician. University College Hospital, London

(so different from "proving" the role of any particular one among multiple causes, none of which may be necessary). Koch's postulates are the prime example and, defying clinical tradition and public health practice alike, direct chemotherapy proven effective against tuberculosis in the worse-than-slums of Madras.[21] Such situations however are little evident yet in the chronic non-communicable diseases; though a few have been mentioned and the inborn gene-enzyme errors of metabolism may be cited, deficiency of light in miner's nystagmus, the X factor in the leaves of the cotton plant which is necessary for byssinosis. Cigarette-smoking surely is the enviromental, behavioural agent of the modern epidemic of lung cancer, and there is reason to hope for similar discoveries in other cancers. *Necessary* series or *sets of causes,* is perhaps a more logical notion: heavy smokers have a low probability of developing lung cancer during the normal life-span (even greater causes of health are operative); the majority who survived Hiroshima and Nagasaki were fortunate not to have the necessary set of causes for developing leukaemia (or, a more hopeful way of looking at it, the body's defences, their resistance, saved them).

To label all the causes which are not necessary as "contributory factors" is not helpful. So we need another kind of model. Most obviously, the chronic diseases are products of the interaction between people and their place in the world, of causes jointly in these, the "ecological" view:

$$\text{causes in host} \rightleftharpoons \text{environmental causes}$$

Dispositions in the host, in human needs, potential and limits, are *inborn* through various genetic mechanisms and *acquired* in previous experience and current life-situations. Environmental causes occur in the *natural* world; and in *society,* its living conditions, technology, human groups and institutions, social networks, values, culture. There could be general causes and specific agents in any of these. "Interaction" comprises such manifold processes as the realising of genetic potential; the way the individual perceives the environment and therefore how stressful it is to him; the satisfaction of "human needs" in society. The model is, has to be "open" or "open-ended", because usually there is little evidence of a necessary agent to close or lock the system. It admits of qualitative "yes-no" factors, and the more common quantitative, deals in probabilities, in a context of chance and accident; it is concerned as much with defences and supports, "causes of health", as with pathogens.

To proceed. Causes in personal dispositions or the environment often cannot usefully be distinguished because of *individual habits and behaviour* that derive from both, as do a person's customary diet or exercise, his social roles and family relationships. Thus, there is a "field":

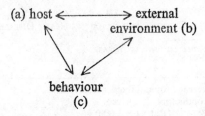

(b) and (c) are described as *ways of living,* together as the *mode of life or life-style.*

Cardiovascular Disease in Middle Age

As relief, I hope, from this theorising: causes and defences can be postulated in (a), the family history, age and sex, blood group, body-build, the blood pressure, cholesterol and glucose levels; in (b), ranging from the stage of development of the country and the rat-race to the hardness of the local water supply; and in (c), in smoking behaviour, for example, and the exercise that is taken in leisure-time. Or, (a), there evidently are individual variations in metabolising fat and car-bohydrate; which can, or cannot, cope with (c), the ordinary food being eaten; which, in turn, is dependent on the prevailing standard of living and plane of nutrition, on local culture-patterns and on family behaviour (b), as well as on personal tastes (a). In any situation all three contributions may be plain and, anyhow, should be kept in mind. Characteristically, the behavioural mainly are studied today, as in Table 7.8 where an "additive" effect of these two postulated causes is indicated. In Table 7.9, there is summing again, here of a positive, protective factor and the pathogenic high blood pressure. In Table 7.10, on page 179, the effects of occupation — a dangerous physical environment — together with smoking habits, indicate a multiplier effect, "synergism" between them, and not simple addition, as indeed is hinted also in Table 9 (B). We are back again to whole-man medicine and to ecology.

TABLE 7.8
EXERCISE, CIGARETTE SMOKING AND IHD
Incidence of Fatal Myocardial Infarction
Age-adjusted Rates per 1,000 per Year

	More Active	Less Active
Not Cigarette Smokers	0·69	2·57
Cigarette Smokers	1·30	5·18

Health Insurance Plan of Greater New York.
Shapiro, S., Weinblatt, E., Frank, C. W. & Sager, R. V. (1969) *Amer. J. publ. Hlth* **59,** Pt II, 1–101.

TABLE 7.9
BLOOD PRESSURE, EXERCISE AND ISCHAEMIC HEART DISEASE[28]

(A)

TEN–YEARS INCIDENCE OF ISCHAEMIC HEART DISEASE
London Busmen[22]

Casual systolic BP (mm Hg) At Entry	Average Annual Incidence of IHD	
	Conductors	Drivers
	(Rates per 1,000)	
—129	6·7	12·6
130–149	9·1	9·9
150–169	11·2	15·4
170–189	12·7	21·0
190+	22·6	27·8

Ages 40–65, standardised.   664 men free of IHD on entry.
90 first clinical attacks, all forms.

(B)

PREVALENCE OF ISCHAEMIC MYOCARDIAL FIBROSIS
National Necropsy Survey [23]

Clinical and Pathological Evidence	Physical Activity of Occupation		
	Heavy	Active	Light
	(Prevalence of the scarring per 100)		
Essential hypertension present	2·2	9·4	24
No record or evidence of hypertension	3·7	3·8	6·6

Ages 45–59.
1,349 men. Deaths from other than IHD (accident, cancer, etc.).

(C)

ISCHAEMIC CHANGES ON ELECTROCARDIOGRAM
Civil Service Executive-Grade Officers[24]
Prevalence rate per 100

Casual Systolic BP (mm Hg)	Q/QS, ST–T, T Wave Changes Reported	
	Vigorous Exercise*	No Report**
—129		6·6
130–149	3·8	10·4
150+	6·8	16·5

Ages 40–65.   Point prevalence.
*125 men, **384 men. Age distributions are quite similar.

TABLE 7.10
SMOKING HABITS IN 370 ASBESTOS WORKERS: DEATHS FROM LUNG CANCER

Smoking Habits of Workers	Deaths from Lung Cancer	
	Observed	Expected*
Never smoked regularly	0	0·05
History of pipe/cigar smoking only	0	0·13
History of regular cigarette smoking	24	2·98
Total	24	3·16

The men in the three groups otherwise were similar.
*On basis of general US mortality data.
Selikoff, I. J., Hammond, E. C. and Churg, J. (1968) *J. Amer. med. Ass.*, **204**, 106.

Variations on the Theme

The same physical, mental and social cause — tuberculosis, syphilis, cigarettes, alcohol* — can be associated with many diseases: the notion of "specific cause-effect" is inapplicable. Smog killed by cor pulmonale and by coronary heart disease. Coxsackie B virus is involved in a variety of disorders. Radiation produces multiple mutations, the steroids manifold toxic reactions.[25] The (boring) stereotypes of the unconscious are manifested in a multitude of disorders. Inducted to the same military depot, some 18 year-olds end up twice the men they were, a few will have a psychotic breakdown, and in between there is likely to be a great variety of positive – negative physical, mental and social adaptations.

Conversely, different causes can be involved in the same disease, depending presumably on the other personal dispositions and on the rest of the environment. The pathological repertory of the body is not unlimited, in inflammation, liver necrosis, the "organic brain syndrome" dyspepsia, depression, etc. There are many causes of septic or aseptic meningitis. A variety of known causes produce the same type of leukaemia (though in most cases that occur there is only a question mark). Different external causes acting on the growing embryo at a critical time can cause the same deformity, and different genes may also do so. The same cell-type of lung cancer is found with quite different external causes, cigarette smoking, uranium, nickel. There are many known causes of "industrial" dermatitis. The same symptom or piece of (disordered) behaviour can originate in many motivations.

Finally, particular causes may be effective in some situations and inoperative in others, this part of the concept seems to be the most

*"Drunkenness maketh him have the throat of a fish, the belly of a swine and the head of an ass. Drunkenness is hurtful to the body, the cup kills more than the cannon, it causes dropsies, catarrhs and apoplexies, it fills the eyes with fire, and the legs with water and turns the body into a hospital."
The Vicar of Kirdford, in Willard B. (1965). *Sussex*. London.

difficult to live with: a negative finding may apply only to its particular situation. As seen, simple proof and customary logic help only with the necessary cause; if this fails to pass a test the hypothesis is falsified. But the reality of multiple causes cannot be tested by such methods of "affirmation and demolition" . . . Cigarettes seem now to be the leading cause of chronic bronchitis; but last century there was a lot of the disease — and no cigarettes. The driven, striving entrepreneur surely was familiar in Victorian England, but it seems he rarely suffered from ischaemic heart disease. Such refutation does not dispose of these hypotheses. Different *patterns of causes* presumably were operating last century, the *epidemic constitution* was different. The cigarette, or the personality type, are not biologically necessary causes of bronchitis or IHD; they are determining, but incomplete.[26] Conceivably there is no indispensible cause of either. . . Half the men who develop ischaemic heart disease are in the top quarter of blood-pressure distribution, but half are not, and most with high blood pressure don't suffer from heart-attack (we may or may not understand why). Hypertension, moreover, does not seem to lead to IHD in populations, like the Japanese, with low average plasma cholesterol values. High blood pressure, nevertheless, is a major cause of IHD . . . Simple environmental control can prevent the expression of inherited dispositions — scurvy, rickets, goitre, for example. Social class, its known and unknown components, manifestly is "causal" in reproductive performance. But the last two columns of the simple analysis in Table 7.11 show the *social* factor overwhelmed in a particularly favourable *biological* situation (young mothers who are not "primips") and particularly unfavourable ("worn-out multips"). In an intermediate group not specially favourable or unfavourable by age and parity, mothers in their late 30's bearing a third child, the social class range in stillbirth was widest, from 14 in class 1 to 33 in class 5. The situation seems to be the same in Fig. 7.3: the rate of lung cancer among heavy smokers is similar at all levels of the "urban factor" (air pollution possibly).

THEORY AND ACTION: HEALTH AND PREVENTION

To sum up: it is obligatory in the chronic diseases to think of their multiple causes, variously combining and of varying moment, of the explanation provided and of the predicted gain should causes be removed. Multiple causes offer multiple possibilities of action. In conditions as common as cardiovascular disease, the numbers at stake must be remembered: cigarettes seem far less important as a cause of heart-attack than of lung cancer but far more deaths are involved; the softness of the local drinking water may be involved in a large number of cardiovascular deaths during middle age even if these are only a fraction of the very large total of these deaths. Such dialogue between theory and practice is essential. It is a classic situation in

TABLE 7.11
BIOLOGICAL AND SOCIAL CAUSES IN STILLBIRTH[27] [28]

1949–50
England and Wales
Rates per 1,000 Total (Live and Still) Births

Social Class	MOTHERS		
	Of All Ages and All Parities	Aged 20–24 Bearing Second Child	Aged 40+ Bearing Sixth or Later Child
1	16	—	—
2	19	11	52
3	21	12	56
4	23	12	56
5	26	13	56

Single, legitimate births.
—Nos. too few.
Lancet (1955) **1**, 343, 554.

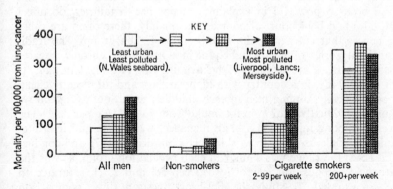

Fig. 7.3 Two postulated causes of lung cancer: cigarette smoking and 'urban' environment (air pollution). Estimated annual death rates, men aged 35–74, 1952–5. (Rates are standardised for age.) Areas in N.W. England and in N. Wales.

Mortality in moderate smokers (100–199 cigs. per week) was highest in the most urban — most polluted — area, but there was no trend with degree of 'urbanisation'.

Stocks, P. (1957) *Suppl. to Part II of the 35th Ann. Rep.* of the British Empire Cancer Campaign, London.

Public Health that useful action can be taken, and will often have to be attempted, on the basis of what is known at the time and without waiting for fuller understanding; which imposes particular responsibilities on monitoring and research. The immediate hope in the chronic diseases is to learn enough of the pattern of causes for an acceptable regimen to be stated that will make good sense in terms of health and achieve some primary prevention, at a known and bearable cost.

EPIDEMIOLOGY OF PERSONAL BEHAVIOUR

The last section raises a fundamental question for health and prevention today. Evidence multiplies that the epidemic chronic non-communicable diseases which beset us are associated with the mode of life — yes, but often in the domain of personal habits and behaviour rather than the impersonal external environment. The Schneeberg-Joachimsthal cancer of the bronchus was due to the industrial process, the modern epidemic follows from the twentieth century curse of cigarette smoking. It remains true that within wide limits communities determine their own death rates.[1]

Knowledge about many aspects of personal behaviour is scanty. Getting the facts to relate to health and disease is proving difficult and expensive, often it hasn't yet been attempted. This is now a key area for research, for example to devise adequately reproducible and valid estimates of the great variety of *exercise taken in leisure-time.* And there are far more emotive and less "researchable" areas than exercise.[2]

The factors that are the stock-in-trade of epidemiology, social-occupational class, income level, area of residence and so forth, and have been so powerful in explaining major health failures, do affect attitudes and behaviour, of course; but, plainly, there often are other influences that cut across the membership of such groups The traditional categories often are unhelpful in studying the chronic diseases insofar as these are diseases of behaviour. This is evident in *diet,* its *fat content,* say, in a country with high earnings and till recently cheap food. Typically, among men in early middle age in South England we found individual variation in fat intake from 73 to 216 g per day.[3] The average among middle-class bank managers was 125 g. and in white-collar bank clerks 133g; in working-class bus drivers 127g and conductors 124g; the range was similar in each occupation group, as was the fatty-acid composition, narrowly between 5:1 and 2.5:1, saturated to polyunsaturated. To study the diet-heart question, direct comparison of individuals eating less than 100 g, 100-125 g, etc., has to be made. The imprinting of eating patterns among the family in childhood, variation with particular personality traits including health consciousness, subcultures, these might be sensible first investigations.[4-7]

References on page 300.

TABLE 7.12

(A) ADULT MALES SMOKING
Average Weekly Consumption of Cigarettes
Britain
1970–1

Social Class	No. of Cigarettes
1	47
2	67
3	75
4	73
5	84

Statistics of Smoking in the United Kingdom (1972). London.

(B) YOUNG PEOPLE SMOKING
Average Weekly Consumption of Cigarettes
Britain

	No. of Cigarettes			
	Boys		Girls	
Age	1968	1971-2	1968	1971-2
13	0·7	0·8	0·4	0·2
14	2·4	2·6	1·6	1·6
15 at school	3·4	4·4	2·0	2·0
left school	19	21	7·8	15
16 at school	7·8	6·9	2·3	3·7
left school	24	26	14	23
16-19	63	62	37	43

Statistics of Smoking in the United Kingdom (1972), London; and Todd, G.F. personal communication.
"Since (tobacco) is so hurtful and dangerous to youth . . . shorteneth life . . . breedeth many diseases . . . I wish it were known by the name of youth's bane . . ." E.D. (1606). (Bewley, T., personal communication.)
See: Bynner, J. M. (1969). *The Young Smoker;* Bewley, B. R., Day, I. & Ide, L. (1973) *Smoking by Children in Great Britain*. HMSO, London.

(C)
PERCENTAGE OF SMOKERS BY PARITY AND SOCIAL CLASS
Perinatal Problems (1969) Ed. Butler, N. R. & Alberman, E. D. Edinburgh, p. 73.

Cigarette smoking, on the other hand, is strongly social-class tied. The middle class/working class divide is plain, Table 7.12 (A); and so, (B), is a miserable future ordained for the less educated, and the continuation by modern means assured of the historic social-class trend of disease. But this analysis tells us little that helps. Doctors, and to a smaller extent other men in social class 1, have responded to the new information on smoking. Why they? Which needs were gratified by such a change in behaviour? Did their situations favour it? What

professional roles, and *middle-class* aspirations and goals? Whose opinions did they respect? How much did their physiological knowledge and medical experience — their interest in prognosis and the data on ex-smokers — count?[8] And how much was fear?

The upshot is that we want a fresh look at our categories in social medicine. We want new categories and better understanding of the old — like "occupation" or "class". This is another area where the help of the behavioural sciences is essential: to describe relevant patterns of behaviour, their formation and what needs they meet, and how to influence desirable change.[9-12] There is good evidence that the attitudes and example of parents and peer groups are influential in starting children to smoke, so the educational system and the family represent hopeful points of entry. Thereafter, physiological addiction, reinforced by most of the social signals, is harder to overcome. Parental models we may guess are crucial also for habits of eating and exercise; if patterns of obesity are laid down in childhood and adolescence this may be the only hope.

PERSONAL PARTICIPATION IN HEALTH AND PREVENTION

It is one of the changing characters of health problems, the new "sanitary idea" (though as old as the Greeks), the 18th century pioneers had plenty to say about it, and twentieth-century "maternal and child welfare" is in the same tradition, that prevention of disease is likely increasingly to be a matter of personal decision and personal participation. The general as well as the specific rules for healthy living that are beginning to be formulated, in eating, exercise, smoking, drinking, will entail quite a change in their style of life for many. There still are abundant "environmental" problems to be solved, but the point has I hope been taken. Compare the Victorian programme for laying drains and today's campaigns for washing the hands; the prevention of undernutrition and of obesity; fencing machinery, and the Highway Code; fluoridation of water supplies, old type, and goodness knows difficult enough, and not eating sweets, new; the modern responsibility for seeking help from health services and of sticking to the — effective — medicinal and other regimens that increasingly can be prescribed.[13-16] Today's world problem in social medicine is that of over-population, due in part to the imbalance between environmental death-control and personal fertility-control. The environmental causes of pollution are plain enough, but don't we as people consume, litter too much? (Two cars and now a second house.) Many are still attached to domestic coal fires and cheap coal.

We look forward therefore to greater personal responsibility for health; but a new kind of partnership also needs building in place of the old where, so often, it was enough for the community to do things for the individual. Behaviour patterns derive from environment as well as host. In health, do we need more appropriate culture patterns; goals and models for young people of what the individual ought to be doing for his own and the general good? It's fashionable for women to be slim; why not generate such a movement for men? And not merely encouragement: what about the provision of facilities? For enjoyable exercise? Access to the country? We need "new styles of architecture" as well as "a change of heart". It also remains elementary Public Health (Community Health we now say) to deter, to reduce the invitations to mischief; why not ban any public advocacy of smoking? From the production of safer cigarettes, all the way to blocking of the opportunities for crime, there is plenty of scope for community action. And seat-belts are no different from crash-helmets.

Of course the new responsibilities are onerous. What so often prevents prevention today is people: we refuse to be bullied, won't be persuaded, are slow to learn, don't — can't — act, lack the moral fibre; we are unlucky in our dispositions and motivation. Bad habits seem more contagious . . . It is clear that finding the causes of chronic diseases is easier than communicating the knowledge and translating it into changes of behaviour before "habits turn to diseases". The doctor–patient relationship, our pastoral role, standing in the community — and what we know about people, are great assets but, how obviously, far from enough. The help given up to now by the behavioural sciences is disappointing. Why? Are they getting enough support? How much research, social policies and services, health education, do we devote to the changing of behaviour? In a free society how much ought to be? Should not the main thrust be pushed back to M & CW and school health?[17-20]

TABLE 7.13
VIGOROUS EXERCISE IN LEISURE TIME

Married Men

Active Recreations	Professional	Social Class Skilled workers	Semi- and unskilled workers
	(%)	(%)	(%)
Swimming	34	20	8
Football	6	8	5
Tennis	8	2	0
Squash, etc.	7	2	0
Athletics	2	1	0
Av. No. Sports	1·1	0·6	0·3

At least monthly.
Young, M. & Willmott, P. (1973) *The Symmetrical Family*. p. 214, London.
Sample, London Metropolitan Region, 1970. 591 men.
The trends are the same at 40–59 years (Willmott, P., personal communication, 1974).

Uses of Epidemiology

There is much to do, particularly by experiment. New diagnoses of community health in lean body-mass, blood carbon monoxide levels, cardiovascular fitness, have to be related to changes in caloric intake, cigarette smoking, and exercise habits of sundry behaviour groups. Table 7.13 points to the same as the smoking, but there are many other ways of taking adequate exercise in leisure-time; the whole field of leisure is open to action research. . . We do not yet know whether a direct approach to the casualties of young people is worthwhile, or whether an appeal to youth culture, perhaps to society as a whole is required. Even limited trials could be instructive.

BRONCHITIS (CNSLD)[1-4]

The great London smog of December 1952 (Fig. 7.4) started an epochal revival of interest in bronchitis and the relationships of atmospheric pollution to health. Many of the 4,000 deaths of that disaster were in elderly sufferers from chronic bronchitis. On the "onion principle", the increasing control over pulmonary tuberculosis and pneumonia should have drawn attention to refractory respiratory disease, chronic bronchitis in particular, so it is hard to understand why it was so long neglected. (For what will they criticise us?) The burden on the community is only too easily documented. Bronchitis is a major cause of death in middle- and old age and of admission to hospital, and the leading certified cause of sickness-absence and chronic disability in the working population.

The main components, or stages, of the disease can tentatively be described like this:[5]

(1) *Chronic, Productive Cough.* — Subjects have excess mucoid bronchial secretion, with expectoration and irritant cough, but otherwise are little troubled.

(2) *Bronchitis with Infection.* — After recurrent illnesses, infection may become established with irreversible damage to lungs and bronchi. Cough is increased, and the sputum becomes purulent. Incapacity for work is common, and death from pneumonia may occur.

(3) *Bronchitis with Generalised Airways Obstruction.* — At first the narrowing of the bronchi and reduction of ventilatory capacity are demonstrable only by physiological tests ($FEV_{1.0}$ and $FEV_{10.}/FVC$), but later, and with advancing years, there is increasing dyspnoea and cyanosis, repeated hospital admissions and persisting disability. Respiratory crippling may ensue, alarming

References on page 300.

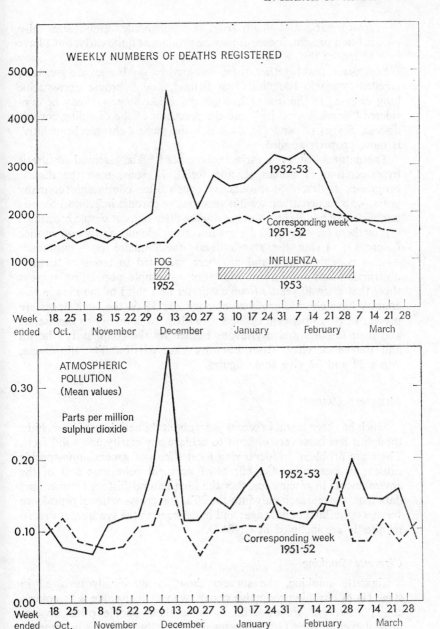

Fig. 7.4   The great fog, or 'smog', of December 1952. Weekly numbers of deaths registered in Greater London (*upper fig.*), in relation to levels of air pollution indicated by SO$_2$ (*lower fig.*). All causes of death; all ages; both sexes. The 1953 influenza epidemic is also shown.

Rep. Publ. Hlth med. Subj. No. 95 (1954). HMSO, London.

emergencies, and death from cor pulmonale. Emphysema also is often present, indeed it may be prominent quite early, but I have to ignore this aspect.

Separately, and together, these and kindred syndromes are generally labelled "chronic bronchitis" in Britain, and "chronic non-specific lung disease" in the rest of Europe and USA. Stage (1) may be considered "simple bronchitis" and the precursor of the disabling chronic disease, Stages (2) and (3), to which the name "chronic bronchitis" is more properly applied.

The natural history is variable, however.[6-9] The essential feature is hypersecretion of mucus (Lynne Reid). In some men the disease progresses as described, productive cough often continuing for many years, with recurrent winter illnesses, before chronic infection becomes established in middle age. But the disease often halts at simple bronchitis (1); or there may be rapid decline into complete incapacity and cardiac failure (3). Using the standardised questionnaire on symptoms[10] — this is reproducible and has been validated in terms of airways obstruction and subsequent mortality — sample population surveys show that after 40 years of age a quarter to a third of the men in this country have chronic productive cough. By 55–64 the later stages are present in 10–15 per cent of men who often are a misery to themselves and their families and a grievous burden on the community's health and welfare services, from intensive care to disability allowances. Pages 29 and 32 give some figures.

MULTIPLE CAUSES

Much has been learnt in recent years about the aetiology of bronchitis, though it has been very difficult to achieve any clarity and solid facts. There are problems in identifying local effects of general, non-specific causes; in integrating the effects of personal behaviour and of the environment; in piecing together the long natural history from cohort data that, as yet, reach only into the 20's, and cross-sectional prevalence surveys describing middle age; and in delineating the syndromes that so manifestly are included in CNSLD.

Cigarette Smoking

Cigarette smoking, the surveys show, is specifically involved in stage (1) of chronic productive cough, whose other name is "smoker's cough". Surveys are essential, because these people often do not present even to their GPs (Chapter 6). Simple bronchitis is uncommon in non-smokers, less common in pipe smokers, commoner in heavy than in light cigarette smokers, and usually stops when smoking is stopped. Productive cough also occurs more often in men than in women, but this seems to be a function largely of sex differences in smoking habits.[11] *Pathologically,* smoking is associated with hypertrophy of the mucus glands and goblet cells in the bronchial walls and with cilial statis; later, atypical cells with squamous changes of the epithelium appear.

Unhealthiness of Towns

Living in towns (Table 7.14 overleaf) was important in the progression to the infective and obstructive disease illustrated. And cigarette smokers in London and the county boroughs of England and Wales (the large towns, mostly) had about twice as much of the chronic disease as smokers living in rural districts. Within each smoking category, pulmonary function — peak flow — was lower in town-dwellers than country people and the volume of sputum greater.

Chronic *air pollution* from domestic and industrial burning of coal is the urban-environmental factor under most suspicion; local density of population, and with it the opportunity for cross-infection, seemingly is not so important.[12-14] In an elegant piece of "clinical epidemiology", seeking to overcome the limitations of indirect "ecological" study, exacerbation of symptoms in individuals with chronic bronchitis was found to accompany acute increase in local intensity of smoke and sulphur dioxide — mini versions of the smog episode.[15-17] In postmen doing similar outdoor work across the country, sickness-absence and invaliding on account of bronchitis were associated with an index of local fog.[18] [19] Mortality in the county boroughs correlated highly with another crude index of pollution we developed — the amount of coal burnt in domestic fires (Fig, 7.5). Respiratory disease was responsible as seen for most of the historic *urban/rural* differentials in mortality. Taking the analysis of page 186 a step further, from "respiratory disease" to the *mortality from bronchitis* (c), by degree of local air pollution, we find even steeper gradients:

Rate per 1,000	England & Wales	Rural Districts	County Boroughs		
			Clean	Intermed.	Dirty
M 1·2 =	100	52	80	126	176
F 0·27 =	100	59	71	132	186
Ages 45-64[13]					

In the agricultural, "truly rural" districts (data are not available) the ratios are surely below 52 and 59, so the picture is probably an understatement. In two-factor studies, disabling bronchitis was prevalent among all smokers, but reached a peak in late middle-age among the cigarette smokers living in heavily polluted areas.[20] [21]

Environment, Quality of Life

The results of the Clean Air Act of 1956, latest effort in 700 years of campaigning, are in many places quite splendid;[21] [22] a Londoner is

TABLE 7.14
BRONCHITIS IN TOWN AND COUNTRY

Prevalence at Ages 40–64
Rates per cent

	Type of Area								
	Rural Districts			Urban Districts and Municipal Boroughs			London and County Boroughs		
	No.	%B	%SD	No.	%B	%SD	No.	%B	%SD
Males	158	12	3	355	15	7	274	23	13
Females	170	8	2	332	7	2	280	9	6

College of General Practitioners (1961). *Brit. med. J.* **2**, 973.
  B=Bronchitis present on clinical diagnosis.
SD=Bronchitis diagnosed on standard questionnaire.

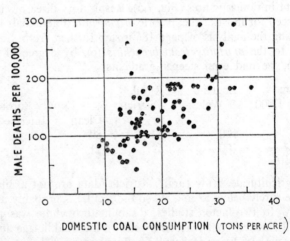

Fig. 7.5 Mortality from bronchitis, in relation to an estimate of chronic air pollution in county boroughs of England and Wales. Death rates of men aged 45–64 in 1948–54.[12][13] The correlation in women was similar.
  Registrar General (1956) *Quarterly Return* No. 432, Appendix D. *Brit. J. prev soc. Med.* (1959) **13**, 14.

entitled to feel expansive about clean air. During the London fog of 1962, the "extra" deaths were less than a quarter of those in 1952; SO_2 concentrations were similar in both episodes but there was far less smoke in the later, page 67. (Many bronchitics had also learned to stay indoors, however.) "The hellish and dismal cloud of fuliginous and filthy vapour" is now abating. In the "dirty", most heavily polluted, officially "black" areas of Britain, about 70 per cent of dwellings now are covered by smoke-control orders.[23] Average winter sunshine in London has been raised from about 1·2 to 1·7 hours per day.

There seems to have been a fall in *hospital admissions* for bronchitis (p. 81), crudely 13 per cent fewer in 1972 than in 1962. (These data have to be treated circumspectly as epidemiological indicators, because of changing fashions in diagnosis, etc. But even a small decline while admissions as a whole rose by close to a third would be remarkable.) When I mentioned this to clinician friends from Sheffield and London, two areas whose smoke-control programmes are almost complete, both remarked they were now seeing far fewer patients in extremis with cardiac and respiratory failure from bronchitis. *Death rates* also are beginning to fall, particularly in London; and there no longer are exacerbations of chest symptoms or of bronchitis mortality in relation to the minor increases of basically low pollution levels. These, indeed, now seem to be lower than the necessary threshold, or "floor", for damaging health.[24-26] But in some places, and sadly in the North, progress in cleaning the air has been slow, because of miners' claims to concessionary coal and for similar reasons.[23] Comparative study of local health-statistics is now obligatory.

The Childhood History

Studies in children show a strong tendency for symptoms of bronchitis to vary with the degree of local air pollution, overleaf. How does this affect the principle of "permissive" legislation whereby local authorities virtually set their own pace in cleaning the air?

In the Medical Research Council's Annual Report for 1973/4, Mill's classic "canons" of scientific proof are applied to the epidemiological evidence implicating *air pollution* as a cause of *bronchitis*. The results add up to a convincing picture in terms of *time-sequence* of the two; their *distribution by place;* the *strength of the relationship; consistency with other evidence* (there isn't very much from the laboratory); and the *weakness of alternative explanations* for the statistical associations.

Standard of Living

The "epidemic constitution" of bronchitis begins, however, in the social structure, Fig. 7.6, page 193, for example. In the great cohort study in Newcastle-upon-Tyne, bronchitis and pneumonia during the first five years of life were only about a tenth as common in social class 1 as in the poorest group.[27] Again, when the two factors were studied together, both "class" and atmospheric pollution were found

TABLE 7.15
AIR POLLUTION AND RESPIRATORY TRACT INFECTIONS IN CHILDREN
National Cohort Born in March 1946
Rates per cent
Various Areas of Britain

| Morbidity | Degree of Pollution in Area | | | |
	Very Low	Low	Moderate	High
Infection of *Upper Resp.* *Tract* at 6–7 years	13·7	15·8	13·6	14·8
Infection of *Lower Resp. Tract*				
Attack at 0–2 years	19·4	24·2	30·0	34·1
Hospital admission under 5 years	1·1	2·3	2·6	3·1
Rales and rhonchi at two or more special school examinations	0·5	2·1	2·5	2·7

Douglas, J. W. B. & Waller, R. E. (1966) *Brit. J. prev. soc. Med.*, **20**, 1.
Social-class composition in the areas was similar.

TABLE 7.16
DEATH RATES FROM BRONCHITIS BY SOCIAL CLASS
England and Wales
1949–53

| Mortality | | Social Class | | | | |
Ages 45–64 per		1	2	3	4	5
Ages 45–64 per	Men	0·40	0·62	1·1	1·2	2·1
1,000 population	Married women	0·07	0·11	0·22	0·28	0·37

Registrar General: *Decennial Supplement on Occupational Mortality*. HMSO. London.

to be producing effects.[28] If numbers had permitted three and four-way analysis of the data, including for example the mother's age and the size of her family, the range of Fig. 6 might have been even wider — we cannot say what happens at the extremes of such distributions. As every schoolboy ought to know (but it was disappointing recently to hear both panel and audience of the leading middle-brow radio quiz programme quite oblivious of such elementary facts of life), mortality from bronchitis in the "working classes" during middle age is far higher than in the middle classes (Table 7.16), The General Practitioners' Morbidity Survey gave similar results and later mortality data indicate little if any progress.

Poverty may be effective by lowering general resistance, and through such special factors as *overcrowding,* and *inadequate convalescence* from acute respiratory illness. *Jobs* in social classes 1 and 2

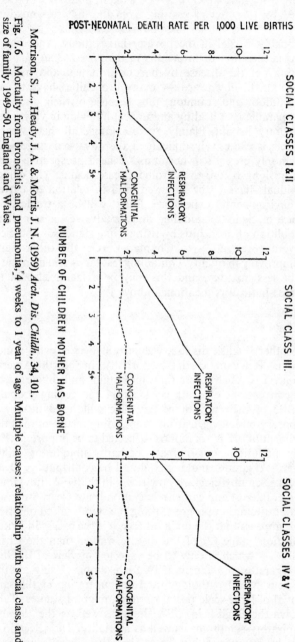

POST-NEONATAL DEATH RATE PER 1,000 LIVE BIRTHS

NUMBER OF CHILDREN MOTHER HAS BORNE

SOCIAL CLASSES I & II

SOCIAL CLASS III.

SOCIAL CLASSES IV & V

RESPIRATORY INFECTIONS

CONGENITAL MALFORMATIONS

Fig. 7.6 Mortality from bronchitis and pneumonia, 4 weeks to 1 year of age. Multiple causes: relationship with social class, and size of family. 1949–50. England and Wales.

Morrison, S. L., Heady, J. A. & Morris, J. N. (1959) *Arch. Dis. Childh.*, 34, 101.

differ manifestly from those in classes 3–5; as said, outdoor workers in heavily polluted towns suffer excessively from the disease, and dusty work, in foundries for example, may be a specific cause.[29-30] *Cross-infection* is probably crucial in the poverty–large family syndrome of Fig. 7.6. The concentration of bronchitis in the *lower social classes* is due to "breeding" of the disease by bad environment and personal behaviour, and "drift" downward — many bronchitics have to give up customary outdoor and strenuous jobs because of their disability. This is another paradigm of healthy and unhealthy living in very recent if not contemporary Britain. Plainly, to disentangle all these various causes and effects is excessively difficult at the advanced stage when bronchitis commonly presents in hospital. We need prospective population study from long before the chronic disease begins. The careers of many individuals have to be followed, and in relation to current personal and environmental experience. But it will be a tragic irony if the persistence of cigarette smoking, and its adverse social pattern, prevents the abolition of bronchitis by rising living standards and clean air and its overdue relegation to Chapter 1. (On the other hand, cigarettes are improving in quality, containing less tar — and nicotine — so they may be less noxious; and this may be a factor also in the improving disease-indicators mentioned above.)

ENGLISH DISEASE

Rickets, the other English disease, was also associated with atmospheric pollution. Relevant certified mortality in North America and in Scandinavia is much lower than in Britain, and differences in diagnosis and conventions of death certification and coding probably account for little of their advantage.[31 32] The childhood history of many contemporary middle-aged Britons, including recurrent infection and an environment of urban squalor, is suspected to be important;[33 34] continuing air pollution, our climate perhaps, ubiquitous winter viruses, and heavy cigarette smoking could all be contributing. Death rates from CNSLD-emphysema are now rising in the USA, how much because of greater interest and earlier recognition is not clear. Studies in a number of countries are in progress, using the standardised questionnaire,[1 18] and it appears that the main difference is the excess in Britain of chronic infection, stage (2) of the disease, rather than the earlier simple bronchitis — which is only to be expected in view of the high prevalence of cigarette smoking in USA for example. Using another technique of geographical pathology (and demonstrating at the same time the potential of large-scale postal surveys), migrant studies (Table 7.17) have shown the English in USA doing as well as the "locals", for serious respiratory symptoms as well as mortality. The selection of emigrants may be a confounding factor, but these results are most encouraging.

TABLE 7.17

DEATH RATES FROM CHRONIC NON-SPECIFIC LUNG DISEASE IN NATIVE-BORN AND MIGRANT POPULATIONS

Age-adjusted Rates per 100,000

Population	Men	Women
US subjects born in USA	24	4
British subjects in UK	125	24
migrants in USA	23	4
Norwegians in Norway	10	4
migrants in USA	9	2

Reid, D. D., Cornfield, J., Markush, R. E., Seigel, S., Pederson, E. and Haenszel, W. (1966) *N.C.I. Monogr.* **19**, 321; Reid, D. D. (1971) *Isr. J. M. Sci.* **7**, 1569.

PREVENTION IN CHRONIC NON-SPECIFIC LUNG DISEASE

The indication from current work is that many causes are contributing to incidence and prevalence, disability and mortality, and differently at different stages. Only a minority of persons exposed to these many insults suffer and, characteristic of the whole field of chronic disease, we know little of what is involved in this immunity — though there is a genetic clue now in emphysema, and the important suggestion that the scene for adult bronchitis is set in childhood. However much remains to be discovered, there is plenty of indication for trial and experiment, and for special and general measures that make good sense in terms of health and give some hope of control as well as relief.[35] By a general *reduction of cigarette smoking* in the population, by explaining to "chesty" youngsters why not to start, helping smokers to give up the habit when they begin the "precursor" cough and a fortiori when the disease is established. By *cleaning air* at least to levels where bronchitic symptoms are unaffected. By *early treatment of respiratory infection* throughout life; possibly, by change of residence and job (I haven't been able to deal with occupational aspects) for adults with persistent infection. By attempting to *reduce disability* and maintain working capacity in the vulnerable people with established disease: anticipating trouble in cold weather, fog and 'flu epidemics, possibly prescribing antibiotics through the winter to prevent more tissue destruction, though results at this stage are disappointing; and by spotting the men whose sickness-absence is lengthening — say at 3 months — and mobilising the resources of industrial as well as medical *rehabilitation*.

REDISCOVERY OF BYSSINOSIS[1-5]

During the six years following the introduction of the compensation scheme in 1941, 39 men of some 15,000 cotton workers-at risk were certified as "totally disabled" by byssinosis. In Lancashire the disease was considered a small and diminishing problem; modern methods of dust control were generally believed to be successful and the few men developing byssinosis thought to be victims of environmental conditions long since past. Chronic bronchitis however still plagued the air-polluted mill towns, and local people regarded the little byssinosis

References on page 301.

that was recognised as part of this prevalent chest disease aggravated by exposure to an irritant dust. Unexpectedly in 1947 a new interest was aroused in the health of cotton workers. The *British Medical Journal,* on the basis of occupational mortality rates, suggested that they suffered excessively from hypertension and heart disease, and Schilling carried out a field survey to explore this idea. He found little of interest in the blood pressures: instead, a quite unexpected amount of respiratory disease was exposed. Of 131 typical middle-aged card and blowroom workers examined, two-thirds suffered from "Monday feeling", the characteristic symptom of byssinosis — a tightness of the chest, which may be exceedingly unpleasant, after the weekend break; and 12 per cent were severely disabled. The common impression that byssinosis had been conquered seemed altogether too sanguine, relating to the tip only of an iceberg.

Schilling next made a survey focusing on respiratory disease and since there are no characteristic X-ray findings in byssinosis he took particular care to standardise the clinical "history" and devise a questionnaire that was repeatable and valid. The table shows good agreement between observers:

Prevalence of Byssinosis: Comparison of Gradings by Two Observers
183 Male Cotton Workers aged 40–59

		OBSERVER A			
		Normal	Grade 1	Grade 2	Total
		79	67	37	183
OBSERVER B	Normal	78	72	6	0
	Grade 1	70	6	47	17
	Grade 2	35	1	14	20
	Total	183			

Complete reproducibility in $72 + 47 + 20 = 139$ (76%); agreement on the presence or absence of byssinosis in $139 + 14 + 17 = 170$ (93%).

Normal = no evidence of byssinosis.
Grade 1 = chest tightness and/or breathlessness on Mondays only.
Grade 2 = chest tightness and/or breathlessness on Mondays and other working days.

Half the men (98), the observers thus agreed, were suffering from the disease — and none of the "controls" questioned in a local engineering works gave the pathognomonic history. In addition, a test of ventilatory capacity was used and it was found that among men of the same age the forced expiratory volume ($FEV^{0.75}$) was lowest in those with a grade 2 history, intermediate in the presence of grade 1 disease, and highest in cotton workers who were "normal" by the questionnaire. The more objective test, i.e., confirmed the validity of the classic symptom.

More Uses

By now it was clear from the population studies that the clinical picture of byssinosis is quite different from that of chronic bronchitis. In early byssinosis there is little cough or spit and no chest infection but, instead, a fall in ventilatory capacity, tightness of the chest and shortness of breath. In the late stages the clinical picture does become confused, both conditions causing fibrotic changes in the bronchi and respiratory crippling. Cotton workers frequently suffer from both these common conditions, with cor pulmonale only too often at the end — which resulted in the misleading occupational mortality statistics of "heart disease". Extension of the survey to Holland confirmed the distinction between the two diseases. Byssinosis is almost as common in Dutch as in Lancashire mills spinning similar types of cotton but chronic bronchitis is of course the "English disease".[6]

By leaving the hospital with its concentration of advanced and complicated cases, and moving into the cotton mills and the community, Schilling was able to detect the disease from its beginnings and to follow its natural history. He could also complete the clinical picture in other ways. Thus, the absence of byssinosis in women was illusory: most of the women disabled by it presented themselves to chest clinic or GP as Lancashire housewives suffering from "bronchitis", and the diagnostic lifetime occupational history was not taken. The same is true of the reputed immunity of old men: i.e., the clinical picture of byssinosis based on hospital experience was as wrong in its way as the mortality statistics: wrong about sex and age, wrong also on the natural history and, above all, seriously wrong on the size of the burden on the population. How it came about that so much was missed is another of those mysteries, a peg on which to hang any number of texts on medical education, the strategy of research, standards of local health services, information systems to some purpose, clinical and community medicine, etc., etc. For the individual operative in middle age the prospect of a job in his home town apart from cotton often was bleak, and there was a reluctance to probe, and draw the lessons, by management and Unions in a contracting industry chronically beset by economic difficulties. The contrast, however, with Welsh miners and their pneumoconiosis, and the public issue they made of it, remains remarkable. The difference in political traditions obviously was another factor. In Lancashire, understatement of the symptoms may also be connected with the peculiarity of an industry in which men and women work alongside each other doing similar jobs.

". . . the limits of resistance are different in each culture. The 'impossible' effort, the 'unbearable' pain . . . are less individual functions than criteria sanctioned by collective approval, and disapproval . . ."[7]

MULTIPLE CAUSES

As expected, cigarette smokers are vulnerable to byssinosis, these operatives for example:

Prevalence of Byssinosis: Smokers and Non-smokers

Female Card-room Workers

	At-risk	Affected With Byssinosis	Median Age	Mean Years of Exposure to Cotton
Non-smokers	144	62	39	14
Smokers	82	52	28	9

$X^2 = 7.87$, $P < 0.01$.

The frequency of byssinosis in Holland, Africa and the USA (the disease, so highly prevalent, was described there astonishingly late[8]) rule out suggestions that the climate of Lancashire or local air pollution are important causes. The role of bronchial infection is still unclear.

In Search of the Agent

To incriminate the specific cause in cotton manufacture would be invaluable for prevention, and some progress has been made. Surveys of different mills showed that the disease was commoner where medium and coarse grades are spun. Next, a strong and direct relationship was shown between the prevalence of symptoms and proximity to the carding engines, the dustiest process. These figures for female workers with similar years of exposure are typical:

Prevalence of Byssinosis and Type of Work
Women aged 40–59 Years

Occupation	No. at Risk	No. with Byssinosis
Near card engines	109	51
Distant from card engines	109	25
Ring spinners	61	2

Such findings removed any doubt that there was a specific cause in the local working environment. (Incidentally, because more women than men work in the card rooms more women in fact suffer from byssinosis.) It was now possible to begin to define the *risk*, in terms of dose-response relationships between current fine dust exposure during the working shift and prevalence of disease (grade $\frac{1}{2}$ = occasional chest tightness on Mondays. For example:[9]

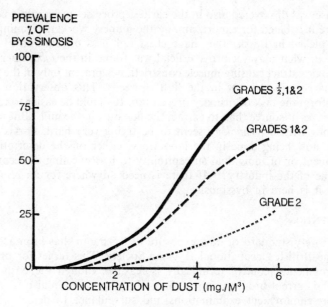

Fig. 7.7

At a concentration of 1 mg/m³ the early and mild manifestations of the disease begin to be seen, the more severe forms from higher levels (2 mg/m³).

Field Survey and Laboratory Experiment[1] [9] [10]

In the advance of medical knowledge the three main methods of learning — clinical observation, laboratory experiment, population survey — each make their characteristic contribution, raising questions also for study by the other two and testing notions derived from them. The recent exploration of byssinosis illustrates a fruitful collaboration between laboratory worker and epidemiologist, clinicians having described the disease for them well over 100 years ago.

Field studies, continuing those described, showed that exposure to fine particles of the vegetable dust lowered ventilatory capacity in the cotton operatives, suggesting that a specific substance in the dust produced bronchial constriction or mucosal swelling. The *pharmacologists* confirmed that extracts of cotton dust do indeed contain a histamine-like substance that contracts smooth muscle preparations in animals and isolated human bronchial muscle. *Geographical* study then showed that this extract is unlikely to arise, as had been suggested, from bacterial or mould action on the bales of cotton (which commonly lie for months in damp warehouses in Liverpool). The disease was discovered also in the earliest processes of handling cotton, before it is baled for export, among the ginnery workers cleaning it as it is picked in Egypt; they have chest tightness on Saturdays!

Next, what may yet prove crucial was found in the *laboratory:* that the toxic extract causing muscle constriction is present only in the leaves of the cotton and not in the fluff or seeds. This observation could transform the task of primary prevention. It should be easier to remove the leaves at source than to extract the fine dust in the mills. But neither US nor British *technology* seem to be trying very hard, nor is much work now being done in the laboratory, either on the description of the agent or of individual susceptibility to it. Reflecting the economic decline of the industry?[10] If there is need anywhere for an *ecological* view it is here in byssinosis.

PREVENTION[12]

A safety standard of dust exposure of 0·5 mg/m^3 has been accepted by the British Occupational Hygiene Society. This target for primary environmental control technically is feasible, though the costs seem beyond current profit margins. "Secondary" prevention also is advised — pre-employment examinations and surveillance to detect workers with the beginnings of "Monday feeling" or of impairment in ventilatory function. And, of course, this is no place for smokers.

A Dangerous Trade

Latest prevalence surveys give rates of 20–50 per cent with byssinosis in the card room and by no means negligible figures among other workers; the available exhaust ventilation often still fails to capture the finer particles.[12] New disability pensions, 1,172 in 1960–2, were granted to only 215 in 1970–2. Certified deaths continue fairly uniform at around 30 p.a. Numbers-at-risk are of course fewer now but this is inadequate to explain the decline in compensated cases.

CANCER IN THE REPORTS OF THE GENERAL REGISTER OFFICE*[1-6 26]

Over 100,000 deaths per year are certified to malignant diseases in England and Wales. Since William Farr's days, death certificates have been much used as an *instrument for learning* about causes, and in cancer, as in other fields, interesting and important data have been gathered. The tables that follow are all taken direct from the Registrar General's publications or calculated from data these provide. The

*Now absorbed in the Office of Population Censuses and Surveys.

References on page 302.

great majority of human cancers are now considered to have major causes in the mode of life, in personal behaviour and the environment, and such statistics of the occurrence in various population groups and environments, and the often rapid ups and downs of frequency, may provide the first clues. I try to illustrate the range of information and some of the highlights; needless to say, there is no attempt to be comprehensive about what is now a substantial literature.

Sex and Age

Analysis of mortality by sex and age is an admirable introduction, so many questions immediately arise, and any theoretical model of carcinogenesis must be consistent with the patterns observed in human populations. Considering the "force of mortality" with *age* in *women* (Table 7.18), the rate for cancer of the cervix rises sharply till the late forties, in breast and ovarian cancer till the early fifties, and in cancer of the corpus uteri till the late fifties; thereafter the rates in this country tend to level off. This "biphasic" pattern may be related to hormonal function (a figure on log scale would have shown it better). In neoplasms with a major cure rate, *mortality* data are inadequate

TABLE 7.18
MORTALITY FROM CANCER AT DIFFERENT AGES

1970–2
England and Wales
Death Rates per 100,000 per Year

Sex and Site	Age						
	40–	45–	50–	55–	60–	65–	70–74
Men							
All Sites	67	134	249	461	770	1156	1608
Stomach	6·0	13	25	50	89	137	188
Lung, etc.	20	53	110	213	369	528	685
Prostate	0·1	0·8	2·8	8·6	23	55	116
Bladder	1·4	3·0	7·0	15	27	49	77
Women							
All sites	93	166	243	340	448	573	738
Stomach	3·3	6·2	9·9	19	33	52	91
Lung, etc.	7·6	17	32	45	62	73	81
Breast	33	54	70	89	100	110	120
Cervix uteri	8·4	15	21	20	20	20	22
Corpus uteri	0·8	2·1	4·3	7·7	12	14	18
Ovary	10	18	25	31	37	42	45

to describe the incidence with age. In fact, in all these examples the *incidence* rates in cancer registers tend to peak several years earlier.[7] The age pattern for cancer of the stomach is quite different, and other patterns can be identified for other sites.[7] Age, the summation of biologic and social experience, is of such importance in cancer that to regard it as a "cause" seems again sensible.

In *men*, total cancer mortality quadruples, broadly speaking, from 35–44 to 45–54, trebles from 45–54 to 55–64, then doubles from 55–64 to 65–74 years of age. In cancer of the stomach (? strongly behavioural, environmental) the trend of mortality with age is steeper; in prostatic cancer (? largely hormone-dependent) there are scarcely any cases at all till the late fifties when the death rate soars.

HISTORICAL STUDY

Cohort Analysis. — "The danger when studying age-specific death rates", writes Case, "is that it is easy to be misled into thinking that the rates for consecutive age groups in any given year, say the age groups 45–49, 50–54, 55–59, and so on, form a series of rates that reflects (only) the effect of age on susceptibility to cancer, an error that may sometimes cause serious misunderstanding. The people in the age group 55–59 in 1960 are, of course, the survivors of those who were in age group 50–54 in 1955, who are in turn the survivors of those in age group 45–49 in 1950, and so on: that is to say, they are the survivors of those born in the years 1901–05. If we wish to study the effect of age on the death rate we must, therefore, go back into the past and study the age- specific death rates of a group of people born within a fairly small defined number of years, and the survivors of that group through the ensuing years, so including the effects of experience as well as those of ageing itself. An environmental cause may have begun to operate at a particular time, so that in any given year the mortality in consecutive age groups reflects such factors as well as the effect of age."

A group of people defined at birth or at the beginning of a specified period (rather than by death or other event at the close of it) is called a "generation", or "cohort"; and study of the future history of such a group, of what happens to them as they "march through life", is called "cohort analysis" (the notion has already been introduced in Chapter 6). The method makes it possible to associate changing age-specific death rates with long-term environmental changes that have occurred during the lifetime of survivors of different cohorts. "Cohort analysis thus offers better chances of distinguishing between nature and nurture, and of correlating changes in the death rate with the social history of the period."[8] [10]

For example: Table 7.19, studying the death rates from lung cancer of the male cohorts born in successive 5 year periods from around 1880–81 onwards (the centres of each cohort being spaced five years apart), we see that the changes in mortality accord with the common use of the cigarette, now postulated to be the agent of the modern epidemic of the disease. Since smoking of these in any quantity began in the trenches and factories of the first world war, men born around the turn of the century will have been maximally exposed, the first generation to smoke to saturation — they were able to start smoking cigarettes in their teen's — whereas previous generations could develop the habit only later in life. In consequence, exposure increased progressively among cohorts born during the latter part of the nineteenth century, reaching a maximum in those born in the twentieth. The Table, covering the span of middle age, shows a rising mortality from lung cancer at each age of death in the cohorts born up till the turn of the century, and a levelling of these death rates, at a high ceiling, in later cohorts — conforming with the history of the cigarette habit. *Women* began to smoke cigarettes in quantity only during the second world war, and there is no sign yet of levelling of the rising death rates among them.

I find the "cohort" concept difficult to apply and have misgivings that elsewhere, in Chapters 1 and 2, and this section, age and age-specific death rates have been discussed without due allowance for possible interactions between the survivors of successive generations and the

TABLE 7.19
COHORT ANALYSIS OF LUNG-CANCER MORTALITY IN MEN
Age-Specific Death Rates from Lung-Cancer per 100,000 Men Born Around 1881, 1886, et seq.
England and Wales

Men Born Around	Age at Death				
	40–44	45–49	50–54	55–59	60–64
	Death Rates per 100,000 per year				
1881	2·7	7·6	26	59	102
1886	5·2	19	43	88	172
1891	8·7	27	60	135	255
1896	15	30	95	200	332
1901	*19*	*54*	*122*	*232*	*368*
1906	*24*	*58*	*125*	*230*	*373*
1911	*25*	*59*	*123*	*222*	
1916	*25*	*56*	*115*		
1921	*22*	*52*			
1926	*21*				

The last *figure* in each column is the age-specific death rate for 1966–70, the second last for 1961–5, etc.
Rate for 1971:

20	*53*	*111*	*206*	*369*

From Registrar General's Tables.

changing mode of life. For a start, it might routinely be recalled that those who passed critical periods of their lives during the Great Depression and/or World War 2 have a very different history from their predecessors or those who followed them. At the same time, cohort analysis permits more sophisticated forecasting.

Recent History of Cancer Mortality. — To return to the more conventional, Table 7.20 brings out the encouraging fact that, lung cancer

TABLE 7.20
RECENT HISTORY OF MORTALITY FROM CANCER[7] [8]

Ages 55–64
England and Wales
Death Rates per 100,000 per Year

Site	1921–30	1960–1	1970–1
MEN			
All Sites	467	602	611
Lung, bronchus	13	288	288
All, less lung, etc.	454	314	323
Mouth, tongue, etc.	46	5·7	7·9
Oesophagus	38	12	16
Stomach	106	86	70
Colon	51	31	34
Rectum	48	26	25
Liver, etc.	30	9·8	3·2
Pancreas	13	23	27
Prostate	16	15	15
Bladder	13	20	22
Brain	10*	14	12
Leukaemia	5.1*	11	11
WOMEN			
All Sites	417	350	391
Lung, bronchus	5	31	51
All, less lung, etc.	412	319	340
Stomach	67	34	26
Colon	51	33	33
Rectum	25	15	15
Liver, etc.	33	7·6	1·1
Pancreas	7·5	12	15
Breast	78	79	95
Cervix	22**	20	20
Corpus uteri	3·9**	13	10
Ovary	16	33	34
Bladder	48	5·0	5·4
Leukaemia	3·7*	7·9	6·8

*1936–8   **1940–4.

TABLE 7.21
MORTALITY FROM LUNG-CANCER IN METROPOLIS, TOWN AND COUNTRY

1950–53
England and Wales
Standardised Mortality Ratios*

Population	Men	Women
England and Wales	100	100
London County	156[†]	149[†]
Conurbations	126	121
Urban Areas		
Population 100,000+	111	101
„ 50-100,000	95	89
„ -50,000	84	86
All Rural Districts	64	76
"Truly Rural" Districts England	48	67
„ „ „ Wales	33	56

*All ages; the ratios are adjusted for age composition to the
national experience.
†1950–2. Hewitt, D. (1956) *Brit. J. prev. Soc. Med.,* **10,** 45.
Registrar General, *Area Mortality, 1951.* HMSO. London.

apart, mortality from cancer in men is lower than in the 1920's (after
rising before then for many years). Age 55–64 has been chosen for
illustration to complement the earlier discussions in the book. The
diagnosis 50 years ago will be less valid, e.g. in liver, pancreas. Total
death rate from cancer in women is indeed less, a modest advance
in health . . . The rate to be watched now is for *cancer of the stomach;*
mortality recently began to fall in this country, mysteriously, and
somewhat later than in America. [2] [5] [6] Amidst the anxiety over food
processing and additives in relation to carcinogenesis, this downturn,
it is evident now in many countries, is reassuring. Improvements in
diagnosis and treatment are unlikely to be responsible, perhaps improvement in food processing, preservation? . . . Most disappointing in
women's mortality is the high persistence in *cancer of the breast,*
during a period that has seen much attention to it and heroic adjustments
in therapy. (The 1970–71 rate is *not* an error.) The figures raise acutely
the issues broached at the close of Chapter 6. About 1 in 20 women
in this country may be expected to suffer (p. 100), and two-thirds
of these to die of breast cancer. In the famous New York study, earlier
diagnosis and prompt treatment reduced mortality by a third in
seven years of observation. Studies are under way in several centres of
the UK; we ourselves are comparing, validating and costing, physicians'
and others' clinical examination and X-ray mammography[13-14] . . .
What useful high risk groups can be described?

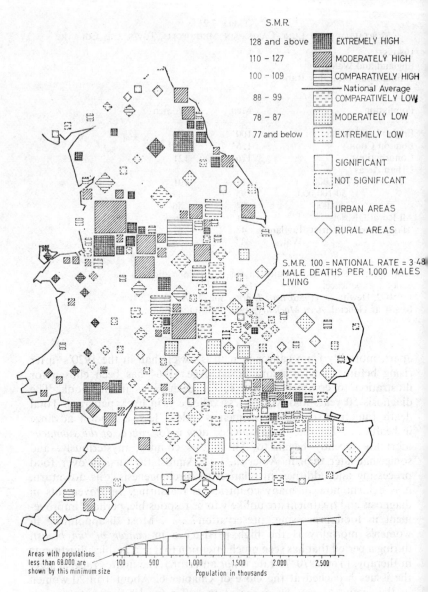

Cancer of Stomach: Males

Fig. 7.8 Local differences in mortality in England and Wales, 1959–63. All ages; the local rates are standardised by the national average for differences in their age-composition. The size of the 'squares' (representing urban areas) and of the 'diamonds' (rural) are proportional to the populations-at-risk.

Howe, G. M. (1970) *National Atlas of Disease Mortality in the United Kingdom*. Nelson, London.

In Different Places

Table 7.21 describes the mortality of lung cancer in relation to the density of population, or "urbanisation", another classical mode of analysis. The rate for men in London was three to four times that in the "truly rural" districts of England. An active search is under way for carcinogens (? polycyclic hydrocarbons) in the atmospheric pollution that follows from urban-industrial living. But, of course, they also smoke fewer cigarettes in the country, and smoking started later there.[15] A well known "exceptional instance" to emerge from this kind of elementary geography is Stocks' observation of an excess of cancer of the stomach in North and West Wales[16] (Fig. 7.8). This persists significantly year after year and is still unexplained. Have the inhabitants a special genetic composition? More blood-group A non-secretors (that particular trail was revived here)? Dietary habits of their own? What of the local geology of soil and water? Are there special diagnostic problems in the area? Etc. Numbers are small in these counties, which presents its own problems of validity.

Social Class

Two trends are very clear among the women (next page). The strong association with "poverty" in cervical cancer cannot be accounted for simply by the higher fertility rates of social classes 4 and 5. The higher mortality from cancer of the breast in upper socio-economic groups is a world-wide phenomenon and in this country it was even more pronounced in 1930–32. Speculation on connections between mode of life and endocrine function is in order.

Cancer and Fertility

Accepting the death rate at 45–64 years of age among married women who have borne a child as 1, the differing ratios for these four cancers in Table 7.23 are striking. . . The association of cervical cancer with the married state, and with the bearing of children, like the social class distribution, support, if rather remotely, the hypothesis previously stated.[18-20] There are several "clues" to cancer of the breast which is far and away the leading malignancy among women.[11] The steep rise in mortality is coterminous with the child-bearing period; the disease is less common among married women, in particular among women who have borne a child. An international collaborative study has now shown that the risk of breast cancer is directly related to the age at which women bear their first child: at the extreme, women who do so before the age of 18 years are at only a third the risk of those who do not have a child till they are 35 or later, or have no children.[21] The risk was found to be unrelated to breast-feeding; and the familiar social-class

TABLE 7.22
MORTALITY FROM CANCER IN THE FIVE SOCIAL CLASSES

1949–53
England and Wales
Standardised Mortality Ratios at 20–64 Years
All Classes = 100

Site	Social Class				
	1	2	3	4	5
Men					
Stomach	57	70	101	112	130
Lung	81	82	107	91	118
Prostate	128	99	102	93	102
Testis	164	121	92	98	90
Married Women					
Lung	119	95	102	98	96
Breast	137	110	104	84	85
Cervix uteri	64	75	98	105	134
Corpus uteri	110	93	110	85	95

Registrar General, *Decennial Supplement on Occupational Mortality,* HMSO, London.

TABLE 7.23
FERTILITY AND CANCER IN WOMEN

Mortality of Other Women Proportionate to that of Fertile Married Women
1950–53
England and Wales
Ratios at Ages 45–64 Years

Site	Married and Fertile*	Married and Infertile	Single
Breast	1	1·2†	1·4†
Cervix Uteri	1	0·7	0·4
Corpus Uteri	1	1·6	1·3
Ovary (and Fallopian Tubes)	1	1·7	1·4

*i.e. who have borne a child.
†1948–9; estimated.

Registrar General, Commentary vols. and personal communication.
Logan, W. P. D. (1953) *Lancet,* 2, 1199.

distribution was confirmed and shown to be independent of child-bearing. This part of the field is only one example of the as yet largely unrealised potential of record-linkage in the long natural history of cancer...[22] By way of "foresight", the reader might reconsider the implications for community medicine, and its strategy for health and prevention, of the trends in sex mores described on pages 62-64, for the future incidence of cancer in women, in cohorts dated by the changes in behaviour evident from the mid-1950's. For cervical cytology services, and for new ventures in the early diagnosis of breast cancer?

Working of Health Services

Research into death-certification, as a step towards its improvement, plainly is worthwhile: appraisal, for example, of how accurate the certificates are, how complete, and so what inferences may safely be drawn from them.[23] The General Register Office has made several studies.[23-25]

MORBIDITY — AND THE NATIONAL CANCER REGISTRATION SCHEME[3] [7]

Epidemiological data of absorbing interest are becoming available from the NCRS which includes about three-quarters (why $\frac{3}{4}$?) of the malignancies now recognised in England and Wales and links the disease recognition with mortality records. Table 1 in Chapter 4 is a successful product of the scheme. Readers working in British hospitals might examine how the records are completed in them (in their name), and consider also how the report forms could be improved to yield more information for aetiological research as well as clinical control. Cancer is highly suitable for registration: "The patient will usually seek medical care for the condition, the diagnosis is relatively specific and definitive, and good co-operation can be obtained because the condition is widely recognised as of major importance" But greater rigour and standardisation of diagnosis often are needed. In all, corresponding to the 100,000 deaths, about 150,000 new cases are encountered annually, seven or eight in the "average" general practice of England and Wales.

GEOGRAPHICAL PATHOLOGY[1-8]

Britain is a small country yet striking differences have been found within it in the incidence of cancer of the stomach and cancer of the lung. By tradition, the term "geographical pathology" is used for the comparative study of countries, or between ethnic and national — not merely social — groups within them. In the search for clues to causes, the geographical method has been particularly fruitful in atherosclerosis-ischaemic heart disease [9-13] and in cancer.[14-19]

One of the solid facts about ischaemic heart disease is that the half or two-thirds of the world which is very poor suffers little from it. This generalisation has stimulated much enquiry, and it is a main plank of today's leading dietary hypothesis: that the low incidence of IHD among peoples at an early stage of economic development is associated with their low mean concentration of plasma cholesterol, and this, it is postulated in turn, reflects the plane of nutrition and, in particular, low intake of animal and dairy (saturated) fats. Table 7.24, from the International Atherosclerosis Project, supports the hypothesis, but mainly for total fat: correlations were weaker with animal fat (and with sucrose). Genetic causes also may be important in the contrasting susceptibility of populations. So — in another tradition — it was established that mortality from IHD among the (selected) middle-aged Japanese emigré men in Hawaii is higher than among their counterparts in Japan and, a move further West, among Japanese men in the USA is higher still and resembles that of white Americans.[20] [21]

An equally challenging "international" fact: death rates during middle age are substantially higher in the USA than in Sweden, the English rates lying in between; ischaemic heart disease is much involved and, indeed, cardiovascular mortality in American men under 65, is almost as great as total mortality in Sweden (Table 7.25). Perhaps we can achieve some prevention of heart-attack without scrapping the Western mode of life and going back to nature.

Sweden as well as USA is over twice as rich as the UK, and health-service expenditure per person in 1969 was about 6½ per cent of GNP in both countries against 4½ per cent here (since then rising in all three). USA has substantially more doctors than the other two countries, but the most interesting figures are for general hospitals. Overall, both Sweden and USA had a 40 per cent higher admission rate than England and Wales; average length of stay in the US hospitals was 9·3 days, in England and Wales 11·1, and in Sweden 12·6 days. Perhaps important. (But what do we expect of "medical care"? Among middle-aged men of this country, heart-attack and stroke, plus lung and stomach-cancer, account for 60 per cent of deaths, p. 65; and much of the 40 per cent remainder is as intractable). Alcohol consumption is similar in the three countries; of tobacco per adult in 1970, 9·4, 5·9 and 4·5 lbs, in the order of the death rates. (Maxwell, R. (1974) *Health Care: The Growing Dilemma*. New York) . . . I add that animal fats are eaten in similar quantities in the three countries. Sweden, however, is substantially lower on calories than the other two, 200–300 less per day. FAO *Food Balance Sheets, 1964–66*, Rome. This, together with the higher level of physical activity in that country of which a traveller can tell, should also be worth following up.

Cancer Variation

Cancer is apparently common in all countries, though localisation of the malignant growth shows marked differences, the reasons for which are increasingly being sought in differences of environment and personal habits. Higginson, of the International Agency for Research on Cancer, has estimated that some 90 per cent of all human cancers probably arise from removable causes in these.[22] Table 7.26, on page 212, shows the range of incidence in ten populations advanced in social development (including their health-information systems). Aggregate differences

TABLE 7·24
ATHEROSCLEROSIS IN "DEVELOPED" AND "DEVELOPING" COUNTRIES

Prevalence of Advanced Lesions of Aorta and Coronary Arteries;
Levels of Total Serum Cholesterol; and
Consumption of Fat in Different Populations
Men and Women Aged 25–64

Location– Ethnic Group	Athero- Sclerosis (a)	Ranking of Serum Cholesterol (b)	Per Cent Calories from Fat (c)
Oslo	2	2	1
New Orleans White	1	1	2
Manila	4	6	8
Caracas	5		9
Jamaica	6		7
Puerto Rico	7	4	4
Cali	8	8	14
Sao Paulo White	9		3
Lima	10	10	6
San José	11	11	15
Santiago	12	5	13
Bogotá	13	9	11
Guatemala	14	12	12
Durban Bantu	15	7	10

Rank order correlation coefficients, r, (a) and (b), 0·688; and (a) and (c), 0·755;
both highly significant.
Scrimshaw, N. S. and Guzmán, M. A. (1968) *Lab. Investig.*, **18**, 623; *The Geographic Pathology of Atherosclerosis* (1968) Ed. McGill, H. Baltimore.

TABLE 7·25
DEATH RATES: ALL CAUSES AND CARDIOVASCULAR DISEASE

1970
Rates per 1,000

	Men				Women			
	45–54		55–64		45–54		55–64	
	All	CVD	All	CVD	All	CVD	All	CVD
USA White	8·8	4·1	22·0	11·5	4·6	1·3	10·1	4·1
England and Wales	7·0	3·5	21·0	10·2	4·3	1·2	10·2	4·1
Sweden	5·4	2·0	13·9	6·8	3·4	0·7	7·8	2·7

National Center for Health Statistics, Washington, DC;
Registrar General; World Health Organisation.

TABLE 7.26
INCIDENCE OF CANCER IN TEN "DEVELOPED" COUNTRIES

Standardised Rates per 100,000 Population-at-Risk
All Ages
Early 1960's Mostly

Site*	Highest Rate		Lowest Rate	
Males				
Tongue	Connecticut	3·2	Israel, All Jews	0·3
Oesophagus	Finland	6·6	Alberta/Sweden	2·0/2·7
Stomach	Finland	45	Alberta	14
Colon	Connecticut	27	Finland	6·8
Rectum	Denmark	17	Norway	6·8
Lung	Birmingham	73	Norway	17
Prostate	New Zealand European	40	Israel	13
All Sites**	Connecticut	258	Norway/Alberta	175/176
Females				
Breast	Connecticut	62	Finland	29
Cervix	Denmark	31	Israel	4·9
Corpus uteri	Connecticut	15	Scotland	7
All Sites**	Connecticut	220	Scotland	159

Rates are standardised on a model "world" population.
*7th Revision of the ICD (*International Statistical Classification of Diseases, Injuries, and Causes of Death*) (1957). WHO, Geneva.
**Excluding skin cancer.
   From UICC: Cancer Incidence in Five Continents. Ed., Doll, R., Muir, C. S. & Waterhouse, J. (1970) Vol. II. UICC, Geneva; Higginson, J. & MacLennan, R. (1973). In *Modern Trends in Oncology – 1 Part 1: Research Progress.* Ed., Raven, R. W. London; Waterhouse, J. (1974). Personal communication.

are smaller than the astonishing variations in site frequency. This is a traditional arena for generating new ideas and testing the old: to survive, an hypothesis on aetiology *must* be consistent with such facts of life. The higher rate of lung cancer in Finland than Norway can be explained by past differences in smoking habits. The Israeli experience in cancer of the cervix confirms findings among Jews in New York and supports the hypothesis on sexual behaviour. And so on.

Some of the contrasts with less developed populations are even more striking. There are enough clinical impressions and travellers' tales, and hospital figures are liable to be biased, cf. page 124. But incidence rates are now becoming available. In these two *African populations:*

Men

	Oeso-phagus	Colon	Liver	Testis	ALL
Bulawayo	76	8·0	48	0·0	300
Natal	41	2·0	28	0·1	206

The highest rate for liver cancer among the ten "developed" countries was 2·5 in Sweden, and the lowest for testis cancer 0·8 in Finland.

In women

	Breast	Cervix	Corpus uteri	ALL
Bulawayo	36	80	3·6	369
Natal	12	49	4·7	161

Nitrosamines are being intensively investigated in cancer of the oeso-phagus; in cancer of the liver, aflatoxins.[24]

Disorders of the Large Intestine; Economic Development; Food Processing[25]

Burkitt brings together the non-infective disorders of the bowel, uncommon in poor developing countries living in a traditional manner and on a largely vegetarian diet, but widespread health problems of the "West". I paraphrase:

> Constipation ("normal" in the West)
> Appendicitis (the commonest abdominal emergency)
> Diverticular disease (present in perhaps quarter the population after middle age)
> Polyposis (reported in one-fifth of necropsies after age 20)
> Carcinoma of the colon (cancer characteristic of developed countries)
> Carcinoma of the rectum.

He associates these conditions not merely in their geographical distribution but in the date of their emergence in particular communities: appendicitis, he thus suggests, begins to increase several decades before the others. Searching for causes in the "western" mode of life, this is the postulated chain of events:

An increased consumption of fibre-depleted carbohydrate foods, and of sugar and highly refined flour in particular, results in reduced intake of fibre which, in turn, leads to prolongation of intestinal transit times and the passage of small, firm stools. The muscular effort of the colon required to propel the viscid faeces raises intra-luminal pressure, forcing out diverticula . . . Raised pressure in the appendix, distal to obstruction . . . Stasis is believed to enhance the formation and increase the concentration of potential carcinogens in the faeces. . . [25] [26]

A grand hypothesis like this needs testing by all the ways of learning in medicine. . . Meanwhile, the British *population* data show no fall in fibre intake since early this century, though less of it comes from cereals.[27] Recent *hospital-admission* and *mortality rates* do not show a rise in appendicitis or bowel cancer.[28]

Colon Cancer of "Western" Countries and the High-Fat Diet

Williams and his colleagues [29] have found that where there is a high incidence of *cancer of the colon,* as in the U.K. and U.S.A. by comparison with African and Eastern countries, people have higher concentration of bile salts in their stools, and local anaerobic bacteria (bacteroides and certain clostridia) are more capable of degrading the bile salts: these steroid bile-acid derivatives, it is postulated, are carcinogens or co-carcinogens. This mechanism, they think, may link the high rate of colon cancer in "developed" countries to the fact that these have a high national fat-intake.[30] [31] Laboratory and epidemiological research is actively under way.

World Medicine

"Experiments of opportunity" are being recognised on a world scale in contrasts of genetics, mode of life, and disease prevalence. The low rates of breast cancer in Japanese women was for nearly 50 years ascribed to protection by lactation, which tends to be prolonged among the Japanese, before refuted.[32] MacMahon is leading a world-wide enquiry whose main finding on the protection by early child-bearing (or, anyhow, by the second half of pregnancy) has already been reported . . .[17] In Kerala, S. India, there is high background radiation: What of the incidence of congenital malformation, leukaemia, etc?[33] There is less hypertension at high altitudes, and in lowlanders living in the high Andes there seems to be actual reduction in blood pressure levels.[34] Can this be related also to other changes in the mode of life? To exercise, or to diet? . . . The Masai in Kenya eat a high animal-fat diet, how come they have low blood cholesterol levels and IHD?[35] [36] Yemenite Jews, like many others, are experiencing the effects of abrupt exposure to a Western mode of life; since all have immigrated to Israel there is a unique opportunity for family genetic studies to be done concurrently with environmental.[37-39] Table 7.27 about a polymorphic trait illustrates the kind of study of population genetics made possible in Israel by the "ingathering of the exiles".

Disease clusters are legion; for an inveterate list-maker this is a dangerous opening. Amyotrophic lateral sclerosis in Guam,[40] betalipoproteinaemia in the Lebanon,[41] cerebrovascular disease in Japan,[42] diabetes in the Pima Indians,[43] eclampsia unknown,[44] favism in Sardinia.[45] Or, cancer of the mouth in India, pharynx in Sweden, oesophagus in the Caspian littoral, and Brittany, stomach in Japan, liver in the Bantu, pancreas in the US Negroes, small intestine nowhere,

TABLE 7.27
FREQUENCY OF GLUCOSE 6 PHOSPHATE DEHYDROGENASE DEFICIENCY
Males of Some Jewish Communities in Israel

Continent: And Ethnic Group		Per Cent Affected*
Europe:	Ashkenazim	0·4
Asia:	Non-Ashkenazim	
	From Yemen	5·0
	From Cochin	10·0
	From Iraq	25·0
	From Kurdistan	58·0

*The gene is carried on the X chromosome so that the *percentage of males affected* is the same as the gene frequency and is a direct measure of the prevalence in the community. Random sample studies.
Sheba, C., Szeinberg, A., Ramot, B., Adam, A., Ashkenazi, I. (1962) *Amer. J. publ. Hlth.*, **52**, 1101; personal communication.
Genetic Polymorphisms and Geographic Variations in Disease (1962) Ed. Blumberg, B.S. New York.

colon in Canada, and rectum unknown.[2] [14] [15] [18] [24] [46] The historic description by Burkitt, O'Connor and Davies of multiple malignant lymphoma among children in Uganda and later by virtuoso map-making in a defined if large area of tropical Africa (Fig. 7.9), next page, led to the hunt for an arthropod vector that could explain the distribution and a viral agent. Malaria and its consequences, it now appears, are related [47] [48] and the E.B. virus is strongly suspected.

INTERNATIONAL COLLABORATION

Adapting the words of WHO,[49] the essential prerequisites for co-operative international study is to standardise nomenclature, definitions, techniques. That accepted, the following categories of inquiry may be rewarding and justify the labour involved.

(1) Problems for which world experience is the unit of knowledge. Such are population, the genetic description of populations, pollution, the diseases of a world on the move, health services.

(2) Diseases in the study of which the contrasts between countries might be stimulating; as illustrated.

(3) When numbers of cases, or of persons exposed to a suspected cause, in any one country are too small. For example, studies of persons exposed to certain ionising radiations (women treated for cancer of the cervix uteri, patients given thorotrast), or the investigation of asbestos-mesothelioma have required the assembly of data from several countries in America and Europe.

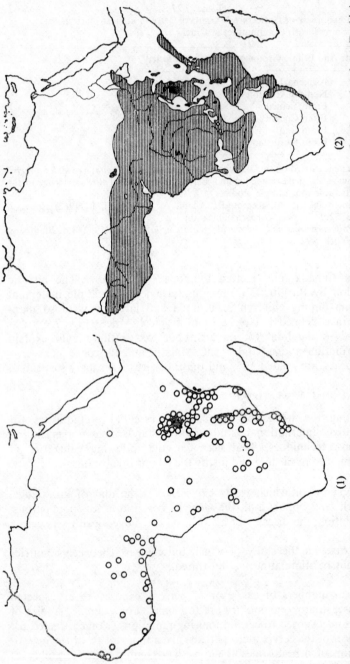

Fig. 7.9 (1) 'A tumour safari' in East and Central Africa: the circles represent areas of known distribution of *malignant lymphoma* (Burkitt). (2) Climate: the shaded part of the map represents areas of Africa where the temperature does not fall below 60°F (15°C) and the annual rainfall is above 20 inches (Haddows, A. J.).
Burkitt, D. (1962) *Brit. J. Cancer* **16**, 379; (1961) *East Afr. med. J.* **38**, 511; (1963) *Cancer: Progress*, (ed.) Raven, R. W., p. 102. Butterworth, London.

(4) Conditions of limited distribution intensive study of which can illumine thought in other fields, for example Chagas' aortic disease or Balkan nephropathy, high cadmium intake in rice-eating countries, and specific genetically determined conditions (Huntingdon's chorea or acatalassemia).

(5) When there have been substantial migrations of populations. Thus, among Japanese emigrating to the USA, the high risk of cancer of the stomach and the low of cancer of the colon and cancer of the breast which are characteristic of the home country, appear to change sooner or later towards the American — "Western" — pattern: evidence for environmental, behavioural causes.

The preamble contains the main point: useful collaboration depends on common language and the comparability of data.[50] *Joint expeditions* are one answer, for example the studies of ischaemic heart disease by Keys and his associates.[13] *Parallel studies* in several countries under central control and using the same protocols are another;[51] and the international study of schizophrenia and its diagnosis, for example.[52][53] *Standard methods* are another — [54] uniform questionnaires, records and registration systems, X-ray and biochemical reference centres, the use of model case-material.

The Appropriate Universe in Physiological Studies

The opportunity is now opening up for international study to define the healthy, the normal in that sense (the word will not go away) and not merely the common or average. Western populations, as said, have high mean levels of plasma cholesterol and a steep rise with age. What are the normal — healthy — ranges? What is universal and what locally specific? What are the inherited and acquired, biological and social factors that produce a country's characteristic lipid profile? This is to ask what is the appropriate universe for physiological study, next page. . . My own introduction to such a "cross-cultural" approach was the other way round, by the laboratory technician in China who believed that what he was seeing all the time and we call mega-loblastic degeneration of the bone marrow was "normal".

And in Behaviour

Observation how people behave (and what is approved) in different cultures, how others imagine is the right way to run a family or bring up children, has transformed the world-view of what is the human predicament and what merely our kind of society (or even Vienna).[55-57] Every medical student used to read Margaret Mead: "A number of related forces," she wrote, "have combined to make the adolescent in America (and I add Britain) stand at the point of highest pressures and difficulty, just as another set of forces place her at the lowest point of pressure in Samoa,"[58] Whatever the validity of the particular

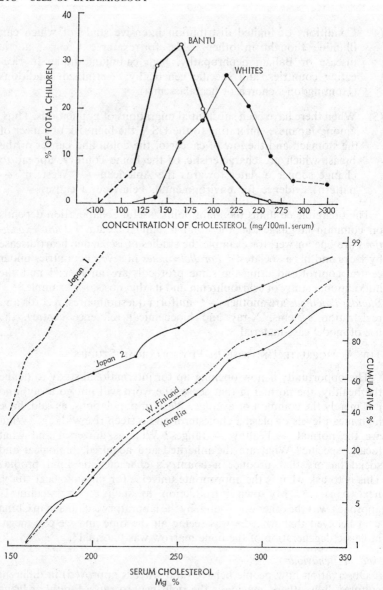

Fig. 7.10 Serum cholesterol in several populations. *Upper figure:* Distribution in Pretoria (South Africa) children of 7–11 years. 322 Bantu, 464 White. *Lower figure:* Distribution in men of 40–59 years. Numbers ranged from 112–240 in each five-year sample. Japan 1, fishing; Japan 2, farming; both Finnish are rural and small-town populations.

Upper: Duplessis, J. P., Vivier, F. S. & DeLange, D. J. (1967) *S.A. med J.* **41**, 1216; see also ibid (1969) **43**, 1516. *Lower:* Kimura, N. (p.231); Karvonen, M. J., Blomquist, G., Kallio, V., Orma, E., Punsar, S., Rautaharju, P., Takkunen, J. & Keys, A. In *Acta med. Scand.* (1967) Suppl. 460. (p.169).

example, it plainly is misleading to diagnose social behaviour and mental functioning on a sample of one culture only.

MULTIRACIAL SOCIETY[59-61]

The massive immigration into Britain in the 1960's from the West Indies, India and Pakistan, Cyprus, Malta, Africa (on top of the customary flow from Ireland and the old Dominions) means that these frontiers are here now at home. Appreciation of the cultural differences in family structure and child care, in the attitudes to health, in short and long-terms goals — as well as in the diseases the immigrants bring with them or acquire here — have suddenly acquired a new significance for Britain, for all of us in medicine and for social policy. And there is a new cultural "distance"—between overseas doctors and native patients.

ECOLOGY OF MENTAL DISORDERS[1-9]

The title pays tribute to Faris and Dunham whose study in Chicago in the 1930's opened the modern era of the epidemiology of psychosis. Examining mental-hospital admissions for schizophrenia, they found a striking excess from the deteriorating centre of the city, from skid row and the slums near the railway termini with their lodging houses and population of transients and down-and-outs. Conversely, the lowest admission rates were found among the more stable population of the outer residential tracts.[10] In recent years there have been many such observations: mental disorders, it is evident, are strongly connected with the mode of life, with social class and community structure. Equally evident, multiple causes, genetic as well as environmental, biological and social, are somehow involved. Major advances on causation have been made only in mental disorders with a physical basis and specific agent, for example in GPI, pellagra, the severe subnormalities. In *suicide*, possibly, we can begin to think of preventive programmes: treating depression; combating isolation especially in the old and bereaved; specific befriending by telephone helpers; clinical alertness to warning signals in alcoholism and in the modern epidemic of self-poisoning; the use of North Sea gas or ordinary gas with less CO— these measures may already be disrupting the pattern of final disaster.[11-14]

It is scarcely surprising that so little has been learned of aetiology, so intractable is the nature of much of the material. Earlier, p. 44, I have remarked how troublesome it is to agree on what is a "case" and to achieve a reproducible diagnosis merely on history and clinical observation.[15-19] Recognition may be simple only when there is gross disorder of mental function and social relations and manifest disability.

References on page 304.

When disorder is less severe and does not involve the whole personality, or is accompanied by little distress and/or disability, it can be very troublesome to agree criteria on which a person is to be regarded as sick or not. Moreover, his social network, rather than the individual, often may be the meaningful unit of study — and that again presents special difficulties. Definition of what is "healthy" or "unhealthy" in human behaviour is usually quantitative, but over a great range. Diseases and syndromes often are poorly defined and investigators have to fall back on listing of symptoms, mood and behaviour. This of course may be rewarding, symptoms have meaning; but various and even contrary meanings. That a person is anxious tells nothing about aetiology. A family may be peaceable because in harmony, or just conforming and liable to crack under the first strain; how discern what lies beneath the surface? Or, again, the same psychological forces can be manifest in diverse mental, social and physical effects. There are many outlets for aggression; a complete clinical picture of depression may be unattainable. The same kind of overprotective family situation seems to be found as often as it is looked for, preceding a multitude of disorders. . . Be all this as it may, there is a sad dearth of hard fact on the causes of major as well as minor mental disorders, and so on how to prevent them. But what I hadn't appreciated till scanning again the mass of literature that accumulated since the last edition, was the dearth of epidemiological work *in search of causes*, a situation somewhat obscured by the communicativeness of psychiatrists and social scientists. Lack of ideas? Methods? Money? Investigators? Is the "medical model" of disease entities, and their causation, misleading? It wants airing. Of course, the popular trend open-endedly to hand over to psychiatry (and to social work), in hope or in resignation, the whole of the human condition is no help.

Faris and Dunham's observations touched off a controversy that is still echoing, though the actual problem is relatively simple. Is it that the multiple deprivations of the social environment which they described *breed* an excess incidence of schizophrenia? Or, interesting enough but telling us far less about "causes", is it merely that the victims of schizophrenia, perhaps in the early stages of the illness or precursor disturbance, *drift* into these areas of the city? . . Classically, in the old, blighted city centres, there is, or was as in Chicago, a clustering of physical, mental and social pathology, of crowding, squalor and poverty, unskilled occupations and unemployment, multi-problem families and neglected children, violence and crime, prostitution and venereal disease, tuberculosis, hard-drug addiction, alcoholism, mental disorder. (And, very likely also, an army, if never enough, of social-medical workers.) Table 7.28 is an illustration from a district nearer home where our unit worked for many years. Group relationships are liable to be weak, isolation common, and standards of behaviour ill-defined; there is "a high tolerance of psychological pathology of all

TABLE 7.28
SOCIAL DEPRIVATION, SOCIAL PATHOLOGY[21]
1960's

POPULATION	SOCIAL CLASS	HOUSING			HEALTH			CHILDREN			OLD PEOPLE
	SC 4 & 5 (%)	Households no hot water tap (%)	Shared WC (%)	Over-crowding (%)	Infant mortality (‰)	TB cases (‰)	Mental hospital discharges (‰)	At school at 16 (%)	Received into care (‰)	Juvenile delinquency (‰)	Pensioners living alone (%)
	(1)	(2)	(3)	(4)	(5)	(6)	(7)	(8)	(9)	(10)	(11)
England and Wales	26	12	6	3	18	7	4	36	5	20	20
Inner London Borough of Tower Hamlets*	37	35	21	8	17	12	6	20	25	37	27
One ward in this borough*	43	55	32	10	22	27	9	16	27	46	42

*Population, 1966, 200,000; of the ward, 11,730. Age-compositions are unremarkable.
Power, M. J., personal communications.

Notes to Table 7.28

Col. (1) Per cent all personal service, semi and unskilled manual workers (in Social-Economic Groups 7, 10, 11, 15; SC 4 & 5) as proportion of all economically active and retired males over 15 years. Census 1966 *Summary Tables*. Gt. Britain (E & W); County Report Greater London; Enumeration District Tables.

Col. (2) Per cent households, no hot water tap, of all households. Census 1966 (as Col.1).

Col. (3) Per cent households, sharing inside or outside WC, of all households. Census 1966 (as Col. 1).

Col. (4) Per cent households, density of over 1·5 persons per room, of all households. Census 1966 (as Col.1).

Col. (5) Rate per 1,000, deaths under one year of all live births – R.G., *Stat. Rev.,* Pt. 2, 1967. *Annual Report,* Tower Hamlets, MOH.

Col. (6) Rate of cases on Register at 31.12.67 per 1,000 of total population. Personal communication, DHSS. *Annual Report,* Tower Hamlets, MOH.

Col. (7) Rate, per 1,000 population over 15, discharges from Mental Hospitals to East London, 1967. *Report of Psychiatric Rehabilitation Assn.* London.

Average general hospital beds occupied per 1,000 in 1970; E & W, 4; Tower Hamlets, 9·3. (Ashley, J. S. A., personal communications).

Col. (8) Per cent at 16 years, boys at school, of all boys of this age. *Education Statistics,* 1966. HMSO, London. *Annual Abstract Greater London Statistics, 1966.*

Col. (9) Rate of receptions into care, 1967/68, per 1,000 of all under 18. Home Office *Child Care Statistics* 1966/67. Childrens Officer Tower Hamlets, personal communication.

Col. (10) Rate of first court appearance (case proven) per 1,000 boys, ages 10–17 years, in 1967. Home Office *Supplement. Crim. Stats.* for 1967. MRC Social Medicine Unit. (A typical year.)

Col. (11) Per cent all males, 65+, and females 60+ living alone, of total population of this age group. Census 1966 (as Col. 1).

By tradition, Tower Hamlets receives immigrants. During the 1960's they constituted c. 9% of the population of the borough and the ward, many of them latterly coming from the new commonwealth.

sorts". Does the personal chaos of schizophrenia derive from this social disorganisation which deforms the thought patterns, communication and interpersonal relations of the child (genetically) predisposed to the disease? Or is there a high prevalence of schizophrenia in these areas for the same reasons that bring others there who are unable to cope, are at odds with society, who need to withdraw from close emotional involvements? In brief, is there social generation of the disease, or social selection and segregation by it? How important it is to find some aetiological answers is plain in the personal misery of which every reader will know — and in health-service statistics: close to half of all patients in mental hospitals, about a seventh of the patients in all hospitals, are labelled "schizophrenic". About 1 per cent of the population may be expected to become schizophrenic between 15 and 45 years of age.

The answer to this key question from a pair of studies seems clear enough — at any rate for this country and what is or was recognised here as "schizophrenic" disorder.[20] [21] Goldberg made a direct *clinical study of a consecutive series of young men admitted for schizophrenic disorders to a typical metropolitan-district mental hospital.* This assured uniformity in diagnosis, the considered assessment of currently practising specialist-psychiatrists; and the clinical situation permitted fuller social study than is possible on a mass scale. She found that the paternal occupational careers were quite unremarkable (this applied also to grandfathers, uncles, and sibs): there was nothing unusual in the social circumstances of the children's upbringing, last 2 cols. of (A), next page. On the other hand, the failure of the young men themselves was striking. Sometimes at school, but commonly in late adolescence, as the case-histories showed, they were unable to make the grade. Some did not start at all on the jobs that were envisaged for them; some retreated after a while into routine or unskilled work carrying little responsibility; others in whom the illness developed more acutely dropped out of the labour market altogether. Thus, as the tragedy unfolded and they had to be admitted to hospital, the occupation, and "social class", of the patients was often well below that of their families. In studying the aetiology of a condition that is so liable to change the mode of life, the sequence of events and the "incidence" again are the crucial facts. It may be inordinately difficult to date the onset of "schizophrenia", but definition of "first attack" by first admission to mental hospital is manifestly too late to be useful.

Morrison complemented these case-studies by *documentary survey of national samples of individual first admissions to mental hospitals.* He found the customary excess of young men diagnosed "schizophrenic" in class 5, Table 7.29 (B), the miscellaneous labourers, kitchen hands, etc. Then he confirmed from the birth certificates of the young men that their fathers were quite ordinarily distributed by social class. The

TABLE 7.29
SOCIAL "DRIFT" AND SCHIZOPHRENIA[20] [21]

(A)
Social Class of Consecutive Sample of Male Patients Under 30 Years of Age Admitted to a Mental Hospital in Greater London; and of Their Families
1958–62

| Social Class | Patients | | Fathers Main Job | Other Male First-Degree Relatives Main Job |
	At First Admission	Last Known*		
1 and 2**	8	1	15	54
3	21	15	25	129
4	7	11	5	21
5	14	7	7	24
No occupation	—	18	—	11
?	2	—	—	26

*After 2-4 years' follow-up.
**Including students.

(B)
Social Class of National Sample of Male Patients Aged 25–34 Years Admitted for the First Time to a Mental Hospital; and of Their Fathers when These Patients were Born
1956
England and Wales

| Social Class | Patients | | Fathers | |
	Observed	Expected*	Observed	Expected*
1	12	12	14	8
2	21	44	42	42
3	178	203	192	191
4	52	55	66	68
5	90	39	55	59
?	18	—	2	—

*"Expected," on the national distribution at the relevant Census.

sons, that is, were not born disproportionately into social class 5 but themselves had drifted subsequently into it.*

Colleagues thus established in independent studies, at different levels of enquiry, that movement downwards was responsible for the well known social concentration of schizophrenia. (Contrariwise, manic-depressive psychosis, which often leaves the personality relatively intact between episodes does not lead to such mobility and, indeed, in the original studies in Chicago the residential distribution among the

*This is another example of the use of official, administrative records for medical research: two routine documents (the mental-hospital admission card and the birth certificate) were linked to provide valuable data on the familial aspect of disease. The information used is simple, valid enough to be used, and there is plenty of it.

census tracts was rather uniform.) The correct answer was obtained by direct enquiry, and by asking not merely in what social class patients were found (patients representative of the disease and of the population), but how they came to be there. Both studies depended on hospital data with their multiple biases. But there was nothing in the clinical series, in the social distribution of patients with relatively early disease for example, to suggest that selection of patients for admission to mental hospital was responsible for the deficit from classes 2 - 3 or the excess from class 5.

Schizophrenia is widespread through the population, the classical florid disease seems to be common the world over — which points to an organic basis and to heredity, confirmed in the high incidence in first-degree relatives — and/or to environmental causes different from those so far considered.[22-25] The possibility that a peculiar disorder of early family relations and communication is a cause of the disease has attracted intense public interest,[26] though as stated the hypothesis is very hard to test — one of the numerous major issues now confronting social medicine that can be clearly defined but taken little further. Meanwhile, as well as the genetic disposition, it is clear that general, non-specific, traumatic life-situations can precipitate breakdown with schizophrenia also, initial and recurrent,[27 28] and in view of the effectiveness of early and prompt treatment of acute episodes this offers an opening to the community physician.

"Culture of Poverty"[29-34]

Multiple genes evidently are involved in *low (measured) intelligence,* in the "slightly subnormal" end of the distribution curve. It could be that an element of foetal brain damage also sometimes is present. But, it is becoming clear, the relatively poor performance of deprived groups, ethnic as well as social-economic, in meeting the demands of the "culture", is compounded by multiple denial of elementary psychological and physical needs, including nutritional, very likely in the developing countries. Children in these circumstances are likely to suffer from lack of environmental stimulation (input), of opportunity to exercise intellect and communication, retarded growth from the wasting away of that which is not used. Their lower "IQ" will also be a result of the lower aspirations, the inferior self-image of these underprivileged groups, "the self-fulfilling prophecy of the city slum". Of course some also will have drifted there because. . . The same process of retardation and frustration is apparent in the inferior "educability" of lower working-class children, by comparison with better-placed children having similar inherited intelligence, Table 7.30.

TABLE 7.30
PSYCHOLOGICAL AND EDUCATIONAL DEFICITS; SOCIAL MALADJUSTMENT[35-47]
LOWER WORKING-CLASS CHILDREN
Britain
Reports from Cohort Studies, 1940's to 1970's

INFANCY
First words and sentences spoken later than average

DETECTED IN EARLY CHILDHOOD
Behavioural unresponsiveness
Lower IQ
Cognitive skills:
Restricted linguistic code
Less and later grasp of writing
                       reading
                       drawing
                       numbers

DETECTED IN LATER CHILDHOOD
School attainment at apparent same level of ability:
Slower learning
Less improvement
Fewer good certificates gained
More school absences
Earlier school leaving
More dropouts, failures
Social adjustment, competence:
Disturbed behaviour reported more often
More often brought before the Courts

YOUNG PEOPLE
Fewer university places gained; more wastage
More teenage pregnancies, marriages

Multiple causes implicated in "lower working-class":
Low wages — Unfit housing — (Nutrition —) IQ means and distribution — Large
families — Disorganised, single-parent homes — Coloured immigration — School
opportunities; utilisation — North regions — Inner city blight — Perinatal injury —
Physical and mental handicap — Parental occupation; education; communication,
interest, stimulation; mothering — "Transmitted cycle of deprivation" — Heredity

(B)
Heights and Weights of Glasgow Children by Social Class
Averages 1970

| | Boys | | | | Girls | | | |
| | 5 years | | 13 years | | 5 years | | 13 years | |
Social Class	Ht	Wt	Ht	Wt	Ht	Wt	Ht	Wt
1	43·8	43·2	61·6	101·8	43·6	43·6	61·9	107·2
3	42·6	42·2	60·0	96·5	42·4	41·2	60·2	101·2
5	41·9	41·0	59·9	91·9	41·6	39·7	59·3	98·7

Inches and pounds.
cf. Table 1.2, page 6.

Early experience and personal relationships seem to be crucial in personality development: "The complete disruption of *mother-child* relationship by death or serious illness is much less common now than it was 50 or even 30 years ago," wrote Carstairs. "But what of the quality of that relationship when it is not interrupted? Bowlby claims that a child experiencing maternal deprivation in infancy may become peculiarly susceptible to psychiatric disorders in later life (and that) maternal deprivation occurs when mother and child fail to establish a 'warm, intimate and continuous relationship in which both find satisfaction and enjoyment. . .' It is difficult to believe that maternal care of this quality was very common in the slums of our large cities either in the early years of the century or during the depression of the 1930's — or even today. Close family ties can exist in spite of overcrowding and poverty, but on the whole the younger children of a large slum family are unlikely to enjoy relationships with their harassed mothers in which both find satisfaction and enjoyment. . .[48] Supporting data on the possibility of long-term consequences for human relationships of such social pathology, in emotional disorder and in psychopathy, are conflicting as well as scanty, but the hypothesis makes good sense. Much study is now in progress in search of what hopefully is a "general cause" of mental health, study ranging from problem families to the ethology of animal development, and including some epidemiology.[49-52] The recent rediscovery of the "cycle of deprivation" (disadvantage breeding disadvantage) is an opening to population study and, even more, to action research. It complements Table 30 (A) and (B) and the discussions of juvenile rheumatism, perinatal and postneonatal mortality, et al.

MODERN WORLD

Epidemiological enquiry should also be making a relevant study of contemporary social life: helping to define where it provides supports and new sources of health; what are the prevalent social stresses, the new frustrations; how the rising expectations of personal fulfilment are working out; and whether this "epidemic constitution" is resulting in discernible changes in mental health and in the frequency, character or presentation of mental disorders. (Of course this should be done together with behavioural sciences, though they do go on about alienation, to misquote Auden.) I have previously referred to this classic and most difficult of questions, one that has often been asked since the upheavals of the American and French Revolutions,[53] but there are few answers. Simple answers only in such new phenomena as cortisol, dialysis, LSD and insecticide psychoses; methadone addiction. There is surprisingly little evidence of lesser or greater "mental illness" in response to the upheavals of modern Britain, the changes in its family life, and the weakening of social bonds and institutions. Perhaps wider

TABLE 7.31
PRESCRIPTIONS IN GENERAL PRACTICE
National Health Service
England and Wales
Millions

Year	Hypnotics 1	Tran-quillisers 2	Anti-Depressants 3	1+2+3	Other Prescriptions
1962	18	6·6	2·0	27	170
1964	19	9·0	2·8	31	179
1966	20	13	3·9	36	226
1968	21	16	5·3	42	225
1970	20	17	6·5	44	223
1972*	19	20	7·3	46	229

Joint Pricing Bureau; and personal communications.
*Estd.

study of behaviour patterns, of old, as of young people, would be useful. In 1972, the 22,000 general practitioners issued 46,000,000 prescriptions for hypnotics, sedatives, tranquillisers, Table 7.31; comparable data on alcoholism and its apparent changing character should also be given. Evidently, there is a great deal of (minor) depression and widespread emotional difficulties across the social classes;[54] recall the opening pages of Chapter 2 and Table 3.10. Among the highly vulnerable middle-aged men, nothing specific in psychological disturbance has so far been identified. Research in the USA[55] is relating heart-attack to a behaviour pattern of competitive striving dominated by deadlines, the victims never having "a day to call their own".* This hypothesis in terms of the "system", of society producing the kind of characters it needs to run itself, then destroying them in the process, is being confirmed in prospective study. It remains the only preferred explanation of the high US rates of coronary disease. History may well repeat itself, the study of disease leading to the discovery of social stresses, and not vice versa. The approach through *vulnerable groups* and *social casualties* is surely applicable in this time of troubles.†

*"An illness, sclerosis of the vessels of the heart . . . It is a disease of the most modern times. I think its causes are spiritual . . ." (Pasternak).

†"You see, I understand what it is when the lonely person begins to feel like an animal. When the night comes and he feels like howling from his window like a wolf" (Bellow). "He died from solitude . . . Solitude from mere outward condition of existence becomes very swiftly a state of soul . . . In our activity alone do we find the sustaining illusion of an independent existence as against the whole scheme of things of which we form a helpless part" (Conrad). "Isolation" can be studied epidemiologically in terms of personality, family cycle, social roles, locality, demographic trends, housing policies, industrial mobility, medical pathology, and so on.

The Average, the Healthy — and the Approved

To take up this theme again: deviant behaviour is that disapproved either by society in general or by its influential forces (the "establishment"). Norms therefore are different again and, even more than in regard to mental health or illness, they are *relative* (student rags vs. others' hooliganism), often *contradictory* (public attitudes to motoring offences and to crimes of property; or to neglect of children and of old people), and *shifting* (growing permissiveness in sexual behaviour but illiberality towards drugs). I am writing of Britain in the early 1970's. Labelling as "deviance" is commonly aimed to protect cherished values of the society; a line is drawn ("qualitative") because of the presenting dangers, but taboos may derive from widespread and deeper consensus about what is right or natural. That said, the factors, personal, in family and in the larger society, that place people on a "continuum" of behaviour are very little understood.[56-58]

Socially acceptable and socially disapproved behaviour, needless to say, are not the same as medical models of healthy and unhealthy.[59] Sometimes, those deviant and/or rejected plainly also are ill, can't help themselves, are suitable cases for treatment. But how much the illness is cause of the non-conforming behaviour, or its consequence, may not be so plain in the chain reactions, e.g. of alcoholism or the maimed character of the chronic delinquent. A degree of alcohol-dependence that will worry the far-sighted personal doctor may be approved sociability and an accepted means of relieving tension. Equally, for society to cast out and criminalise will often strike the doctor as poor treatment, unlikely to be helpful.

Epidemiology could help with badly wanted value-free analysis of incidence and prevalence of such human variation;[58-61] definition of syndromes; completing the clinical picture by study of kindred phenomena, the reactions to social frustration in terms not merely of lawlessness, but also of respectable functional disorder or mental illness, "geographical pathology":

"The United States is variously reckoned to have between 200,000 and 400,000 narcotic addicts while Britain has less than 3,000 known narcotic addicts — giving the US a pro rata prevalence approximately 18–36 fold that found in this country. The pro rata prevalence of alcoholism in the USA must be at least 200–300 per cent greater than the most inflated British estimate. In America there are about 2 million arrests for public drunkenness each year: the annual total for England and Wales is just over 80,000 drunkenness arrests.

But again it is necessary to look at the wide context. In New York last year there were 1,691 murders, in London 113: there were 78,202 instances of robbery in that American city and 3,167 in the British city of comparable size. (Anyone familiar with the problems of criminological research will of course interpret these comparisons with due caution. Differences in legal definitions, police practices and rates of detection must all affect the outcome.) Background merges with foreground: in New York narcotic addiction is intimately related to the problem of crime on the streets: in London that is not the case . . . That the two countries have markedly different drug problems and different national responses to those problems, can be viewed therefore as nothing of a surprise. William James (1911) even suggested that the fundamental temperament of the "bottled-lightning" American differed inexorably from that of the typical Englishman with his 'dull look and cod-fish eyes' . . ."

Edwards, G. (1973) Anglo-American Conference on Drug Abuse, Royal Society of Medicine, London.

Table 7.32, on the distribution of official delinquency in the schools of East London, is straightaway a hopeful approach: it seems as well as personal and familial causes, there are environmental causes of such misbehaviour, and eventually often great misery, in the education system; the schools with little delinquency show low rates even among their children living in "bad" areas. Exhaustive search has failed to find reasons for this remarkable and consistent distribution in factors outside the school, such as police practice, or the immigrant complement, sex composition, religious affiliation, buildings or size of the schools or yet in the selection of pupils. Here is an urgent lead to further enquiry, in the hope not merely of better understanding but of achieving some *prevention* by social-environmental change. No one will claim that once they have been recognised, *treatment* of the delinquents by the law, social work, child guidance, anything, offers better prospects.

SOCIAL GROUPS

The last theme I want to take up in this section follows from "delinquent schools" — that of the *social group* and its influence on behaviour and mental health. Many of the "populations and "groups" I have been considering in this text are aggregates, collections of individuals defined ad hoc for study. Thus the shape of 8,400 busmen was investigated, or a sample of young men admitted to the country's mental hospitals for schizophrenia was drawn from the records. By "aggregate" the point is intended that either there are no emotional bonds between the individuals who compose it (any contact between these schizophrenics obviously was contingent) or, if there is such interaction (as there must be among the busmen) this, so far as present thinking goes, is not relevant to the question at issue.

Groups in which feelings are invested and, through one mechanism or another, interaction occurs between the members, are true *social groups;* unfortunately, there is no better name that avoids the ambiguity in the word "group", and the meaning has often to be inferred from the context. The social group thus is different from — greater or smaller — more or less healthy — than the sum of its parts, its members. Whatever their ostensible purpose, the social groups to which people belong, the family; ethnic group; neighbourhood; work, including research teams; classes at school or university; friendship groups and gangs; peer groups; fellow-sufferers; the hospital ward; deviant groups, these are of great moment in the mental life, in forming behaviour patterns and meeting the needs for security and personal fulfilment. What individuals feel and think (and complain of), how they

TABLE 7.32
DELINQUENCY IN EAST LONDON SCHOOLBOYS[21]

(A)
First Court Appearances (Case Proven)
in the Five Years 1958/9–1962/3
Ages 11–14 incl.

School Attended	Average Annual Incidence Per 100 Boys
J	0·6
R	1·1
B	1·3
N	1·9
D	2·3
P	2·3
G	2·8
O	3·4
L	3·5
F	3·5
C	3·6
E	3·8
S	3·9
T	3·9
H	4·6
U	4·8
W	4·9
A	5·9
Q	6·3
M	7·7
Average	3·1

At these ages, mostly stealing and truanting.
Smallest school: 80 boys aged 11–14, on average on the roll; largest, 577.
Tower Hamlets Childrens' Dept. Juvenile Court, Police, Probation Service, Inner London Education Authority.
Power, M. J., Benn, R. T. & Morris, J. N. (1972). *Brit. J. Criminol.*
Power, M. J., Ash, P. M., Shoenberg, E. & Sirey, E. C. (1974) *Brit. J. Soc. Work*, **4,** 1.

(B)
Chronic Offenders: Boys making a Third Court Appearance (Case Proven)
1958–68
Ages 11–16 incl.

School Attended	Incidence Per 100 Boys (Table A)	No. of Boys Making First Appearance	Per cent of These Boys Making Third Appearance*
J–D	0·6–2·3	117	27
P–F	2·3–3·5	159	31
C–H	3·6–4·6	314	34
U–M	4·8–7·7	251	44
All	0·6–7·7	841	35%

*As juveniles, i.e. up to 17th birthday. During 1958–68, four out of five boys attending these schools, left during their fifteenth year.

At 15 and 16 years much of the "delinquency" by now is disorderly and aggressive misbehaviour of various kinds.

(C)
Studies of girls at 11–14 show an equally wide range between schools, though at far lower levels (main offences, shop-lifting and truanting); work in progress.

see the world, the kinds of relationships they have with others, all, it may be postulated, are potential in inheritance, developed in the family, and continuously modified through experience in the changing social groups to which they belong. Modes of perception, norms of behaviour, including health and prevention-related behaviour, values, morale, are properties of social groups. These groups have to be studied. It must be expected that the incidence, and the form of mental disorders — and, so important, how these are coped with — will be related to the nature of group life in the social environment, and epidemiological studies have to pay greater attention to this. Psychic "epidemics" have long been recognised,[62] they were obvious to the Greeks, and sundry psychological mechanisms can be postulated. Analogies with the propagation of infectious disease are plain in the spread of drugs, neurosis or delinquent behaviour. In contrast, the potential therapeutic role of a hospital — or prison — institution is also beginning to be utilised. We are coming to appreciate better how much mental health too is catching. The notion of "mental health" is a particularly nebulous one and I fancy that the right approach at present is through social groups.

Social Relations in Industry. — I have already referred to the role of occupation in physical health. However boring, work also plays a key part in the psychological equilibrium of the individual, attaching him firmly to reality (Freud). The work-group in our society is the principal social group after the family, and work a principal social role. (That was the last edition. Today, the work-ethic is in decline, and many would disagree.) Figure 7.11 illustrates a correlation between the nature of the group and its functioning. Communication, the ease of creating personal networks, quality and quantity of social involvement and participation — for example, what safety precautions are observed? — will vary with the group and possibly its size; the accidents may be regarded as group-traits.[63] Such observations can be the basis of an hypothesis; though in interpreting the findings it has to be remembered that the larger units, with different technology and, possibly, job-satisfaction may also have the more efficient reporting systems, etc. (life is like that, especially for social scientists).

Social groups then are a large part of the social environment that is critical for mental health. There has been far too little systematic study of individual capacity and social wellbeing in relation to the variety of group-membership, and epidemiological methods have been too little applied to these questions. Experiments of opportunity are plentiful. Why can the same kinds of working-class children show vastly different delinquency rates? . . . Recruits may be randomly selected into different military units — but what consequences in health! . . . Local factories engage workers with presumably a similar variety of dispositions: why do they produce such diverse accident-rates, sickness-absence, labour turnover? . . . Similar patients are admitted

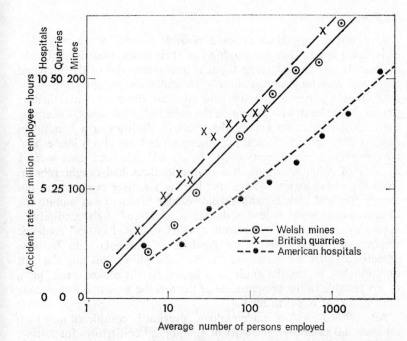

Fig. 7.11 Accidents in employees of Welsh mines, British quarries and American hospitals: the average rate in a recent period in relation to the size of the occupational-social unit.

Revans, R. W. (1960) In *Modern Trends in Occupational Health* (ed. Schilling, R.S.F.). Butterworth, London.

to their district mental hospitals — with what variation in superadded social breakdown, secondary disability? The prospects are bright for the joint enterprise of epidemiologists, students of social structure and of group dynamics.

HYPOTHESES[1-7]

The *search for causes* of the chronic diseases, and so also for means of *prevention,* may be abstracted in a model like this:

(1) Statement of hypothesis
(2) Testing it, and deductions from it
(3) Relating the postulated cause to others — and to the general understanding
(4) Evidence of its effectiveness in practical application.

Straightaway it must be said that in real life such tidy progression is unusual.

References on page 306.

(1) The Hypothesis

How useful hypotheses about a possible "cause" are generated is little understood. They are products of their times, what is in the air, of what is known and being thought important, and of the prepared mind and individual imagination — in epidemiology, immersed in the data, ranging over social life and medical discovery, investigating practical problems; and seizing on the unexpected incidence, discerning the critical connection among the tracts of statistics or a handful of cases. *Where* epidemiological hypotheses come from also is interesting: they emerge — from everywhere. In clinical practice: there were a number of chimney-sweeps, two of the mothers had caught rubella; from the physiological laboratory: linking vigorous exercise and not merely physical activity with cardiovascular health; from monitoring of the environment: is lead a danger to children?; by serendipity: a survey for hypertension in cotton workers disclosed instead epidemic respiratory distress;[9] and from nowhere in particular: do business executives suffer an excess of "stress" disorders? Put so, the last question just makes the grade as a hypothesis: it makes sense (just), is just testable in the present state of the art, the answer is not already known, and it is worth having.

Any of the "uses" of epidemiology" previously considered may turn up clues, all have been the start of aetiological conjectures for testing. *Historically,* does not its abundance early this century show that coronary atheroma is necessary for production of the heart disease, but not its sufficient cause? . . . Rising excise duty helped to focus interest in the increase of lung-cancer on cigarettes; and men (who smoked them) showed a disproportionate rise in mortality. Cohort study suggested that rising delinquency after the second world war was related to the particularly traumatic experience of that generation during it, a hypothesis with convenient built-in test: the passage of time and a further rise of delinquency in the late 1950's refuted it.[10] *Community Diagnosis* is always raising aetiological questions . . . The excess of pernicious anaemia in the less prosperous north and west of Britain[11] prompted a generalisation about the environment: Could this be related to the incidence of atrophic gastritis? And can the distribution of parietal antibody be mapped? . . . The excess of cancer of the stomach in North and West Wales started a search for trace elements in the local soil and revived the study of blood groups and disease.[12]

(2) Test; and Deductions

Stating a hypothesis, we must first try to prune it to essentials. Nutrients are complementary, a high animal-fat diet is usually high also in animal protein; can situations be found of one but not the other? In a dynamic "system" like the family, to abstract one element then try and put it back into context again may be the only way of making progress (however traumatic for the psychiatrist).

The proposition and deductions from it should now be tested in as many, as different, as distant, and as independent situations as possible. Any single investigation is liable to be limited and biased as well (save us from our preconceptions), but a lesson may be drawn from the consistent behaviour of pieces of evidence that are none of them in themselves as convincing as could be wished. This is what we attempted when stating a hypothesis relating physical activity of occupation to coronary heart disease, and what we are now seeking to do with the later hypothesis. If vigorous exercise in leisure-time is efficacious, preventive, this should be evident also among the unrecognised clinical cases of CHD and the silent ones (Chap. 6, section 1), and also in early ischaemic disease (section 2) . . . Table 7 (C) on p. 166 confirms the hypothesis: there are unrecognised and silent infarcts as well as patients among the 11 major Q/QS changes; the minor, mainly ST-T segment and T wave, changes that were accepted may be regarded as "early" ischaemic disease, and there was twice as much of it in the men not reporting VE . . . If cardiovascular fitness is the mechanism, what are the expected manifestations of that? A slight advantage in prevalence of tachycardia among the men reporting vigorous exercise was not borne out in the numbers with *slow* pulses — the simplest evidence there is of cardiovascular "training". Plainly, we have not identified a group of athletes among these middle-aged civil servants (it is most unlikely such a group exists). If the hypothesis on VE is confirmed, it may refer to exercise short of the amount/intensity required to produce "fitness" (and far less than the daily routine of the bus conductor).

Direct Test, and Indirect

The testing of a causal hypothesis should include a direct study of representative persons, categorised for example in terms of their smoking habits: their mortality from cancer of the lung is then analysed. This is a superior method to the indirect study of the lung-cancer death in countries, say, or social classes, which have been graded by the average amount of cigarettes smoked in them. How wrong a way — how diminishing, that can be of asking the right question, Table 7.33 (A):

Mortality from Lung Cancer in the County Boroughs of England and Wales
Males Ages 45-64

Average No. of Cigarettes Smoked in Towns*	Annual Mortality from Lung Cancer per 100,000**
–10 per day	127
10–14	141
15–19	145
20+	155

*Information from trade sources. 1952-5. Estimated.   **1948–54.

But the shallow gradation did verify an obvious deduction from the hypothesis. Smoking is a cause in personal habits and behaviour where individual differences are crucial and it has to be studied as such. On the other hand, in dealing with properties of the external environment, "indirect" "ecologic" study is the first and may be the only practicable step:

The "Water Story"
Drinking Water and Local Death Rates per 100,000 in the Large Towns of England & Wales[16-18]
Ages 45–64

Local water calcium (P.P.M.)	Cardiovascular disease & Bronchitis		Other causes		All causes of death	
	M	F	M	F	M	F
100+	634	261	626	415	1260	680
70–99	754	306	699	437	1453	743
40–69	786	335	742	448	1528	784
20–39	799	328	691	436	1490	765
10–19	914	378	726	461	1640	840
–10	926	394	762	471	1688	866

1958–64.
Number of towns at each level of water-hardness varied from 7–15.

The harder the water supply, the lower the annual death rate. Calcium is the main cation in hardness, and the negative correlation with cardiovascular disease (and bronchitis) meanwhile is strongest with that. We have to assume that unless there is some confounding difference in the amounts that people drink, of which there is no sign, the variations between towns will be reflected among the individuals in them. But towns differing in their water supply differ also in many other respects, and the trouble is to know what really is being found. Correlation, association, does not necessarily mean "cause": the commonest statement in epidemiology. The softness of the local water, I dug out of repressed memories of schooldays, was one of the reasons the cotton industry, and the industrial revolution, started in Lancashire. Is the correlation with drinking water merely a roundabout way of describing a more important connection between cardiovascular disease and social-industrial conditions? There is no *statistical* answer to the dilemma, "when does association mean cause?" but sometimes the possibility of an *epidemiological* answer, in a natural experiment, or a deliberate one — and to explore by every means what actually is happening. In this instance, painstaking search revealed only minor correlations between water-quality and numerous social-environmental indices: size of town, prevalent industry, housing conditions, wage-levels, history of unemployment, availability of medical services, etc. Allowing for these scarcely affected the values of the correlations between water-calcium and cardiovascular disease.[16-18] (Though Birmingham, with its own soft water piped in from Wales in the midst of a hard-water region, yet with the low death rates of the surrounding area, remains a "sore thumb".) There are numerous examples in classical epidemiology, from the water and bowel infection; in fluoride and dental caries; in goitre; in malaria and in tuberculosis where elementary ecologic observations have opened up new territory, led to viable hypotheses, and provided highly relevant evidence in support — or otherwise.

Experiment of Opportunity[19-23]

Snow showed that mortality from cholera in persons happening at the time to have clean up-river water was lower (i.e., some prevention was achieved) than in a similar population drinking a down-river contaminated supply, (p. 144). The epidemiological imagination will seize the opportunity presented by such an "experiment" . . . The effects of social-cultural change on individual physiology and pathology are being studied (too little and sometimes already too late) in the new nations, notably in Israel. A hypothesis about radiation was confirmed, if the appellation is not blasphemous, by subsequent leukaemia in Hiroshima and Nagasaki. The mass movement to switch to filter cigarettes should give an answer to that particular question. Occupational mortality statistics of physicians have been followed with particular care: many of them were quickly health-educated by recent discoveries to give up cigarettes (unlike their patients, the public). It would be heaven-sent to find a comparable population of children not exposed to (violent) TV . . . Snow's was the perfect *experiment of nature* (the alternative name) though, as often, man-made. It was as near a controlled experiment in the laboratory as could be desired. Those studied had in effect been "randomised" between the two water supplies. In his words, they were "divided into two groups without their choice, and, in most cases, without their knowledge", there was no self- or other selection of the drinking water by "rank or station, condition or occupation", characteristics that might themselves be associated with the cholera. The experiment of opportunity often falls down on this essential criterion, and the proof it can provide is thus by no means "incontrovertible".

CASE-CONTROL AND COHORT STUDIES[24-31]

Table 7.33 (B) is taken from a study of large numbers of patients with cancer of the lung, Figure 7.12 summarises the results of the quite different and independent study of British doctors; to demonstrate such dose-response relations is progress to the formulation of scientific laws.

There are two main ways of testing directly a hypothesis on causes. The first starts with *cases* of the disease, patients who already have it, and looks backwards, compares them *retrospectively* for history of the suspected cause, smoking say, with appropriate *controls,* usually patients with other diseases. The larger the series of cases the better, and they should be as typical of the disease as can be defined and found. The assumption is that the controls belong to the same original population as the cases, differing only in terms of the disease-in-question, so they too must be drawn carefully. Sources of bias are endless, all the selective influences on hospital admission for a start, and the safest course may be to study as unselected a series of cases as possible, and to take for controls as large a sample of as random a collection of patients as practicable, matching only for sex and age and any other attributes not being studied. That way, there will be less chance of biasing the controls with patients who are suffering from diseases having their own systematic connections with the suspected cause.

The second method starts by defining a population free of the disease, each individual of which is characterised by the postulated cause(s), smoking for example. The whole *cohort,* as it is called, is then followed to see who develops the disease as defined, and how this is associated with smoking habits: the *incidence* is observed, and compared in smokers and non-smokers, heavy, moderate and light smokers etc. The approach is *prospective,* looking ahead, "time future contained in time past", a method already advocated for study of the natural history of disease . . . There is much to be said for and against each of these methods.

Case-control studies, typically, are easy to mount, there may be only too many patients with cancer of the lung in local hospitals, and a study can often be done quickly if necessary (for example, recently, to show whether oral contraceptives increase the risk of breast or cervical cancer; meanwhile, not at all). Something like 100 per cent co-operation is common, and much information can be obtained from each patient. This is the method of choice, therefore, in the early stages of enquiry. As seen, first hunches on possible causes of disease have often come from clinical observation (smoking and lung cancer,[32]

TABLE 7.33
SMOKING AND CANCER OF LUNG

(B)
Retrospective Study of Patients of Various Ages with Lung-Cancer and of Matched Controls

| Average No. of Cigarettes (or Equivalent in Pipe Tobacco) Smoked Daily Over 10 Years Before Illness | Proportions in Each Group | | | |
| | Males | | Females | |
	1357 Cases %	1357 Controls %	108 Cases %	108 Controls %
Non-smokers	0·5	4·5	37	55
– 5	4·0	9·5	15	23
5–14	36	42	22	17
15–24	35	32	13	5·6
25–49	22	11	13	—
50+	2·8	0·9	—	—
Total	100	100	100	100

Doll, R., & Hill, A. B. (1952). *Brit. med. J.*, **2**, 1271.

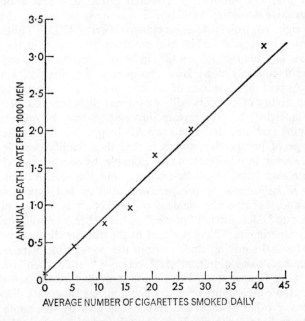

Fig. 7.12   Smoking and cancer of lung (C). Death rate from lung cancer by number of cigarettes smoked daily at the start of the 10-year period 1951–61. Rates are standardised for all ages. Men smoking pipes or cigars as well as cigarettes are excluded.

Doll, R. & Hill, A. B. (1964) *Brit. med. J.* **1**, 1394, 1460.

oxygen excess and retrolental fibroplasia,[33] irradiation and leukaemia),[34] and formal case-control studies followed. The trouble with
retrospective studies lies in the validity of the information that is
obtained: remembering and forgetting are meaningful, biased. Patients
with chest illness often feel guilty about smoking, a history of alcohol
consumption is notoriously unreliable, mothers racking their brains
for what might have gone wrong will recollect — something, battering
parents may deliberately mislead, old men forget — selectively
. . . Moreover, "blindness", in conducting the survey, may be
impracticable, and pressure by the investigator (of which he may be
unaware) to elicit an answer, a particular answer, may be greater with
the cases under suspicion than with the controls, and these, too, may
differ in their suggestibility. *Cohort,* prospective "longitudinal" studies
overcome many of these difficulties. Since all questions are asked in
advance of the occurrence of the disease under investigation, there
should be less such error, conscious and subconscious, in the investigator who is asking the questions and the subject giving the answers.

In some situations the prospective is the only way of getting satisfactory information. Study of the characteristics of men dying suddenly
in their first heart-attack, an essential group to know about, must
be prospective. Questioning widows is not the same; and, anyhow, who
are the right controls? More generally, suffering IHD is liable to lead
to changes in exercise habits and smoking-behaviour, in the work a
man does and his outlook on life, in blood pressure level and plasma
cholesterol concentration: How reconstruct the situation before the
event? A postulated cause, of course, precedes its postulated effect
. . . The ability of patients with emotional disorder, and of controls
not so suffering, to give private information may be quite unequal;
questioning before the event could help . . . The other great
advantage of prospective studies is that they readily provide disease
incidence rates, in non-smokers, for example, by comparison with light,
moderate and heavy cigarette-smokers, and the scale of the *risk on
average to individuals.* So prospective studies do test hypotheses more
strictly and, because the element of prediction is strong, plausibly.
But cause and effect are not "proven" as in algebra, symbolic logic or the
planned experiment. Thirty per cent of the doctors did not participate
in the classical smoking study; within the population of respondents,
some smoked, some didn't, subjects were not "randomised" (the magic
word again). It cannot yet be said for sure whether this self-selection
indicates some inheritance or experience connected also with dispositions
to cancer or other disease, and responsible also by this route for the
associations found with smoking; though intensive search along these
lines has been distinctly unrewarding.

In the study of chronic diseases, prospective cohort studies may
mortgage energy and resources for years ahead. Even with so common
a condition as ischaemic heart disease, huge numbers exposed-to-risk

are likely to be necessary for multiple-cause analysis, and all ought then to be kept under observation, not merely for new events, but for changes in "exposure", smoking more or less for example... It is expecting too much, in the present state of the art, to mount prospective studies relating events in the teens and, a fortiori, in early childhood experience, to adult personality, psychosexual or whatever; "lapses" and losses from the population would ruin the best designed study. And prospective studies are unsuitable for conditions of low incidence, however important, like multiple sclerosis or heroin addiction, schizophrenia or precocious IHD; unmanageably large cohorts would be needed. Prospective studies, finally, are not for prospecting: before embarking on them there should be strong indication that gold is there to be found, and where it should be looked for.

Many, many hypotheses do not survive the testing. The idea wasn't good enough in the first place. Methodology is inadequate. Findings cannot be repeated. Correlations are shown to arise by chance. Apparently distinct causes turn out in fact to be the same. It is some third factor that is producing the correlation. Some hypotheses however do come through, they explain and predict something, deductions from them "work", and they make sense: this is one of the main criteria, adapting again from Mill's "canons" of scientific proof.[1][3][4] Common sense, and sense in terms of what else is known and thought in epidemiology, in clinical medicine, in laboratory experiment; they are consistent with and add to the general understanding.[35-38] (Though, of course, *un*conventional wisdom, not to fit, may sometimes be even more important.)

(3) "MULTIVARIATE ANALYSIS"[1-3][39]

To continue the discussion from page 182: the search for causes of chronic diseases is push and pull between isolating single causes and description of their patterns. In our infant mortality work, a collection of largely "independent" biological and social causes were confirmed, alerting health-workers to simple vulnerable groups — and contributing to a theory of healthy reproduction. The main were *maternal age* (physiological and social efficiency?), *birth rank* of the infant/*size of family* (risks of deprivation and infection), the two causes described on page 55; and paternal *social class* (with its correlates of quality of present and past environment), also previously noticed. Others identified were: *intervals between childbearing* (personality and ecology plainly are involved as well as physiology); *loss by the mother of a previous child* (specific responsible pathology accounted for a small minority); the *region* of the country (introducing biological variables, perhaps, as well as climatic and social); and *place of delivery* (availability of specialist skills in emergency). Various combinations of these "causes" yielded ranges in stillbirth from under 10 per 1,000 to nearly 100, and in postneonatal mortality from 3 or 4 per 1,000 to twenty times that.[00-05] Such "inevitability", at the wrong end of distributions, is familiar in the clinical situation, in ischaemic heart disease, psychoneurosis and delinquency also, in which there is saturation with so many adverse circumstances, such overdetermination, that the unfortunates "just didn't stand a chance".

Computer Revolution

In a context of "multiple causes", anything, it sometimes seems, may go — but does the postulated cause matter? By how much? The advent of the computer eases the search for significant patterns among multiple factors. The best known technique, "multiple regression", was used in an attempt to account for some of the gross variation

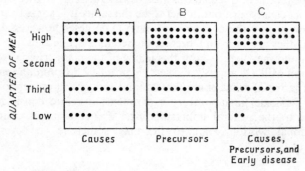

Fig. 7.13 Incidence of ischaemic heart disease, all forms, London busmen during 5 years, by risk factors present at initial examination. Quarters of men identified by risk factors present, using linear discriminant function analysis, a technique similar to that used in Table 4.6, page 106. Each dot represents a first clinical episode of coronary heart disease.[46]

Risk factors: (X_1) Age (in years) at first examination.

(X_2) History of parental mortality in middle age (negative 0, positive 1).

(X_3) Stature (cm).

(X_4) Skinfold thickness at suprailiac crest (mm).

(X_5) Occupation (conductor 0, driver 1).

(X_6) Current cigarette smoking (non-smoker 0, smoker 1).

(X_7) Casual systolic BP (mm Hg).

(X_8) Total plasma cholesterol (mg per 100 ml).

(X_9) Electrocardiographic abnormality of the kind described (absent 0, present 1)

A CAUSES (X_1–X_6); $P < 0.01$.

B PRECURSORS (X_7-X_8); $P < 0.0001$.

C CAUSES, PRECURSORS, and EARLY DISEASE (X_1–X_9); $P < 0.0001$.

593 middle-aged men initially free of recognised coronary heart disease.

of death rates between the towns of England and Wales, e.g. Table 2.4, page 51. The causes assembled in Table 7·34 are making several independent contributions, differing in importance to judge by the value of the regression coefficient. Together, they account for a surprising amount of the overall variance.

The need for such an approach was apparent also in the discussion of *chronic bronchitis,* with its multiple interrelated environmental associations. Three in particular have to be unravelled: social-economics, air pollution, and latitude (life in the rugged old-industrial North of England vs. the more affluent as well as clement South). By multiple regression, it is plain that air pollution and bad social conditions are materially related to the death rates; given these, the contribution of latitude is negligible. How much the association of mortality from this cause with water-hardness reflects an overlap of "cardiac" conditions (cor pulmonale and deaths in congestive failure) it is still difficult to say; we suspect quite a lot. Meanwhile, it has not been possible satisfactorily to dissociate water quality from rainfall, another illustration of the point previously made, and an intensive search is under way for districts with soft water and *low* rainfall, etc.

In our studies of *ischaemic heart disease* among London busmen, we specified an assortment of six "causes": age, family history, occupation, cigarette smoking, etc. Each of these was "weighted" according to its independent contribution, in the presence of the others, to the incidence of IHD in the men . . . Job, driver vs. conductor, was found to have the greatest effect, cigarette smoking next. Men in the cohort were then scored for the presence of these dispositions and divided into quarters according to their total score; this is how IHD struck among them (Fig. 7.13 (A)). In a theory of ischaemic heart disease, *causes* like these are usefully distinguished from *precursor pathology,* here, notably, high levels of blood pressure and cholesterol (Fig. (B)). In addition, minor, probably ischaemic, Q/QS, ST-T segment and T wave abnormalities on the electrocardiogram were regarded as *early disease,* to make up (C). Combining the 9 factors, it is possible to define a great range of risk. Taking it a little further, there was a sizeable minority of men — 40 per cent — who were virtually immune from heart attack in middle age, p. 106 . . . But most of the group at highest risk in Table 4.6 did not suffer an attack in middle or early old age (they were the "false positives"), and the men in that fifth of very high risk accounted for less than half the total of such clinical disease: these typical findings seriously limit practical application.

Such points systems, including several causes assessed according to their demonstrated individual risks, can include qualitative as well as quantitative factors, black and white and shades of grey, classes as well as numerical gradations; and they can be modified to allow for multiplier and more complex effects as well as simple addition. They represent a major advance in competence. Epidemiology, concerned with all discernible social and biological forces expressed in the health of

TABLE 7.34

Multiple Causes of Mortality in the County Boroughs of England and Wales[17 18 45]

Multiple Regression Coefficients (Standardised) of Death Rates on Local Environmental Factors

Men Aged 45–64

1958–64

Cause of Death	Social Factor Score†	Domestic Air Pollution	Latitude N→S	Long-Term Rainfall	Hardness of Water††	Proportion of the Variance of Mortality between the Towns
All causes	+0·19*	+0·36***	+0·21**	+0·30***	−0·24**	84%
Coronary heart disease	−0·28	+0·32*	+0·31*	+0·41**	−0·22*	53%
Bronchitis	+0·29*	+0·32*	+0·14	+0·11	−0·26*	70%

†Composed of nine indices of unfavourable social conditions: unemployment, house-crowding, low wages, early school-leaving, etc.

††Calcium, p.p.m.

*P <0·05; **P < 0·01; *** P < 0·001.

61 towns with population of over 80,000.

populations, now has suitable techniques for such study and helpful models in field theory, "systems" and cybernetics.[3 39 48-52]

Relative Risk[1 53-55]

This is the simplest way of expressing the contributions of multiple causes: how much extra risk is incurred by individuals exposed to this or that cause in comparison with those not so exposed? The risk of those exposed to particular factor(s) is calculated in proportion, as so much greater, or less, than the risk of individuals not so exposed. The three main relevant "behaviours", overweight, cigarette smoking and taking inadequate exercise in leisure-time, overlapped more than by chance in our population of civil servants only by little; and this was the estimated relative risk for each of them, singly, and in the presence of the other two:[45 56 57]

Incidence of Coronary Heart Disease

	Relative Risk	
Risk Factor	Single factor	Standardised for other two factors
Men not reporting vigorous exercise	2·91	2·72 (P < 0·001)
Smoking cigarettes	2·42	2·46 (P < 0·001)
Very obese	1·83	1·95 (P < 0·05)

214 first attacks of coronary heart disease and 428 matched controls; men aged 40–65; executive-grade officers.

Risk of men not exposed to risk factor(s) is taken to be 1·00.

All three risk factors were present in 11 per cent of the cases and in 3 per cent of the controls; two or three factors in 66 and 36 per cent respectively; one or more in 95 per cent of the cases and 62 per cent of the controls.

A last word. If causes are related in a dynamic way, and one or more has a homeostatic function, simple intervention will not have simple results. Any relevant information on this will be particularly valuable. It is basic to nutrition policy that correcting one of the deficiencies of an inadequate diet, in respect of the B vitamins for example, can make things worse in aggregate. Men who give up smoking may become more nervous, and they often put on weight (the "claw of the seapuss" that gets us in the end?). So it is reassuring that the death rate of ex-smokers is lower than that of men continuing to smoke. A particular effect is most unlikely to be produced without a lot of others, intended or not, and it is prudent to try to anticipate.

EXPERIMENTAL EPIDEMIOLOGY[1-6]

Quite early in hypothesis-testing it may be possible to take the critical step from observation to the *planned experiment* (4), and this may be the only way in the end of cutting through the sisyphean argument about what truly are causes, what mechanisms, and what mere associations not as yet understood. When multiple causes so obviously are involved, and the naturally occurring groups demonstrably are "biased", the preventive experiment may be inescapable before mass education to change the mode of life for better health will have much chance of success. At the same time, the undesired side-effects can be compared directly with the actual benefits.[4] Even then it may not be plain sailing, as is evident again today, for a relatively simple situation, in the frequently tepid or worse response to the splendid results, in benefits gained and safety assured, of fluoridation experiments, Table 7.35. The misery of dental caries is universal, the waste of £ millions badly wanted elsewhere in the Health Service is glaring. And yet. . .[7] As said, we know too little how to influence behaviour, which (it doesn't help it's a platitude) is just as important as knowing what behaviour to influence. In field experiment on aetiology, a postulated cause in the population or environment is tested by removing it under controlled conditions. This will be to achieve some of the confidence of Koch's postulates and the experiment in the laboratory.

There are many successful examples from history:[3] adding iodine to salt as goitre prophylactic; preventing pellagra by improving the diet; the prevention of urolithiasis by fluids in hot climates;[8] Corry Mann's demonstration that giving milk improved the physical growth of under-privileged children[9] (today the interest has shifted to the possibility of so improving mental development). Results of such experiments will preferably be assessed in simultaneous assessment of randomised "treated" and "untreated" groups, as in immunisation; or, where this is impractical, "before and after" in the same population as in many experiments in industrial and road safety or the British Columbian campaign to eradicate cervical cancer. Figure 7.14 on page 248 illustrates a large (heroic, I hope someone will say) trial to test the hypothesis that high plasma cholesterol concentration is a cause of ischaemic heart disease. An experiment to prove that the cigarette is *the* cause of epidemic cancer of the bronchus would involve huge numbers of smokers and their allocation at random into two groups one of which is persuaded to stop smoking. If such an experiment could be mounted, and motivation and discipline maintained for long enough, the results might convince the remaining sceptics. The evidence from observation is so overwhelming, however, that few think such an experiment is necessary, even if ethical in the present state of knowledge. It would also be quite beyond our present skills.

References on page 307.

TABLE 7.35
THE FLUORIDATION EXPERIMENT IN ENGLAND AND WALES
1955/6 to 1964/7

Teeth	Experimental Areas Baseline	Latest year	Control Areas Baseline	Latest year
Average nos. decayed, missing or filled teeth (DMF) per child				
Ages 3–7	5·3	2·4	4·9	4·0
Percentages of children free from dental decay				
Ages 8–10	15	34	16	18
Percentages of children with 10 or more decayed teeth				
Ages 11–14	—	7	—	15

—Not recorded.

The Fluoridation Studies in the United Kingdom and the Results Achieved after Eleven Years. (1969) Previously: *Rep. Publ. Hlth. Med. Subj.*, No. 105. (1962) HMSO, London.

"The Research Committee concludes that the fluoridation of water supplies at the level of 1 p.p.m. is a highly effective way of reducing dental decay and is completely safe."

Experiment in the Prevention of Chronic Diseases[10-13]

In ischaemic heart disease the situation is different. The evidence implicates not one, but an array of major causes which are widespread in Western society. *Observation* shows fairly convincingly that men who don't smoke cigarettes, take adequate exercise and aren't too fat are more likely than others to escape this modern epidemic, among many benefits. *Experiments* on each of these three behaviours singly, as in Fig. 14 (which makes far simpler demands on the participants) would be invaluable — but now look over-optimistic if not naive.[14-16] Multi-factor trials, however, changing these ways of living and main precursor abnormalities, one or all of them, simultaneously as indicated, could still be immensely valuable, even though they did not help much in theoretical "proof" of which individual factor (inadequate exercise, etc.) was itself a cause.[17-21] In such trials the concern is with the total regimen; and the hope is to demonstrate that people at high risk because naturally not so virtuous in their behaviour or lucky in their genes will derive benefit from it. All of these factors are obvious ingredients for a modern regimen of health, and actual evidence of better health, especially a lower incidence of IHD, would be a great help to community control programmes. IHD has a very long-term progression, but the suggestions of a quick fall of the disease in wartime Europe, and, more recently, among those who give up smoking (and the hint of lower

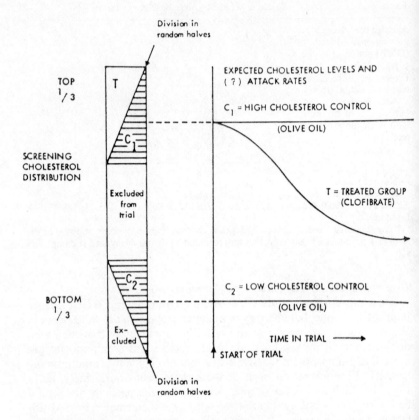

Fig. 7.14 Population experiment in primary prevention: double-blind trial of lowering high plasma cholesterol concentration by clofibrate to determine the effects, if any, on the incidence of coronary heart disease. 5000 men aged 30–59 in the upper third of the cholesterol distribution are the experimental group (T); the other 5000 men in the upper third (randomised) are controls C_1 (receiving a minute amount of olive oil), and an additional 5000 men, half of those in the lower third of the cholestrol distribution (having naturally low levels) form a further control group (C_2).

Oliver, M. F. (1970) In *Atherosclerosis: Proceedings of the Second International Symposium* (ed. Jones, R. J.), p.582. New York.
Heady, J. A. (1973) *WHO Bull.*, **48**, 243.

risks among the obese who have reduced),[22] give reason for hope for quick results from such trials. One obstacle which may yet be serious is that interest and action in an "experimental" population can produce considerable psychological benefit and behaviour change (the "Hawthorne", general, non-specific effect), and a new concern for health may be expressed in mysterious ways. Large enough study-populations, and long enough follow up, to allow for this factor may be unattainable.

Maybe "only nature can do the experiments that you want".[23] It looks that we will have to make the best of less than perfect observation, multifactor trials which give a practical rather than theoretical result, clinical experience, and human and animal laboratory experiment; depend, on i.e., convergence of findings from all ways of learning in medicine . . . The other field now ripe for a strategy that includes such multifactor preventive experiments is the attempt to improve health in older people by care of the middle-aged. Since the interaction of physical and mental health is nowhere more evident than among the elderly, even modest efforts may yield worthwhile results. This would be experimental in two ways that have been considered in the book: in testing notions of aetiology, and in the delivery of better health services.

Three Ways of Learning

In previous editions of *Uses,* much space was given to illustrating how the three main methods of learning in medicine — clinical observation of patients, the controlled experiment in the laboratory, and population study — complement, and supplement, each other in making their particular and characteristic contributions, and how this can lead to greater understanding of benefit to the whole of medicine. By now it is a well-worn theme, so in what follows I confine myself to a few examples of historical interest. Others will readily come to mind; I have found the following can be instructive:

History of great nutritional deficiencies
Ischaemic heart disease: sex ratio; syndromes; physical activity/ inactivity; obesity; mortality
Psychosocial factors: in IHD; hypertension; duodenal ulcer
The diet–heart question
The water story
The salt story in hypertension
Explorations of health: in middle age; old age
Phenomena of ageing
Morbidity: lesions, sickness, disability
Additive and multiplier effects in aetiology
Tomorrow's new health services
Addictions: prescribed medicines; hard drugs; alcohol; cigarettes; food
Toxic effects of new medicines
Recognition of new diseases
Unfolding story of Burkitt's lymphoma.

What struck me most in preparing this section was — a non-event: how backward we epidemiologists are in seizing the opportunities being presented in exploding immunology.

References on page 308.

TABLE TW.1

Sir George Baker's "Consummate Proof" that the Devonshire Colic was Due to Lead Poisoning

Clinical Observation	Epidemiology	Laboratory Study
(1) Baker (1767) recognised that the "endemial colic of Devonshire", commonly ascribed to the acidity of the local cyder that was drunk in large and increasing quantities, often terminated in palsy, especially of the arms, and epilepsy; a recognisable syndrome and "precisely the same disease which is the specific effect of all saturnine preparations" . . . Yet another epidemic from the contamination of food and drink by lead	(2) He observed that the colic was rare in other cyder-producing counties, and commonest in parts of Devonshire where most cyder was made. Suspecting adulteration with lead to be responsible, he found that lead indeed was used in the construction of the presses in Devonshire. The apples were in direct contact with the metal, which was slowly dissolving during grinding or later stages. In other counties lead was rarely so used	(3) "Sine experimentia vanna omnis theoria." Be that as it may, Baker showed by chemical test that the local cyder did in fact contain lead. On his initiative, its presence in Devonshire cyder, and absence in others, was independently confirmed in London. (Baker recognised that he himself was "under the influence of a preconceived opinion")

"In this instance, cognitio causae morbum tollet" (Baker). "Under the influence of his discovery a grievous endemic affliction rapidly became extinct" (Simon), despite local opposition because of the threat to their livelihood.

TABLE TW.2
CAUSES OF CANCERS

Chemical Carcinogenesis; Occupational Epithelioma of Scrotum

Clinical Medicine	Laboratory Experiment	Epidemiology, Occupational Health, Public Health
In 1775, Pott, a leading surgeon of his day, found far too many scrotal cancers in chimney sweepers among his patients and described "a most noisome, painful and fatal disease . . . peculiar to a certain set of people" from puberty on. The chimney sweeps themselves recognised the condition as "soot wart". Pott pleaded eloquently against this exploitation of the "climbing boys" who had often been forced to do this job from 5 or 8 years of age		Beginning in 1788, Parliament passed a series of laws to prevent children being employed as chimney sweeps: this was the first modern official intervention on behalf of children. Enforcement was slowly effective, though Dickens was still writing about the scandal 50 years later
		In 1892, Butlin demonstrated that while still prevalent here, sweeps in other countries do not suffer from scrotal cancer: because they wear protective clothing and because, he

Pott emphasised the long incubation period of the growth. Later, it was observed that the disease may develop many years after exposure to the hazard had ceased

1915-18 Yamagiwa and Itchikawa produced squamous-cell carcinoma of the skin in the rabbit by repeated painting with tar

1924-33 Kennaway and co-workers identified the 3:4-benzpyrene as the carcinogen in tar. This, it is evident, is the responsible agent in the soot. Skin cancer was again reproduced in animals with the benzpyrene. A group of carcinogenic polycyclic aromatic hydrocarbons has been defined

claimed, the nocuous material is removed every day by thorough washing

In 1946, Henry analysed available mortality data on scrotal cancer and followed up the death certificates, taking detailed occupational histories – "shoe-leather" epidemiology. He confirmed that in 1911–39 there was still a gross persisting excess of the disease (nearly 200-fold) in men who had been chimney sweeps. Comparable data are not available for more recent years

Obviously, however, the occupational tumour is now quite rare: methods of domestic heating have improved, soot is removed mechanically, no one climbs chimneys for a living. In general, people are cleaner, and they would tend to wear adequate clothing in such a situation. Moreover, precursor tar warts, should they occur, are likely to be recognised early and cured

TABLE TW.3

CHEMICAL CARCINOGENESIS

Cancer of Bladder in Dyestuffs Workers – and Rubber Workers and Cable Workers and . . .

Clinical Observation	Laboratory Experiment	Epidemiology; Occupational Health
(1) In 1895 Rehn described bladder cancer among a small group of workers engaged in the manufacture of magenta from aniline. He considered inhalation of that to be the most likely agent – whence "aniline tumours"	(2) In 1937 Hueper et al reproduced the tumour in dogs by feeding them β-naphthylamine, an aromatic amine	(3) Ad hoc cohort studies, delayed because of the Second World War and beginning in 1948, by Case and colleagues, soon revealed a gross excess incidence of bladder cancer in dyestuffs workers making and handling β-naphthylamine, α-naphthylamine, and benzidine; though not aniline
		Manufacture of dyestuffs in Britain had been increased when German supplies stopped in World War I. National occupational mortality statistics failed to reveal the problem because the population-at-risk is small and, therefore, included with larger groups
		These tumours characteristically occurred at younger ages ("anticipation") than non-occupational bladder cancer. Their "incubation period" was found to be variable, but mostly between 15 and 20 years
Clinical non-observation has been a serious problem, the occupational origin of bladder cancers being missed. Industrial medical officers, coroners, the staffs of government departments of Employment and Social Security are involved as well as all parts of the NHS		Individual risk of workers developing the disease in conditions prevalent during the 1920's to 1940's was found to be exceedingly high, between 1 in 10 and 1 in 5 (and even up to 1 in 1, one hundred per cent, in a small group of men distilling β-naphthylamine). I.e., it is many times the national average (see p. 101). There is no evidence of any immunity to the industrial disease

The death of a *cable worker* from bladder cancer, the inquest and consequent publicity (1965), the discovery of other such cases, aroused public anxiety and led to new investigations

Serendipity. – During these studies, Case *et al.* discovered a high mortality from the cancer in *rubber workers* who had been chosen as "controls"

Analysis of death certificates over a period of 15 years established that *cable workers* also have an excess of the disease (rubber is used for insulation)

Control of the Hazard. – Manufacture in Britain of β-naphthylamine, the most lethal substance was stopped by 1952. Primary neoplasm of the bladder due to industrial exposure was prescribed as an industrial disease

Exfoliative cytological *screening of individuals-at-risk*, for precursor papillomata, and for cancer, was begun by industry in 1950 and is now widely used. The method may not be sufficiently sensitive

← A carcinogenic group of →
aromatic amines has been defined but is not necessarily exhaustive. Meanwhile, it does not seem likely that a satisfactory method of screening suspected chemicals for their potential carcinogenic activity on bladder and kidney will be found

Surveillance of workers and ex-workers in affected industries continues to be essential. Cases are still occurring in rubber and cable workers; it is not clear if these are residual from known carcinogens that have been controlled, or if other chemicals, or foreign importations (e.g. of rubber for retreading) are responsible. Adequate control of the dangerous chemicals is inadequate in many countries

Perhaps as many as 1 case of bladder cancer in 5 is due to occupation. A high index of suspicion is necessary in *genitourinary practice*, and it is important to take adequate occupational histories: "Of what trade is he?" (Ramazzini)

Epidemiological methods have still to be used to identify high-risk groups, and possibly dangerous processes, and for monitoring the incidence of the disease

TABLE TW.4

HORMONE DEPENDENCE IN BREAST CANCER

Clinical Observation	Laboratory Experiment	Population Studies
1713: Ramazzini noticed that breast cancer was especially common in nuns	A. *Hormones and Normal Mammary Function.* Around the turn of the century, the old theory of "neural" control of	1842: Stern showed that cancer of breast was relatively commoner among single women; and particularly so among nuns
1739: Heister wrote that breast cancer was commoner in nuns, single women, and married women who had borne no children	breast growth and lactation was supplanted by "hormonal" theory. It is now known that many endocrine factors are involved, including oestrogens, progesterone, etc.	1915: Hoffman showed that mortality from breast cancer was close to 10 times higher in England and Wales than in Japan. There was immediate interest in possible hormonal factors
1895: Beatson produced regression of recurrent breast cancer by removal of ovaries	B. *Hormones and Breast Cancer* 1913 Lathrop and Loeb showed that pregnancy protects against experimental	1915: The Registrar General published figures showing that mortality is higher in single women than married; and higher in childless than in fertile married women
Huggins introduced adrenalectomy in treatment (1945)	breast cancer in mice Subsequently, the action of oestrogens in influencing the growth of breast	
Olivecrona introduced hypophy-sectomy (1952)	cancer in animals was demonstrated	Age-trends show a striking levelling at the menopause

Multiple Causes
The synergistic action of *genetic* and *hormonal* factors together with a *virus-like agent* (Bittner) is most effective in producing a high yield of mammary cancer in mice

It was for long further postulated that *prolonged lactation* protects against breast cancer and so partly explains the connections of the disease with marital status, fertility and geography. But a study in USA (1960) found no difference in lactation history between breast cancer patients and controls

A comparative study, using standardised methods, is in progress in several countries. This has shown that it is age at first pregnancy that matters. Lactation does not protect, early age of bearing first child does.

MacMahon and colleagues have postulated altered ratio of oestrogen fractions as possible underlying hormonal lesion; and they are making international comparative studies of this—geographical biochemistry—which are confirmatory

A prospective survey in women of Guernsey aged 35–54 by Bulbrook and colleagues found that low excretion of androgen metabolites is associated with high subsequent incidence of breast cancer. This suggestion of a possible precursor abnormality should be tested in a larger population

TABLE TW.5

A NEW CAUSATION DISCOVERED

Production of Congenital Malformations by Rubella

Clinical Observation	Laboratory Study	Epidemiology; Community Diagnosis; Community Health
Gregg, ophthalmologist, then others in Australia, taking clinical case-histories, connected an unusual frequency in infants of congenital malformations – cataract, heart disease – with rubella early in mother's pregnancy (the rubella syndrome, RS). This was in 1940–1 when rubella had been unusually common after a long period of low incidence. Clinicians recognised the significance of the observation, which opened up a new era of research into possible environmental causes of malformation	*Embryology.* – By animal experiment, and special observation on man, *ethology*, it has been demonstrated that during a critical period of early embryonic life, when organ differentiation and growth are taking place, they are specially vulnerable to damage. The specific malformations associated with rubella commonly are multiple and they are found when maternal infection has occurred during the first trimester, and particularly the 4th to 8th week, of pregnancy; i.e. the period of organogenesis in the human embryo	*Testing of the hypothesis.* – Looking back, and making use of routine official census statistics, a high rate of congenital deaf-mutism was identified in the cohort of births exposed to the epidemics of rubella that occurred in Australia during 1898-9 and other years, as well as in 1938-41
		Serologic Epidemiology. – Surveys have shown that in urban Western populations 15–20 per cent of women of child-bearing age are susceptible to rubella
Other anomalies, such as deafness and psychomotor retardation gradually were added to the rubella syndrome;	*Teratology.* – Congenital malformations have been produced in animals by many different agents, singly or in combination, but always by degree of malnutrition or other damage insufficient to kill the embryo	*Individual Risks.* – Prospective clinical survey by British Medical Officers of Health before virologic and serologic tests became available found these risks *of malformation to infant:*
		567 Pregnant Women with Rubella All these mothers: Risk to infant = 1 in 14

as well as congenital diseases – thrombo-cytopenic purpura, meningitis, etc.

It can be postulated that it is the mildness of the infection, in the case of rubella, which is responsible for the frequent malformation rather than death of the embryo

Virology. – Rubella virus infects the placenta via the blood stream; then invades the foetus where it was isolated 20 years after Gregg. A chronic infection persists throughout foetal life, is present at birth, and may continue up to 3 years of age. Virologic investigations since 1962 have confirmed the observation that RS in the infant can occur even though *the maternal infection is inapparent. Laboratory diagnosis of infected women and infants is* now quite practicable

Maternal rubella in first 12 weeks:
    Risk to infant = 1 in 6
Maternal rubella at 13–40 weeks:
    Risk to infant = 1 in 34
5,611 mothers who did not have rubella:
    Risk to infant = 1 in 36

There was also an excess of abortion, stillbirth, infant death, and low birth weight, in the rubella cases

A later *audiometric survey* of children exposed in utero who appeared normal at birth detected considerable subclinical hearing loss in addition to the clinical deafness

Estimate of proportion of malformation that is due to rubella is difficult to make, but it probably is quite small

Search for evidence of special incidence of congenital anomalies in relation to *other viral infections* in pregnancy has so far yielded little, excepting with cytomegalovirus

Antenatal diagnosis permits termination of affected pregnancies

A vaccine has been developed and immunisation is now being widely used

TABLE TW.6

CAUSES OF GOITRE IN TASMANIA (CLEMENTS); ITS PREVENTION; ECOLOGY

Clinical Medicine	Epidemiology and Public Health	Nutrition; Molecular Biology
Observation in 1949 of high frequency of goitre in Tasmania	A special survey in 1949 during routine school medical inspection confirmed the clinical impressions of high prevalence of goitre among children in Tasmania. Mass distribution of KI tablets was organised, but re-survey five years later showed a further rise of prevalence in the children, i.e. the customary response to iodine was not obtained. Moreover, boys were affected as much as girls, unlike the picture in iodine-deficiency goitre	
	In the period between the two surveys there was considerable increase in milk consumption by children. To meet the demand for	Twenty-five years before, Chesney had demonstrated the goitrogenic action of an agent in brassica seeds (e.g. kale). However, local attempts to isolate

substances from cow's milk with strong enough goitrogenic activity were unsuccessful

milk, production of a forage crop choumollier – a kale – was greatly increased

Selective distribution of the goitre suggested that personal susceptibility was also involved

In due course, incidence of goitre fell but not in some regions where inefficient distribution of the tablets was blamed. So in 1966, potassium iodate was added to bread; and the incidence throughout Tasmania has fallen to that of non-goitrous regions

Modern methods of diagnosis using I 131 up-take studies, T3 resin uptake, etc.

The number of cases of thyrotoxicosis in the island's two clinics quickly more than doubled. Most of the patients were over 40 years of age and had nodular goitres rendering them susceptible to toxic change from rapid increase of iodine intake

Particular efforts were made to ascertain all cases by collaboration between the special clinics and local doctors. During recent years the incidence has fallen, suggesting a cohort effect

The standard Glasgow system of clinical assessment was used, and special studies made to validate current vs. previous diagnosis of thyrotoxicosis

Recapitulation

The epidemiological method is the only way of asking some questions in medicine, one way of asking others, and no way at all to ask many. Several *uses of epidemiology* have been described:

1. To study the *history of the health of populations,* and of the rise and fall of diseases and changes in their character. Useful projections into the future may be possible.

2. To *diagnose the health of the community* and the condition of the people, to measure the true dimensions and distribution of ill-health in terms of incidence, prevalence, disability and mortality; to set health problems in perspective and define their relative importance; to identify groups needing special attention. Ways of life change, and with them the community's health; new measurements for monitoring them must therefore constantly be sought.

3. To study the *working of health services* with a view to their improvement. Operational research translates knowledge of (changing) community health and expectations in terms of needs for services and measure how these are met. The success of services delivered in reaching stated norms, and the effects on community health — and its needs — have to be appraised, in relation to resources. Such knowledge may be applied in action research pioneering better services, and in drawing up plans for the future. Timely information on health and health services is itself a key service requiring much study and experiment. Today, information is required at many levels, from the local district to the international.

4. To estimate from the group experience what are the *individual risks* on average of disease, accident and defect, and the *chances* of avoiding them.

5. To *identify syndromes* by describing the distribution and association of clinical phenomena in the population.

6. To *complete the clinical picture* of chronic diseases and describe their *natural history:* by including in due proportion all kinds of patients, wherever they present, together with the undemanding and the symptomless cases who do not present and whose needs may be as great; by following the course of remission and relapse, adjustment and disability in defined populations. Follow-up of cohorts is necessary to detect early sub-clinical and perhaps reversible disease and to discover precursor abnormalities during the pathogenesis which may offer opportunities for prevention.

7. To *search for causes* of health and disease by comparing the experience of groups defined by their composition, inheritance and experience, their behaviour and environments. To confirm particular causes of the chronic diseases and the patterns of multiple causes, describing their mode of operation singly and together, and to assess their importance in terms of the relative risks of those exposed. Postulated causes will often be tested in naturally occurring *experiments of opportunity* and sometimes by *planned experiments*.

These various uses all derive from the principle that in epidemiology whole "populations" (or representative samples) are studied, not individuals or patients. Information thus gathered by including all degrees of disease and manner of involvement may change our picture of the natural history. Assessment of the community's burden of disease and disability, and of the health achieved, are indicators of the condition of the people and the state of society. Study of groups that are particularly healthy or vulnerable is often the beginning of the search for causes and so of prevention.

Work in Progress
In recent years there has been a notable increase in epidemiological investigation, and it is now being used in the study of health at all levels of organisation from the molecule to the social group. Advances have been recorded in various cancers, atherosclerosis, ischaemic heart disease, hypertension, bronchitis, industrial pulmonary disease, mental disorders, accidents and drug addiction . . . in the definition of factors at conception and during pregnancy and labour, making for the birth of healthy babies . . . New ground is being broken in chromosome studies, the risks of mutation and malformation, population genetics, family studies; in international comparisons by uniform techniques, surveys of morbidity, in identifying individual susceptibility . . . Techniques of investigation are being developed: in population sampling and the assessment of bias, the standardisation of criteria and valid diagnosis, simple tests of physiological function, electronic and other objective screening devices, multiple miniaturised laboratory estimation . . . Computers have opened up new possibilities in multiple factor analysis; in the storage and retrieval of mass-information; for monitoring of new hazards; in health-record linkage; in simulation and model-building; in mapping of health-service and aetiological situations . . . Cohort study is yielding data on historical trends; on healthy, biological variation, the early manifestations of disease, and on risk factors for future trouble; on normal development and on the course of chronic diseases . . . Laws are beginning to be formulated of the action of environmental hazards (e.g. in thresholds and dose-response) and the conditions of health of populations . . . Major developments can be

foreseen: with immunology, in the estimation of health beyond the mere absence of disease, in measurement of disability, in trials of preventive regimens, in service of medical care . . . Nevertheless, medicine needs more of the scientific endeavour of epidemiology, so does *community medicine* and, it may be said, society at large: more of its skills, more of its ways of thinking and looking at the world, and more of its findings.

MEDICINE AND SOCIETY

Medicine as a whole needs more epidemiology, to obtain a true spectrum of disease. Presenting problems are set in perspective and disorders related to total distributions. The physicians' experience can be compared with the health-needs of the population and the patients who are coping with those who do not. Group regularities help to explain the individual instance or its singularity. Measurements can be made of the standards reached by clinical effort and of its efficacy. Epidemiology is fertile with suggestions for clinical and laboratory research, and hypotheses emerging there can be tested in the experience of populations (this indeed may be obligatory before new discoveries can be put into practice). Seeking to comprehend the social and biological forces expressed in the people's health, epidemiology is a "generalist" science, concerned with causes as much as with processes of health and disease.

Epidemiology is the basic science of *Community Medicine*. Using epidemiological methods greater understanding will be sought of population health and necessary information provided for plans to improve it, to prevent disease and deliver medical care. Categories of need have to be better defined. The success of services in reaching stated standards will be assessed, and what in fact are the benefits to health and the relief of suffering in relation to resources consumed. Such a contribution to rationality (and fairness) is an urgent requirement in the management of health services and for ordering their priorities. Epidemiology thus is basic to the training of community medicine specialists.

Finally, one of the urgent needs of highly developed and rapidly changing societies, with their ageing populations, is to determine *ways of healthy living,* the wisdom of body and mind and the principles of social organisation, that can improve the quality of life and lighten the burden of chronic disease. The quest for this knowledge is the main use of epidemiology.

Notes on

Measurements for Uses

The principal measurements used in epidemiology are Incidence and Prevalence for the study of morbidity, and the Death Rate. What follows is concerned in the main with these as they apply in the field of chronic disease. *Incidence* measures the rate of appearance of new cases in a population; *prevalence* is the volume of all the cases. Crude rates refer to whole populations, specific rates to specified sub-populations within them. In practice, these notions may be expressed as follows.

1. The ANNUAL INCIDENCE of a disease =

$$\frac{\text{Number of persons in a population-at-risk during a}}{\text{given year who newly manifest the disease}} \times 1{,}000.$$

The population has to be identified and counted; it may be "specified" by sex, age, occupation and so forth to give the distribution of the incidence, and the persons in it must not have manifested the disease previously. Incidence therefore gives the frequency of *new events, first attacks,* the *onset,* appropriately defined, of the condition being studied. Early manifestations of chronic diseases often are variable, they come and go, and quite different incidence rates for a given period could be obtained by using different definitions. Several situations however are common enough to be generally agreed as the "onset".

(a) In *clinically presenting* disease, the incidence may be accepted as the first appearance of a defined symptom (e.g. characteristic chest pain), or the first absence from work on account of it, as in acute myocardial infarction. In malignant disease the first presentation to hospital services, or the date of diagnosis, is often accepted as the date of onset by cancer registries.

(b) In *subclinical disease,* the detection of signs, like electrocardiographic "ischaemic" change or high blood pressure, however these have been defined, in persons who have not previously shown them, can be taken for the onset. This situation is readily extended to the discovery of silent *precursor abnormalities,* for example cervical carcinoma in situ in women with previous normal cytology.

(c) Such previous knowledge is unnecessary when the natural history of the disease indicates that what is detected very probably is the first attack — e.g. cancer of the bronchus found on routine X-ray.

2.   THE INDIVIDUAL RISK, on average, of developing a disease over a given period of years can often be obtained with enough accuracy by adding the *incidence rates* for the successive intervals within the period. It is usually expressed as a 1 *in X* chance between the beginning and end of the period.

3.   The other main measurement of morbidity is PREVALENCE, which is usually calculated for one *point* or "cross-section" in time. Prevalence depends upon the frequency of a disease and how long it lasts. When recovery is rapid, e.g. many infections, or death is quick, e.g. in several cancers, there is little difference between incidence and prevalence. The more chronic the condition, e.g. osteo-arthrosis or many skin disorders, the greater the difference between incidence and prevalence and the more it matters to have good measurements of the latter.

The POINT PREVALENCE RATE of a disease, therefore =

$$\frac{\text{No. of persons in a defined population at a stated time who manifest the disease}}{\text{No. in that population at the time}} \times 1,000.$$

Sometimes, the *period prevalence* is calculated, say for a year. This is the proportion of the population manifesting the disease over the course of the year: those already showing it at the beginning (point prevalence), plus the new cases and the relapses which occur subsequently. The denominator is the average number in the population, or the part of it being studied, during the same year.

4.   Characteristically, chronic diseases remit and relapse; think of the allergies, manic-depressive psychosis or the episodes of multiple sclerosis.

The ATTACK RATE refers to the number of persons in the population-at risk having a first or later attack during a stated period.

In studying morbidity, information on incidence and some measure of prevalence commonly are wanted, and I hope it is beyond doubt by now how different these are. The *incidence rate* is essential: to give the rate at which the population is being affected and, therefore, the risk on average to an individual; in seeking risk factors — causes and precursors — which lead up to the onset of disease, and in judging the outcome of attempts at primary prevention; to describe the appearance of a new condition and its spread among the population; for historical study — are new cases occurring more, or less, frequently than before? — and to look ahead . . . Since the *prevalence* includes all the cases it is a measure of the burden of a given disease on the community at large and on particular groups, of needs. It may give an indication of the effectiveness of services, e.g. in tuberculosis, and of attempts at secondary prevention by detecting disease early in order to cure or arrest it. Prevalence data thus are useful for describing the natural history of chronic conditions. They are less helpful in seeking causes and precursors because, as so clearly exemplified in acute myocardial infarction, the individual's mode of life and bodily functions are very liable to be changed by the disease. It goes without saying that the causes of incidence of a condition, and of its prevalence, may be very different. This is evident again in IHD; or in cigarette smoking — the social-psychological reasons why this is started (incidence) as against the physiological factors that are so important in addiction (prevalence).

Information for Community Health Services

All the rates described above refer to persons. An individual can appear only once in the numerator and, of course, only once in the denominator. In delivering services, such population data are necessary for the assessment of needs, and in evaluating outcomes in community health and welfare. On *needs,* for example, incidence data will provide intelligence on the changing numbers, frequency and characteristics: of the extremely small babies born, new single-parent families, infants to be immunised, newly ascertained schizophrenics and their family situations, middle-aged men reaching 3-months' sickness absence, persons entered on the Blind Register. Routine monitoring of such notifications can be a first step in "evaluation". Data on prevalence, the build-up of numbers in such categories, and thus of the load on local services, is even more important.

The location and other details of each individual in the numerator often will also be required by services. And if all who have particular needs are to be offered help, sampling of the population which may be adequate for other purposes will be inappropriate and may indeed miss the worst affected — the extremes of distributions or vulnerable small groups and areas.

There is as yet no standard vocabulary of severity of lesions/impairments, or of kinds, degree and implications of *handicap* and *dependency.* Ad hoc definitions are therefore necessary to produce simple information on the *disabled* in the community, in terms of frequency and duration of functional incapacities, interferences with daily living, needs for particular supports and so forth. This is a key field of study and experiment today.

Health-service statistics, however, whether for their own administration or in accounting to the public, tend to deal not in individuals, their needs for and utilisation of services, but in *events:* in *episodes of ill-health* that make demands on services, and in *services delivered.* Thus the numbers are counted of suspect heart-attacks admitted to intensive care units, such-and-such medicines prescribed, spells in hospital or of sickness-absence and their length, out-patient attendances, contacts with GPs — and the cost of these in resources. Since individuals vary widely in the number of such transactions in which they are involved, strict population rates can rarely be calculated direct from the figures. If population counts are required, the "numerators" will be the spells, admissions, prescriptions of various kinds, etc., in a given period, and the denominators are the average numbers of persons-at-risk in the relevant population — of the area health authority for example, or in the hospital's "catchment" area. Hopefully, also, those-at-risk can be specified, say by severity or urgency of illness or disability, related to the needs for the services. In making local or other comparisons the availability of services should be known, because *supply* $\rightleftharpoons$ *demand* $\rightleftharpoons$ *utilisation* $\rightleftharpoons$.

5.   To resume. *Chronic-disease Registers*. — Ideally, these are *personal files* of all in a population with a defined "chronic-disease", and *linking records* of relevant medical and social events as they occur in the registered individual. The registers should be used for surveillance; collated, the information can describe the often long and chequered natural history, and the needs as well as the utilisation of services. Registers of children "at-risk"; or of persons with particular problems, e.g. the ladies over 75 living alone for the first time, and kept with a view to preventing isolation, represent the same principle.

MORTALITY

6.   The DEATH RATE, or mortality, is the proportion of the population-at-risk dying from "all causes" during a given period, commonly a year. The death rate from a particular disease is the frequency of deaths in which the disease, as named in the WHO I(nternational) C(lassification) of D(isease), is taken to be the main or underlying, cause in the chain of events leading to the death. The death rate may thus be defined as —

$$\frac{\text{No. in a population who die (of a disease) during a given year}}{\text{Mid-point population in that year}} \times 1,000$$

When convenient, for example if numbers in the numerator are small, death rates are calculated per 10,000, 100,000 or million of the population instead of the usual 1,000. Similarly, to avoid over elaboration of tables, less common causes of death may have to be coded with the more common. Death, among the aged especially, often involves multiple causes, and these may be mentioned in the several parts of the certificate. *Multiple coding* of the information on the certificate is therefore becoming essential in order to obtain a truer picture of the event. At the same time, this practice will help to demonstrate syndromes and the association of diseases, such as the role of diabetes in heart-attack, or of physical disease in mental disorder of old age. (The same notion is emerging in *morbidity* recording not merely of the ICD diagnosis, but of the *multiple physical, mental, and social problems* that affect the subject.)

Crude death rates are calculated from the total number of persons dying out of a given number living. When comparing death rates to assess the relative healthiness of different populations, or in the search for causes of disease, differences in age structure must be taken into account. *Rates for specific ages* may be used for this purpose; or *age-standardised rates* calculated.

In 1971, 31 per cent of the population of Clacton, a typical "retirement town" in the South-east of England, were 65+ years of age, compared with about 13 per cent in the country as a whole. The crude D.R. in Clacton was 19·2 per 1,000, the standardised rate 11·1, lower in fact than the national figures of 11·6. But, of course, to the community physician, such "correction" of the rate is misleading, since the number of the elderly is the biggest single factor determining community needs and demands for services. On age-structure alone, Clacton requires about 50 per cent more "acute" general hospital beds than the national average.

INFANT MORTALITY refers to deaths in the first year of life. IM= deaths of babies before their first birthday occurring during a given year, per 1,000 live births in that year . . . The STILLBIRTH RATE (of late foetal deaths) and the PERINATAL MORTALITY rate, which includes stillbirths + deaths in the first week of life, are calculated per 1,000 total births, live and stillborn.

Like all the rates that have been considered, mortality can be referred to more specific and relevant populations-at-risk than the simple head-count. These extend from sex and age to occupational analyses, or maternal deaths referred to live births, or deaths in automobile accidents, whether of pedestrians or of people inside the motor, in relation to the number of vehicles licensed or to estimates of the miles driven etc.

7. CASE-FATALITY is the rate of dying among persons having a given disease. The denominator of the rate consists of a defined group with the condition, e.g. cases of asthma, or the hospital admissions for hyperplasia of the prostate (why do I choose these examples?), and the numerator is the number of them who died of it during a stated period. This approach can be extended; for example, to measure the proportion of persons with a given disease who have *remissions* and *relapses* and, with simple Life Table methods, to provide indices of *prognosis* and of various *outcomes* among the sufferers.

8. Locally, the community physician can use all deaths in particular categories among his population to monitor the working of services. Such are the deaths in infancy, and in accidents; and indeed all other deaths that on the face of it might well be avoidable.

Postscript
"Four Cheers for Prevention"*

The years since the war, the 1960's in particular have been great years for health and prevention. We could all make our own lists — so let me recall some of the more obvious achievements in this country in the promotion of health and prevention of disease:

Subsistence poverty reduced
Gross subnutrition in mothers and children virtually eliminated
Seven million new houses built
The Clean Air Act
Maternal mortality at all-time low
Immunisation against polio, measles, rubella
Rh disease conquered
Safety of medicines provision
Several occupational cancers controlled
Institutionalism reduced in mental hospitals and other places
The breathalyser
Crash helmets.

There is, moreover, substantial knowledge waiting to be applied in practice, or applied more fully: about birth control, for example; cigarettes; fluoridation; sugar, dental caries and obesity; seat-belts; in industrial safety; rehabilitation. The message may be as old as the hills, but modern studies on the role of mothering and sensory inputs (and in the poor countries of good nutrition) in the mental development of the young child offer the hope for the first time of a knowledge-based mental health programme and a general "non-specific" preventive psychiatry.

I want to talk about the meaning and nature of "prevention" in the context of today's needs in a "developed" society, indulging little in science fiction if only because it's so hard to keep up with what is already fact. I will be looking only at parts of the field, virtually confine myself to the second half of life and omit, for example, most of the ground on communicable disease and the environment surveyed so magisterially by the Chief Medical Officer.[2] Where we don't know, my concern will be with the "D" rather than the "R" of the Research-Development spectrum. In the foreground are the constraints of social policy and the rationalised Health Service. I have chosen to speak of four principles of attack, four strategies, but of course they overlap. My first is central to a society like ours, its health problems dominated by the "chronic diseases". I refer to the role in prevention of —

*Presidential Address, Section of Epidemiology and Preventive Medicine, Royal Society of Medicine, 11 May, 1972[1]. Amended

References on page 309.

1.   The Quality of Medical Care

In the 50 years of the therapeutic revolution, since the discoveries of insulin and liver, mankind has been blessed by science and technology with a wondrous arsenal of powerful and effective remedies. I am thinking of the treatment of several cancers, adrenal and other hormonal crises, malignant hypertension, shock and haemorrhage, head injuries, respiratory failure, renal failure, hypothermia, depression, haemophilia, heart-valve surgery, life-endangering arrhythmias, asthma, tuberculosis, septicaemia, the care of very small babies, etc., etc., to mention only situations in which lives can be saved and that are directly related therefore to my theme of "prevention". These can be epitomised in the dramatic achievements of emergency surgery — and of resuscitation and nursing and anaesthetics and laboratory investigation and everything else that may be, so often is, vital from hour to hour.

My illustration will, I hope, be familiar. In virtually every condition where hospital treatment is likely to affect the outcome, *case-fatality* is higher in the regional board hospitals than in the teaching hospitals of the National Health Service (p. 88). We first demonstrated this disparity in the Social Medicine Unit, 15 years ago, prompted, as so often happens, to ask the epidemiological question by a clinical observation. At The London Hospital, where we then were settled, there seemed never to be a fatal case of appendicitis in its huge surgical practice; whereas the Registrar General was reporting 800 deaths a year. For a long time we hoped that the Surgeons themselves would take up the question but, apart from a complaint that the public could be unnecessarily alarmed by this kind of investigation, there was no response. So we proceeded to the next step ourselves, together with two teaching and three regional board hospitals, as typical as could be found, and using simple enlargement of the prostate as "marker". Table P.1, overleaf, shows the differences in case-fatality, col. (3).

As expected, this was higher in all the hospitals among the unplanned, emergency, admissions, col. (7) compared with col. (5); fatalities in the planned admissions from the waiting list were remarkably low. But two other features will be noticed in the table: the gross excess of unplanned admissions to hospitals D & E, 180 of 233, col. (6); and the number of deaths in these men, 25, col. (7), sick old men very often with acute retention of urine. Columns (8) and (10) begin to explain where the trouble lay. Compared with D & E, the other hospitals not only admitted fewer emergencies but carried out prostatectomy on more of those they did admit, with consequentially better overall survival figures: the operation, in today's thinking, is indicated in nearly every case. Hospitals D & E had a much heavier load of the most difficult cases, the lowest operation rate and the highest death rate. The other side to the record is that with the greatest requirements, the most crises, hospitals D & E also had the least resources of staffing, buildings, and other facilities, the iron law again. In particular, hospitals

Table P.1

SERIAL ADMISSIONS TO TWO TEACHING HOSPITALS AND THREE REGIONAL BOARD HOSPITALS OF THE NHS, AND DEATHS
Simple Enlargement of Prostate[3].

| Hospitals | All Admissions | | | Planned Admissions | | Unplanned Admissions | | | | | |
| | | | | | | | | Operated | | Not operated | |
	Nos. (1)	Deaths (2)	Case-fatality (3)*	Nos. (4)	Deaths (5)	Nos. (6)	Deaths (7)	Nos. (8)	Deaths (9)	Nos. (10)	Deaths (11)
TH A & B	514	8	1·6%	399	3	115	5	106	2	9	3
RBH C	185	6	1·9%	104	1	81	5	76	2	5	3
RBH D & E	233	26	8·7%	53	1	180	25	123	5	57	20

*Age-standardised on teaching hospital "population".

A, B and C had a specialist urology unit; D & E didn't. The mismatching is seen at its most extreme in the *local admissions* to hospital A and hospital E, which in fact are only a mile or two apart: 71 per cent of the local men over 75 years of age, and 88 per cent of the local cases who were confused and/or in congestive failure, were admitted to hospital E.

In this study, that is to say, we have moved from questions of clinical skills and judgment, the customary context of discussion of quality of medical care, to something else without which these may come to naught. We are considering instead the quality of social organisation: how closely community resources are matched to community needs, which is a question of health services management and priorities in resource-allocation. That technical capability and social provision are so often out of joint is of course at the heart of many of today's discontents, extending far beyond medical care. In that, too often, we fail to relate even ample resources to popular needs determined in any objective way; the inequality, and the injustice done, have proved a most intractable problem throughout the 25 years of the health service — and it was far worse before. A bit more for everybody, which is likely to be the official reaction, cannot itself be the answer to defects in distribution (even if hospitals were the right place to spend more money).

The results of this case-study are disquieting. How common this kind of situation is I cannot say, nor whether it is limited to prostatic hyperplasia: the current boom in geriatric surgery makes it urgent to find out. Coronary heart disease, p. 88, is even more important to elucidate, in view of the much larger numbers of deaths and the general and understandable pessimism over the treatment of acute heart attacks. If produced in a planned clinical trial, such a contrast in coronary death-rates would be regarded as a major achievement. Are some of these "excess" deaths in the regional board hospitals avoidable? I have no idea. In view of the differences in the natural history of the two conditions, factors other than those I've been considering for prostatic hyperplasia must be involved. There could scarcely be a simpler illustration of the need for better health-intelligence systems on a population basis, for systematic information on how health services are affecting the people's health.

2. *"Early Diagnosis"*

But, of course, we are all agreed that far too much of medical care is absorbed in advanced disease, in rescue, reprieve, patching up and lost causes; in marginal benefits and diminishing returns. Somehow, the balance has to be redressed towards a more constructive effort, hopefully turning back the tide of chronic disease, to respond to the plea of the Secretary of State "to turn off the tap". So I now ask today's most fashionable question: Can these chronic conditions, presenting so often in a crisis, be recognised earlier, cut short, or, at the least, their complications prevented? The theory often is ambiguous, the practice, meanwhile, plain disappointing: the successes of early diagnosis in antenatal care and pulmonary tuberculosis are proving hard to emulate. But there are hopes today of averting some of the common breakdowns of old age, of detecting breast cancer advantageously earlier and lowering mortality, of controlling periodontal disease; and we can now make a start on reasonably firm ground with the *control of high blood pressure*. Let us first recall what is here at stake in sickness and death, relative to the blood pressure level in an ordinary population sample, most of whose hypertensive members, typically, had no idea there was anything wrong (p. 105, for example).

Now moderate and severe hypertension can be lowered by today's potent and fairly well tolerated medicines: so the "preventive" question is, can these be used to control hypertension, among people who, mostly, do not feel at all ill, before complications strike the target organs? The trial by the Veterans Administration in Washington[4] lowered the high pressures and yielded a substantial reduction in cerebrovascular accidents, heart failure and renal failure. For public health the main interest lies in the hope of reducing strokes — which was achieved. There is no single medical measure, in the words of the WHO Seminar which reviewed the subject,[5] that would make such a contribution to the quality of life in old age as the *prevention of stroke*. There is another consideration, too: cerebrovascular disease "consumes" something of the order of 10,000,000 hospital and nursing-home bed-days a year in this country, and the figure is rising. Hypertension, of course, is a major factor; and there is a contribution here also to our psychogeriatric predicament.

In any condition as common as hypertension — at 105 mm Hg diastolic blood pressure, a customary clinician's definition, we may be dealing with 3 to 4 per cent of the middle-aged population and perhaps a quarter of a million symptomless and at present untreated cases — any hope for wide adoption of control measures must depend on interesting the consumer, then offering regimens (without too many physical, mental and social side-effects) which can be absorbed by basic health services. This is a miniature of one of the forces now unifying the NHS, to enable *community* preventive programmes to be mounted and followed up in difficult *individual* treatment lasting —"participation"—perhaps for life. . . Our own feasibility study, illustrated in Fig. P.1, is structured on general practice and the team of family doctors; using also public health nurses in case-finding among the total practice population (this will be a big step forward) and for surveillance of the treatment (so will this). A special screening "clinic" has been set up for the study; some retraining of personnel is of course involved. Two local district general hospital physicians are

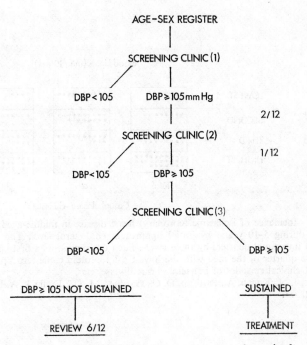

Fig. P.1   Plan of control of high blood pressure in a general practice.[6]

expert advisers and all the facilities of the hospitals are available for the special case. The control of hypertension is likely to be a next major thrust for preventive medicine, and it will represent a sizeable diversion of resources. Many unanswered questions remain, such as how *late* treatment can be postponed, and still achieve worthwhile benefits, and whether women benefit as much as men.

My next "strategy" I have called —

3. *Protecting the Vulnerable Individual*

Pushing further back into the natural history of the epidemic chronic diseases, I want now to be more speculative and fly a kite, to point to dilemmas in our present knowledge and to question whether it is not time to be thinking of another, more physiological, approach to prevention.

Consider the natural history of coronary heart disease in our population. By middle age the underlying coronary atherosclerosis is present in most men. On its basis, about one man in five develops clinical myocardial ischaemia (CHD) by the time he is 65, probably one in four by 70 (good population data peter out in the late 60's). The rate of subclinical disorder is certainly higher. The gene pool for these conditions, that is to say, must be very widespread; moreover,

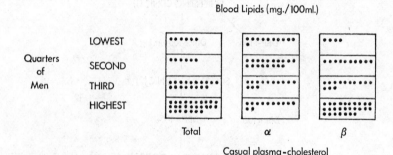

Casual plasma-cholesterol

Fig. P.2 Incidence of ischaemic (coronary) heart disease in middle-aged London busmen during 5–10 years, by initial lipoprotein cholesterol level. The men are classified into equal quarters by these levels. Each dot represents a first episode of IHD: the quarter of the men with the lowest β-lipoprotein cholesterol 'produced' four first clinical episodes of ischaemic heart disease, etc.

Morris, J, N., Kagan, A., Pattison, D. C., Gardner, M. J. & Raffle, P. A. B. (1966) *Lancet,* **2**, 553.

such common, such everyday, occurrences — a mass disorder — cannot be due to wayout behaviour or exceptional stresses, they must be part of everyday living.[7] Many of us cannot take it, cannot cope with the challenges of ordinary life as we like to lead it: they are beyond our limits of healthy adaptation.

Consider next one of the practical facts learned in epidemiological research about coronary heart disease. It is illustrated in Fig. P.2, was first established in Framingham, and is by now beyond dispute.

Food and Health

I want to concentrate on the high plasma cholesterol level, for several reasons. First: it contributes so much to these predictions, it's probably the most powerful of the risk factors yet identified and, conceivably, it may have to be present before the others can "cause" coronary heart disease. In western populations the incidence of CHD rises steeply as blood cholesterol increases above 200 or so mg. per 100 ml. and, as might be expected, with refinement of lipid analysis prediction is more specific, Fig. P.2 for a start. Truly, a major health indicator. Second: taking an ordinary diet, in today's commonplace range of fat intake, many men react with high blood cholesterol values as Fig. P.3 illustrates; diet of course is not the only factor in determining lipid levels. This is human variation again, individual inequality, as

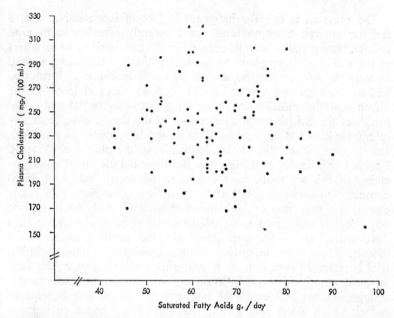

Fig. P.3   Plasma cholesterol concentration in 99 bankmen aged 40–55, in relation to their intake of saturated fat.

Morris, J. N., Marr, J. W., Heady, J. A., Mills, G. L. & Pilkington, T.R E. (1963) *Brit. med. J.*, **1**, 571.

in the requirements for protein and vitamins, for example, or for sleep, or in reactions to medicines, etc.[8-10] Third: it is possible appreciably to lower most high cholesterol concentrations by an acceptable and healthy diet, mainly reducing saturated fat intake, as my colleagues have shown.[11] So the question becomes, can we make use of this information, identify those so vulnerable, and try to protect them? From early in life, when adaptation still is physiological, should we seek to *prevent high blood lipid levels,* for practical purposes, the values at the upper end of the cholesterol distribution? Before atherosclerosis is established, a long time ahead of epidemic clinical disease and while it still may be avoidable — that's the theory — should we try to protect those with such organ inferiority, locus minoris resistentiae? To offer them help, as part of a new individualised modern hygiene for the second half of life, an alternative mode of behaviour. Beginning, say, when young people get married and settle down; though it would be better even earlier, "coronary disease is a paediatric problem". Is there possibly here a new "wisdom of the body and understanding of the heart"? Mightn't this be a very positive activity, truly health-promoting, for the family doctor: through his contact with individuals influencing also the social pattern?[12]

The question is one for judgment in face of inconclusive data, a familiar enough situation (and one I recently experienced in pure culture, though the term could scarcely be less appropriate. As members of the BBC's advisory group on the social effects of television, we had to consider, and recommend, somebody has to recommend, it can't be wished or swept away, what should be done about violence on the screen and the possible long-term dangers to the mental and social health of the British people, no less — in the virtual absence of any relevant evidence at all, anyhow what we would recognise as evidence). Let us return with relief to the simplicities of the plasma cholesterol. This is a question of priorities, too. But there is little doubt about the claims of this metabolic embodiment of advanced, industrial, high-consumption societies. CHD is the paradigm of a disease of many causes, but reduction of high blood cholesterol levels could be one physiological answer to some of the metabolism under strain; thus "preventing" one of the main precursors and, possibly, causes of the disease. Should an intensive, community-based, metabolic-clinical trial be started? Any trial in 20-year-olds wouldn't give us the facts we most want inside another 20 or 25 years. Or do we decide there is enough indirect and collateral evidence on the possible benefits of reducing high blood lipid levels; that there is no reason to suppose this would be harmful; and prudently advise a change of habit? It is high time to be starting a debate on the numerous personal, social — and daunting technical — problems that so obviously arise. Meanwhile, however, the general issue may be forced upon us. One of the mal-nutritions of affluence is the rising consumption of animal and dairy fat, illustrated from the National Food Survey on page 37. The trend now seems to have settled, but are current levels healthy? Healthier than in the mid-1950's? What if the rise is resumed? However confused the story of national diets vis-à-vis coronary disease, to depend more each year on animal and dairy fat makes little sense.

4.   A Healthier Mode of Life

This of course brings me into more familiar territory. How can we influence the social pattern and prevalent life-styles, shift public norms of behaviour? That is far the best way, and if we cannot achieve a more general change, we are likely to fail also with high-risk groups and vulnerable individuals; all three certainly have to be confronted at the same time. The agonising question is how, when popular behaviour is changing so fast and often, as we have just seen, how can we encourage it towards better health? Prevention today is often a matter of individual and family behaviour — in a society too often exerting the wrong pressures. There is no more important or difficult issue for any of us. Few victories for behaviour-change are recorded on page 1 of this postscript to cheer us on our way.

By tradition, I ought now to pause and consider the state of the

nation and the condition of the people, at any rate the major inter-
sections with health. But what can I usefully add to the daily heart-
searching? In community health, the comparison of today's technological revolution is with the first industrial revolution and its
breakneck changes. The cultural changes are truly historic, including
vast subterranean shifts in the balance of feeling and thinking in an
attempt to come to better terms with the irrational, very evident in
the arts where "anything goes", and in the new commitment to human
relations. There is a revolution of rising expectations, spreading across
the social classes, of mental health, personal fulfilment and family
life, and the claim to "happiness" of a secular society. None of these
are based either on knowledge or experience, and they entail wholly
unrealistic hopes of doctors, science and medicine. New sources of
health are perhaps being released in the new freedoms, in the progress
to sexual equality, for example. But how little we understand, still
less control, is nowhere more evident than among young people, the
product of a lifetime of good health and nutrition — and of a revolution
in child care. But this, it seems, frequently is poor preparation for adult
life, to achieve the aspirations of young people either for the world
or for themselves, and too often leads to unhappiness and waste —
whatever the multiple causes of the contemporary epidemics of crime,
self-poisoning, drug abuse, accidents, campus strife, violence, unwanted
pregnancy. More generally, the changes in sexual attitudes and behaviour
have direct impact throughout medicine and public health: an experiment on the health of at least two generations is under way, the reper-
cussions echoing into the distance. In theory, the abatement of guilt
and anxiety which, on balance, may be occurring, could be of mass
benefit, freeing energies for constructive purposes; but the theory is
too slender for any prediction and we must wait and see, hopefully,
wishing them well, while helping in any way we are able, practising
elementary prevention and not merely picking up the casualties. The
loss of "deference" and of young people's respect for "authority"
(so painful to a middle-aged teacher who in his own time was respectful
at least of learning) makes the task no easier.[13] [14]

INGREDIENTS OF A HEALTH POLICY

The main question we have to ask is whether it is possible to describe
any *general causes* of health for today that could take us further than
those responsible for so many of the victories of the past and still to
come in developing countries. It is these "general", non-specific causes in
the mode of life, established in ages of folk wisdom as well as ad hoc
investigation, that so often have been effective in improving health. I
refer to provision of the basic "necessaries of healthy life", to a standard
of living above subsistence, elementary hygiene, adequate living space,
nutritional balance, smaller families (Chadwick, Simon, Thackrah,

Boyd Orr, *et al.*) whose beneficence are exemplified in the health of mothers and children today. Can we advance beyond these to complementary rules for the second half of life? To simple principles of behaviour, for everyone to practice, which would become habits — not interfere with more important matters? That may offer an escape from the trap that the more medical care is supplied the greater is the demand? The answer is beginning to be Yes.

Some principles can be suggested, if not yet with the understanding we would wish. The first is as old as Hippocrates: the *exercise of mind and body.* The exercise of functions is necessary for health, with disuse they wither and waste away. I am referring to physical activity, employment of the mind and faculties, social participation — throughout life. Less than half the sedentary-working, middle-aged, men we are now studying seem to take anything deserving of the name of "exercise", that conceivably is adequate to induce and maintain optimal cardiovascular health. Sedentary living is of course one of the great ecological alterations of modern times, but the consequences in population physiology, musculo-skeletal/haemodynamic/metabolic, and the psychological implications, have yet to be spelled out. Today, the need to apply this notion of health-as-activity is most obvious among the retired. Social forces and personal inclination too often combine to enforce idleness, too forced a disengagement and catabolism. A positive self-image evidently is the key to vigour in old people, and how they react will surely depend on how the rest of society esteems them. Many old people will not want to be too reflective, to re-enact the past, and fewer will want to look forward, so a satisfying life in the present seems a sensible prescription — often made hard to fill. The handicap of those with too little money and too little education is one of the grossest of today's social inequalities.[15]

The control of caloric intake, the second of the "general causes" and today's other great dietary issue in this field, and its role in protecting cardiovascular health is too hackneyed a subject. The fashion for slimming is an unexpected ally. The possibility that over-eating early in life lays down the basis in extra fat cells for later obesity is, of course, of great interest. About *no cigarettes* I will say only that in view of the suggestion on how easy it is to be "hooked", [16] and how soon coughing may begin, stopping youngsters from starting to smoke — again — is the vital issue, and the contradictory signals they receive from Government and society cannot possibly help. Small majorities in the House of Commons we were told are difficult, large majorities even more so; middling majorities we now see are the very dickens. Meanwhile, the infiltration of the cigarette industry into sport creates exactly the wrong kind of image, makes a mockery of "health-education" and is surely the work of the devil.

An even more difficult and confused issue is the *management of social "stress".* To identify characteristic psychic and social stresses liable to be too much for people is our duty both as epidemiologists and as community physicians. And of course this is a challenge also to new social services.[17] It is the prerogative of public health to be simple and direct. So I will illustrate from the kind of piecemeal and practical approach that is immediately open and could be useful, mentioning two different situations: a problem of growth and change; and the pressures put on society's underdogs. It must always be presumed that there will be an imperfect fit between people and their environment, that some or many will be expected to take more stress than is good for them, or more than they comfortably can. Under new or greater pressures, new groups or bigger numbers will break down, the particular expressions, interpersonal, physical, accidents or whatever, depending on a multitude of factors, inborn, in the life-history and in the environment. This is merely to extend the argument from before.[18-20] Whether there is more "stress" generally today than at other periods, and whether we are more or less competent to deal with it — how effective the modern defences are by comparison — are speculations I cannot dwell on here.

"It is changes that are chiefly responsible for diseases, especially the violent alterations" (Hippocrates). Here it is fair enough to mention that extreme case, the bulldozer. I was ashamed recently, when appealed to by local citizens, to discover not merely how little I knew myself but how little data I could find, even short-term and proximate, still less the beginnings of an overall picture, on what happens when sections of the city are torn up to build a highway like the London Motorway Box — to cope with the virtually unrestrained growth of the motor-car. We urgently need information and a public health policy on the possible hazards of *too much change:* For fragile community ties? Mutual aid among families? Gifts between neighbours? Identity in the old? For the chronic, relapsing sick? Those who just will not be able to cope? Anybody's mental health? (How long a check-list?) Should not such be included in "Planning"? And how do they compare with the anticipated benefits?[21] [22]

People in Distress. — Every society creates its own casualties, consigns some of its people, individuals and families, to a life under very special stress; by design or acquiescence, apathy or denial, imposes its own deprivations, frustration and indignities on particular minority groups, denying their human needs and social rights. In our society, they often overlap: the chronic poor in the cities, the abandoned aged, the children who are "finished before they are five", jobless (coloured) youngsters, the hundreds of thousands in substandard housing, the homeless, the middle-aged disabled thrown on the scrapheap, the patients in some long-stay hospitals, the coloured ghettoes, men in and out of the local prisons, the deviants we harrass . . . the catalogue of waste and misery could readily be lengthened. There is only too much scope for preventing the deposit of such groups in the first place; only too much opportunity for us then in our traditional role of protector of the weak and attorney of the poor, for surveillance, to avoid piling stress on top of stress; by social support and personal care to seek to reduce personal and family breakdown, disability, desperation. The cruellest are the most modern of casualties, the accumulating numbers kept alive by health services — by us — but only partly living, grossly handicapped with spina bifida or brain injury, the severely subnormal, vegetating old ladies.

The outlines are emerging of a health policy for tomorrow's community physician in his task as epidemiologist and administrator of services, but also as community counsellor: the reticence of medicine and public health on many of the great social issues of the day does us no credit. Cigarettes apart, we have too often been silent. Where has all the Victorian thunder gone? Do we deceive ourselves that the sources of health lie in medicine?

EPIDEMIOLOGY OF HEALTH

But I want to make another suggestion. The next leap forward, I fancy, is likely to come from a shift in the emphasis of our studies to healthy processes, to the social cultural and economic conditions and sources of the people's good health. So, we might be able more effectively to promote normal functioning, help build up population defences and resistance, more often fulfil potentials for growth and development. It will mean a new partnership with physiology and the behavioural sciences on the scale recently so productive with pathology and clinical medicine. For more useful definitions of health, healthy variation and adaptation, we shall have to rephrase the questions we ask. The stakes are high: quite small shifts in population distributions of blood pressure or blood cholesterol to the left, for example, or of IQ or birth weights to the right (reducing the numbers with seriously abnormal values) could well confer substantial benefits on community health, diminish suffering and lighten the burden on services out of all proportion.

Two challenges for this new epidemiology of health may be mentioned. One is to study ageing and the rate of *ageing* — its postponement, "prevention", and, hopefully, the reduction of associated pathology. We have been too slow, for example, to investigate the remarkable splaying of the distribution, as well as the overall decline, of so many physiological variables that occur with age; to ask how much is due to differential behaviour and environmental effects, contemporary or cohort, and how much is genetic or random. The other challenge is today's grand debate on *environment and the quality of life*. A more systematic epidemiology of human needs, possibilities and limits could enlarge choice in a debate that is at present ill-served by the validity of much of the data fed into it. We could help towards a more rational social accountancy better estimating the costs from economic growth and technology in unhealthy conditions of existence and casualties, as well as what we are gaining in benefits to health. How far, fast, and well people can and do adapt, in what kind of social order, is peculiarly our territory for study.

*　　*　　*

Last Word

The organisation which embodies much of our own activity is now being refashioned. For the first time in history, the formal structure of health services, in certain major aspects, will be designed to meet what we understand to be the needs of the people, and only secondarily in terms of professional and political pressures.[25] I have tried to illustrate some of the avenues open and about to open for *prevention,* agenda for the new health authorities: in bringing to all fair shares of the life-saving potential of modern treatment; in containing wherever possible the havoc of the chronic diseases by catching them earlier; in seeking a physiological hygiene for the vulnerable individual; in reducing avoidable misery by promoting a better society and healthier ways of living. Tomorrow's community physicians will have great opportunities, and greater challenges to face. Let me close with a word to the "academics" among us — we must do our part, too; we must not fail them.

References and Reading

GENERAL

Official Series, England & Wales, Published by Her Majesty's Stationery Office (HMSO), London.
Annual Abstract of Statistics.
Health and Personal Social Services Statistics.
Social Trends.
Department of Health and Social Security, Annual Report.
On the State of the Public Health: Annual Report of the Chief Medical Officer, DHSS.
REGISTRAR GENERAL, Office of Population Censuses and Surveys.
Statistical Review of England & Wales
Part I   Tables, Medical, Annually.
Part II   Tables, Population. Annually.
Hospital In Patient Enquiry (HIPE). Annually.
Population Trends, Quarterly.
Monitors Series.
Life Tables.
Population Projections. Government Actuary.
Adelstein, A. M. (1972) *Hlth Trends,* **4**, 2, 32, 50.

Ackernecht, E. H. (1945) *Bull. Hist. Med.* Suppl. No. **4**, 1.
American Journal of Public Health. Bookshelf Series, annually, Vol. **1**.
Armitage, P. (1966) *Rev. Int. Stat. Inst.* **34**, 27; (1971) *Statistical Methods in Medical Research,* Oxford.
Barker, D. J. P. (1973). *Practical Epidemiology.* London.
Benjamin, B. (1968) *Health and Vital Statistics.* London; (1972) In *Scientific Basis of Medicine Annual Reviews.* London.
Carstairs, V. & Howie, V. (1972). *Health Services in a Population of* 250,000. Edinburgh.
Chronic Diseases and Public Health. (1966) Ed. Lilienfeld, A. M. & Gifford, A. J. Baltimore, Md.
Cohn, A. E. & Lingg, C. (1950) *The Burden of Diseases in the United States.* New York.
Creighton, C. (1894) *A History of Epidemics in Britain.* Reissued 1965. London.
Epidemiological Methods in the Study of Chronic Diseases. (1967) *Wld Hlth Org. techn. Rep. Ser.* No. 365. Geneva.
Epidemiology A Guide to Teaching Methods. (1973) Ed. Lowe, C. R. & Kostrzewski, J. IEA, London.
Epidemiology of Non-Communicable Disease. (1971) Ed. Acheson, E. D. *Brit. med. Bull.* **27**, 1–88.
Farr, W. (1885) *Vital Statistics.* Ed. Humphreys, N. A. London.
Frost, W. H. *Papers of* (1941) Ed. Maxcy, K. F. New York.
Genetics and the Epidemiology of Chronic Diseases (1965) Ed. Neel, J. V., Shaw, M. W. & Schull, W. J. Washington, D. C.
Goldberger *on Pellagra. Collected Papers.* Ed. Terris, M. (1965) Baton Rouge.
Goodall, E. W. (1933) *A Short History of the Epidemic Infectious Diseases.* London.

Gordon, J. E. (1953) In *The Epidemiology of Health*. Ed. Galdston, I. New York; (1963) *Amer. J. med. Sci.* **246**, 354.

Greenwood, M. (1935) *Epidemics and Crowd Diseases*. London; (1948) *Medical Statistics from Graunt to Farr*. Cambridge.

Handbook of Medical Sociology. (1972) Ed. Freeman, H. E., Levine, S. & Reeder, L. G. Englewood Cliffs, N.J.

Health Service Prospects.(1973) Ed. Douglas-Wilson, I. & McLachlan, G. London.

Hill, A. B. (1971). *Principles of Medical Statistics*. London; (1963) *Statistical Methods in Clinical and Preventive Medicine*. Edinburgh.

Logan, W. P. D. (1950) *Popul. Stud.* **4**, 132.

MacMahon, B. & Pugh, T. F. (1970) *Epidemiology: Principles and Methods*. Boston.

McKeown, T. (1961) *Milb. mem. Fd Quart.* **39**, 594.

McKeown, T. & Lowe, C. R. (1974) *An Introduction to Social Medicine*. Oxford.

Morris, J. N. (1955) *Brit. med. J.*, **2**, 395; (1969) *Lancet*, **2**, 811.

Morrison, S. L. (1969) *Lancet*, **1**, 772.

Morrison, S. L. & Last, J. M. (1970) In *A Companion to Medical Studies*, Vol. **2**, 35. Ed. Passmore, R. & Robson, J. S. Oxford.

Occupational Health Practice. (1973) Ed. Schilling, R. S. F. London.

Office of Health Economics. *Series of Papers on Current Health Problems*. London.

Orr, J. B. (1937) *Food, Health and Income*. London.

Paul, J. R. (1966) *Clinical Epidemiology*. Chicago.

Pearl, R. (1928) *The Rate of Living*. London.

Pickles, W. N. (1939) *Epidemiology in a Country Practice*. Bristol.

A Practice of Social Medicine. (1963) Ed. Kark, S. L. & Steuart, G. W. Edinburgh.

Preventive Medicine. (1967) Ed. Clark, D. W. & MacMahon, B. New York.

Le Riche, W. H. & Milner, J. (1971) *Epidemiology as Medical Ecology*. Edinburgh.

Rosen, G. (1947) *Bull. Hist. Med.* **21**, 674; (1948) *Milb. mem. Fd Quart.* **26**, 7.

Ryle, J. A. (1948) *Changing Disciplines*. London.

Serological Epidemiology. (1973) Ed. Paul, J. R. & White, C. New York.

Sigerist, H. E. (1943) *Civilisation and Disease*. London; *On the Sociology of Medicine*. Ed. Roemer, M. I. (1960) New York.

Smoking and Health. (1964) PHS Publication No. 103, HEW, Washington, DC.

Stocks, P. (1934) *Proc. R. Soc. Med.* **27**, 1127; (1938) *J. R. statist. Soc.* **101**, 688.

Suchman, E. A. (1967). *Evaluative Research*. New York.

Susser, M. W. & Watson, W. (1971) *Sociology in Medicine*. London.

Sydenstricker, E. (1933). *Health and Environment*. New York.

Taylor, I. & Knowelden, J. (1964) *Principles of Epidemiology*. London.

Terris, M. & Kogon, A. (Current) *Bank of Epidemiology Exercises*. New York Medical College, New York.

Theory and Practice of Public Health. (1975). Ed. Hobson, W. London.

Trends in Epidemiology. (1972) Ed. Stewart, G. T. Springfield, Ill.

Vernon, H. M. (1939). *Health in Relation to Occupation*. London.

Von Pettenkofer, M. (1873) *The Value of Health to a City*. Transl. Sigerist, H. E. (1941) *Bull. Hist. Med.* **10**, 597.

Winslow, C.-E. A. (1944) *The Conquest of Epidemic Disease*. Princeton.

CHAPTER 1

1. Department of Health and Social Security. *On the State of the Public Health; Annual Reports of the Chief Medical Officer*.

2. Thomson, D. (1966) *Brit. med. J.*, **2**, 427.

3. Morris, J. N. (1951) *Brit. med. J.*, **2**, 548.

4. Morris, J. N. & Titmuss, R. M. (1942) *Lancet*, **2**, 59.

5. Morris, J. N. & Titmuss, R. M. (1944) *Med. Offr*, **72**, 69, 77, 85.

6. *Rheumatic Fever in Scotland*, 1967. HMSO, Edinburgh.

7. *Lancet* (1971) **I**, 897.
8. Thomson, A. M. (1956) *Am. J. clin. Nutr.*, **4**, 647.
9. Harrison, H. E. (1966) *Am. J. publ. Hlth.*, **56**, 734.
10. Berry, W. T. C. (1968) *Proc. Nutr. Soc.*, **21**, 1.
11. Tanner, J. M. (1968) *Sci. Amer.*, **218**, 21.
12. Arneil, G. C. (1967) *Dietary Study of* 4,365 *Scottish Infants,* 1965. HMSO, Edinburgh; (1968) *Lancet* **I**, 803.
13. Morris, J. N. (1973) *Proc. R. Soc. Med.*, **66**, 225.
14. Speizer, F. E. & Doll, R. (1968) *Brit. med. J.*, **3**, 245.
15. Inman, W. H. W. & Adelstein, A. M. (1969) *Lancet*, **2**, 279.
16. Kessel, N. (1965) *Brit. med. J.*, **2**, 1269.
17. *Hospital Treatment of Acute Poisoning.* 1968. HMSO, London.
18. Smith, J. S. & Davison, K. (1971) *Brit. med. J.*, **4**, 412.
19. Wagner, J. C., Gilson, J. C., Berry, G. & Timbrell, V. (1971) *Brit. med. Bull.*, **27**, No. 1, 71.
20. Goldhamer, H. & Marshall, A. W. (1953) *Psychosis and Civilisation.* Glencoe, Ill.
21. Group for the Advancement of Psychiatry. (1961) *Problems of Estimating Changes in Frequency of Mental Disorders.* Rep. no. 50. New York.
22. Sorsby, A. (1966) *Incidence and Causes of Blindness in England & Wales,* 1948–62. HMSO, London; (1973) *Hlth Trends,* **5**, 7.
23. Carter, C. O. (1958) *J. ment. Defic. Res.*, **2**, 64.
24. Goodman, N. & Tizard, J. (1962) *Brit. med. J.*, **1**, 216.
25. Stein, Z. A., Susser, M. W. & Guterman, A. V. (1973) *Lancet,* **1**, 305.
26. Morris, J. N. (1969) *Lancet*, **2**, 811.
27. Heady, J. A., Morris, J. N., Kagan, A. & Raffle, P. A. B. (1961) *Brit. J. prev. soc. Med.* **15**, 143.
28. Morris, J. N., Heady, J. A., Raffle, P. A. B., Parks, J. W. & Roberts, C. G. (1953) *Lancet,* **2**, 1053, 1111.
29. Medical Research Council, Social Medicine Unit and Collaborators. Work in progress.
30. Morris, J. N. (1951) *Lancet,* **1**, 1, 69.
31. Doll, R. (1953) *Brit. med. J.,* **2**, 521, 585.
32. Finland, M., Jones, W. F. & Barnes, M. W. (1959) *J. Amer. med. Ass.,* **170**, 2, 188.
33. Cockburn, A. (1963) *The Evolution and Eradication of Infectious Diseases.* Baltimore.
34. Klainer, A. S. & Beisel, W. R. (1969) *Amer. J. med. Sci.,* **258**, 431.
35. Lewis, A. J. (1962) *Yale J. Biol. Med.,* **35**, 62.
36. Fromm, E. & MacCoby, M. (1970) *Social Character in a Mexican Village.* Englewood Cliffs, N. J.
37. Hoggart, R. (1970) *Speaking to Each Other.* Vol. 1. London.
38. Jenkins, C. D. (1971) *New Engl. J. Med.,* **284**, 244, 307.
39. Marcus, S. (1964) *The Other Victorians.* New York.
40. Trilling, L. (1971) *Commentary,* **52**, No. 3, 39.
41. Gruenberg, E. M. (1967) *In Psychiatry in Transition.* Ed. Stokes, A. B. Toronto.
42. Wing, J. K. & Brown, G. W. (1970) *Institutionalism and Schizophrenia.* Cambridge.
43. Moynihan, B. G. A. (1912) *Duodenal Ulcer.* London.
    Payne, R. T. & Newman, C. (1940) *Brit. med. J.,* **2**, 819.
44. Jennings, D. (1940) *Lancet,* **1**, 395, 444.
45. Morris, J. N. & Titmuss, R. M. (1944) *Lancet,* **2**, 841.
46. Susser, M. (1967) *J. Chron. Dis.,* **20**, 435.
47. Doll, R., Jones, F. Avery & Buckatzsch, M. M. (1951). *Spec. Nep. ser. med. Res. Coun., Lond.* No. 276.
48. Jones, F. Avery (1957) *Brit. med. J.,* **1**, 719, 786.
49. Arie, T. (1970) *In Modern Trends in Psychosomatic Medicine.* Ed. Hill, O. W. London.
50. Pflanz, M. (1971) *Adv. psychosom. Med.,* **6**, 121.

51. Goldberg, E. M. (1958) *Family Influences on Psychosomatic Illness*. London.
52. Carrier, N. H. (1962) In *Society*. Ed. Welford, A. T., Argyle, M., Glass, D. V. & Morris, J. N. London.
53. Benjamin, B. (1964) *J. Inst. Actu.*, **90**, Pt III, 211.
54. Glass, D. V. (1970) *Pop. Stud.*, Suppl. May, p.11.
55. Registrar General, England & Wales, *Statistical Reviews*. Annually.
    Registrar General, England & Wales, *Life Tables*.
56. Woolf, M. (1971) *Family Intentions*, 1967. HMSO, London.
57. Comfort, A. (1970) *Ageing: The Biology of Senescence*. London.
58. Harris, A. I. (1968) *Social Welfare of the Elderly*. HMSO. London.
59. *Our Old People*. (1965) *Socialist Commentary*. London.
    Eyden, J. L. M. (1970) *Soc. Ec. Admin.*, **4**, 3.
60. Ashley, J. S. A. & Klein, R. E. (1971) *Mod. geriatr.*, **1**, 320.
61. Naipaul, V. S. (1972) *The Overcrowded Barracoon*. London.
62. Frederiksen, H. (1966) *Publ. Hlth Rep. Wash.*, **81**, 715.
63. Meegama, S. A. (1967) *Pop. Stud.*, **21**, 207.
64. Newman, P. (1965) *Malaria Eradication and Population Growth*. Ann Arbor.
65. Brass, W. Personal communications.
66. Loraine, J. A. (1970) *Sex and the Population Crisis*. London.
67. Peterson, W. (1964) *Politics of Population*. London.
68. Malthus, T. R. (1798) *Essay in Population*. Reprint (1966). London.
69. Myrdal, G. (1968) *Asian Drama*, Vol. III. New York.
70. Bryant, J. (1969) *Health in the Developing World*. Ithaca.
71. *The State of Food and Agriculture*. Annual Reviews. FAO, Rome.
72. Bridger, G. & de Soissons, M. (1970) *Famine in Retreat*. London.
73. Glass, D. V. (1965) *J. chron. Dis.*, **18**, 1079.
74. Fowler, R. E. & Edwards, R. G. (1970) In *Population Control*. Ed. Allison, A. Harmondsworth, Mddx.
75. Ehrlich, P. & A. (1970) *Population: Resources: Environment*. San Francisco.
76. Pearson, L. B. (1969) *Partners in Development*. New York.
77. Cartwright, A. (1970) *Parents and Family Planning Services*. London.
78. Fox, T. F. (1965) *Lancet*, **2**, 801; (1966). *ibid*, **2**, 1238.
79. Taylor, L. R. (1970) Ed. *The Optimum Population for Britain*. London.
80. Hoagland, H. (1964) *Bull. atom. Sci.*, **20**, No. 2, 2.
81. *Population Policy*. Fifth Report from the Select Committee on Science and Technology. (1972) HMSO, London; *Report of the Population Panel*. (1973) HMSO, London.
82. *Urban Transport Planning*. Second Report from the Expenditure Committee. (1972) HMSO, London.
83. *The Ecologist* (1972) **2**, No. 1; *The Limits to Growth* (1972). Club of Rome. London.
84. Hawthorn, G. (1973) *Population Policy: A Modern Delusion*. London.

CHAPTER 2

1. Department of Health and Social Security. *Annual Reports*. HMSO, London.
   Whitehead, F. E. (1971) In *Social Trends No. 2*, 13. HMSO, London.
2. Froggatt, P. (1968) *Trans. Soc. occup. Med.*, **18**, 89.
3. Halliday, J. L. (1948) *Psychosocial Medicine*. London.
   Lawrence, J. J. & Aitken-Swan, J. (1952) *Brit. J. industr. Med.*, **9**, 1; (1955) *ibid*, **12**, 249.
4. Morris, J. N. (1969) *Lancet*, **2**, 811.
5. Saunders, B. S. (1964) *Amer. J. publ. Hlth*, **54**, 1063.
6. Sullivan, D. F. (1966) *Conceptual Problems in Developing an Index of Health*. NCHS Ser. 2, No. 17. HEW, Washington, DC.

7. Reports European Conferences on Health Statistics, 1963, 1965, 1971. WHO, Copenhagen.
   WHO techn. Rep. Ser. No. 137 (1957); No. 389 (1968); No. 472 (1971). Geneva.
8. Department of Health and Social Security. *Annual Digest of Health and Personal Social Service Statistics. Annual In-patient Statistics from the Mental Health Enquiry.* HMSO, London.
9. *Disease Registers and Their Use.* (1971) WHO, Geneva.
   Wing, J. K. & Hailey, A. (1972) Ed. *Evaluating A Community Psychiatric Service.* The Camberwell Register. 1964–71. London.
10. Abel-Smith, B. & Townsend, P. (1965). *The Poor and the Poorest.* London.
11. Greve, J. (1964) *London's Homeless.* London.
    Bailey, R. & Ruddock, J. (1972) *The Grief Report.* London.
12. *Towards a Social Report* (1969) HEW, Washington, DC.
    Sheldon, E. B. & Moore, W. E. (1968) Ed. *Indicators of Social Change.* New York.
    Bauer, R. A. (1966) Ed. *Social Indicators.* Cambridge, Mass.
    Social Trends. HMSO. Annually.
13. Knox, E. G., Morris, J. N. & Holland, W. W. (1972) *Lancet*, **2**, 696.
14. *Int. J. Epid.*, **1**, No. 4; **2**, No. 1.
15. Dubos, R. (1960) In *Disease and The Advancement of Basic Science.* Ed. Beecher, H. K. Cambridge, Mass.
16. Morris, J. N. (1973) *Proc. R. Soc. Med.*, **66**, 225.
17. Marr, J. W. (1973) *Hlth Trends,* **5**, 37.
    Heady, J. A., Morris, J. N., Kagan, A. & Raffle, P. A. B. (1961) *Brit. J. prev. soc. Med.*, **15**, 143.
18. MRC Social Medicine Unit and Collaborators. Work in progress.
19. Backett, E. M., Shaw, L. A. & Evans, J. C. G. (1953) *Proc. R. Soc. Med.*, **46**, 707.
20. Backett, E. M., Heady, J. A. & Evans, J. C. G. (1954) *Brit. med. J.*, **1**, 109.
21. Ødegard, Ø. (1932) *Acta psychiatr. neurol. Scand.* Suppl. 4; (1956) *Int. J. soc. Psychiatr.*, **2**, 85.
22. Schilling, R. S. F. (1956) *Lancet*, **2**, 261; (1963) *J. R. Soc. Arts*, **111**, 933, 955.
23. Morris, J. N. & Titmuss, R. M. (1942) *Lancet*, **2**, 59.
24. Morris, J. N. & Titmuss, R. M. (1944) *Med Offr.* **72**, 69, 77, 85.
25. Moser, C. A. & Kalton, G. (1971) *Survey Methods in Social Investigation.* London.
26. Armitage, P. (1971) *Statistical Methods in Medical Research.* Oxford.
27. Witts, L. J. (1964) Ed. *Medical Surveys and Clinical Trials.* London.
28. Oppenheim, A. M. (1966) *Questionnaire Design and Attitude Measurement.* London.
29. Walford, J. (1973) In *Occupational Health Practice.* Ed. Schilling, R. S. F. London. p.190.
30. Gilson, J. C. (1959) *Proceedings of the Pneumoconiosis Conference, Johannesburg.* p. 348. London.
31. *American Soldier* (1950) Stouffer, S. A. & Starr, S. F. *Studies in Social Psychology in World War II.* **4**, chaps. 12–14. Princeton.
32. Yerushalmy, J. (1969) *Radiol. Clin. N. Amer.*, **7**, 381.
33. Medical Research Council (1966) *Questionnaire on Respiratory Symptoms.* Dawlish.
34. Rose, G. A. & Blackburn, H. (1968) *Cardiovascular Survey Methods.* WHO, Geneva.
35. Snedecor, G. W. & Cochran, W. G. (1967) *Statistical Methods.* p. 27. Iowa.
36. Heady, J. A. (1961) *J. R. statist. Soc.*, **124**, 336.
37. Marr, J. W. (1973) *Proc. R. Soc. Med.* **66**, 639; *Nutr. Lond.*, **27**, 239.
38. *Times Lit. Suppl.* (1965) Jan. 14, 20.
39. Goldberg, D. P. (1972) *The Detection of Psychiatric Illness by Questionnaire.* London.
40. *Psychiatric Diagnosis in New York and London* (1972) Maudsley Monog. No. 20. London.

41. Goldberg, E. M. (1958) *Family Influences and Psychological Illness.* London.
42. Morris, J. N., Kagan, A., Pattison, D. C., Gardner, M. J. & Raffle, P. A. B. (1966) *Lancet,* **2,** 553.
43. Industrial Health Research Board (1935) *Rep No.* 71. HMSO, London. (Norman, L. G., personal communication.)
44. Stevenson, T. H. C. (1923) *Biometr.* **15,** 382; (1928) *J. R. statist. Soc.,* **91,** 207.
45. Susser, M. & Watson, W. (1971) *Sociology in Medicine.* London.
46. Bottomore, T. B. (1965) *Classes in Modern Society.* London.
   Giddens, A. H. (1973) *The Class Structure of the Advanced Societies.* London.
47. Douglas, J. W. B. (1964) *The Home and the School.* London.
48. Newson, J. & E. (1968) *Four Years Old in an Urban Community.* London.
49. Vernon, H. M. (1939) *Health in Relation to Occupation.* London.
50. *Soc. Rev.* (1972) **20,** No. 3.
51. Morris, J. N. & Heady, J. A. (1955) *Lancet,* **1,** 343, 554.
52. Baird, D. (1969) *Lancet,* **1,** 511.
53. Thomson, A. M. (1958) *Brit. J. Nutr.* **12,** 446; (1963) *Mod. Probl. Pediat.,* **8,** 197; and personal communications.
54. *Perinatal Mortality* (1963) Ed. Butler, N. R. & Bonham, D. G. Edinburgh & London.
55. *Confidential Enquiry into Post-Neonatal Deaths* 1964–66. (1970) HMSO, London. *British Medical Journal* (1973) **1,** 308.
56. Simon, J. (1890) *English Sanitary Institutions.* London.
57. Galbraith, J. K. (1958) *The Affluent Society.* London.
58. Runciman, W. G. (1966) *Relative Deprivation and Social Justice.* London.
59. Miller, S. N. & Roby, P. A. (1970) *The Future of Inequality.* New York.
60. Low Pay (1973) Ed. Field, F. London.
   Jackson, D. (1972) *Poverty.* London.
   How the Poorest Live (1973) A *New Society* Social Studies Reader. London.
61. Myrdal, G. (1952) *Economic Aspects of Health. Chron. Wld Hlth Org.* **6,** 203.
62. Winslow, C.-E. A. (1951) *The Cost of Sickness and the Price of Health.* WHO, Geneva.
63. Wedge, P. & Prosser, H. (1973) *Born to Fail.* London.
64. Davie, R., Butler, N. R. & Goldstein, H. (1972) *From Birth to Seven.* London.
65. Schorr, A. L. (1966) *Poor Kids.* New York.
   Coles, R. & Piers, M. (1969) *Wages of Neglect. New Solutions for the Children of the Poor.* Chicago.
   Birch, H. G. & Gussow, J. D. (1970) *Disadvantaged Children: Health, Nutrition and School Failure.* New York.
66. Davis, K. (1966) In *Contemporary Social Problems.* Ed. Merton, R. K. & Nisbet, R. A. New York.
67. Eppel, E. M. & M. (1966) *Adolescence and Morality.* London.
68. Erikson, E. H. (1968) *Identity: Youth and Crisis.* New York.
69. Fiedler, L. A. (1965) *Partis. Rev.,* **32,** 505.
70. Goodman, P. (1970) *Growing Up Absurd.* New York.
71. *Report of the Committee on the Age of Majority.* (1967) HMSO, London.
72. Adelstein, A. M. (1972) *Hlth Trends,* **4,** 2.
73. Boston Collaborative Drug Surveillance Programme (1974) *Lancet,* **2,** 669.

CHAPTER 3

1. Brotherston, J. H. F. (1969) *Scot. med. J.,* **14,** 130.
2. White, K. L. (1967) *J. med. Educ.,* **42,** 729.
3. *Health Services Research and R & D in Perspective.* (1973) Ed. Flook, E. E. & Sanazaro, P. J. Ann Arbor.

4. *The Application of Epidemiology to the Planning and Evaluation of Health Services.* (1973) WHO, Copenhagen.
   Modern Management Methods and the Organisation of Health Services. (1974) Public Health Paper 55. WHO, Geneva.
5. *Statistics of Smoking in the United Kingdom.* (1972) Ed. Todd, G. F. London.
6. Farr, B. F. (1970) *Seat Belts—The Proportion of Cars Fitted and of Occupants Using Them.* RRL Rep. 342. Crowthorne, Berks.
7. Backett, E. M., Shaw, L. A. & Evans, J. C. G. (1953) *Proc. R. Soc. Med.*, **46,** 707.
8. Backett, E. M., Heady, J. A. & Evans, J. C. G. (1954) *Brit. med. J.*, **1,** 109.
9. Forsyth, G. & Logan, R. F. L. (1960) *The Demand for Medical Care.* London.
   Logan, R. F. L., Ashley, J. S.A., Klein, R. E. & Robson, D. M. (1972) *Dynamics of Medical Care.* London.
10. Matthew, G. K. (1971) In *Portfolio for Health* 1. Ed. McLachlan, G., p. 27. London.
11. Kalimo, E. (1969) *Determinants of Medical Care Utilisation.* Helsinki.
12. McKinlay, J. B. (1972) *J. Hlth. hum. Behav.*, **13,** 115.
13. Kushlick, A. (1972) *Brit. J. Hosp. Med.*, **8,** 161.
14. Parsons, T. (1958) *In Patients, Physicians and Illness.* Ed. Jaco, E. G. Glencoe, Ill.
15. Friedson, E. (1961) *Patients' Views of Medical Practice.* New York.
16. Mechanic, D. (1968) *Medical Sociology.* London.
17. Butler, J. R. (1970) *Brit. J. Sociol.*, **21,** 241.
18. Paul, B. D. Ed. (1955) *Health, Culture and Community.* New York.
    Shanas, E., Townsend, P., Wedderburn, D., Friis, H., Milhøj, P. & Stehouwer, J. (1968) *Old People in Three Industrial Societies.* London.
19. Shaw, L. A. (1954) *Case Conf.*, **1,** 9, *Sociol. Rev.*, **2,** 179.
20. *The General Household Survey.* (1973) HMSO, London.
21. Schilling, R. S. F. (1963) *J. R. Soc. Arts*, **111,** 933.
22. *Employment Medical Advisory Service Act* 1972. HMSO, London.
23. Sidel, V. W., Acton, J. & Lown, B. (1969) *Amer. J. Cardiol.*, **24,** 674.
    Pantridge, J. F. (1970) *Q. J. Med.*, **39,** 621.
    Oliver, M. F. (1968) *Proc. R. Coll. Physns*, **3,** 47.
24. Morris, J. N. (1969) *Lancet*, **2,** 811.
    Morris, J. N. (1970) In *The NHS: Three Views.* Fabian Research Series, No. 287. London.
25. Ashley, J. S. A. & Klein, R. E. (1971) *Mod. Ger.*, **1,** 5.
26. Buckley, W. (1967) *Sociology and Modern Systems Theory.* Englewood Cliffs, N.J.
    The Recognition of Systems in Health Services. (1969) Ed. Chacko, G. K. Arlington, Virginia.
27. Abel-Smith, B, (1967) *An International Study of Health Expenditure.*, WHO, Geneva.
28. Logan, R. F. L. (1968) *Milb. mem. Fd Quart.*, **46,** no. 2, part 2. p. 126.
29. *Lancet,* 1970, **1,** 757.
30. *International Comparisons of Medical Care. Milb. mem. Fd Quart.* (1972) **50,** no. 3, part 2.
31. Kushlick, A. (1967) *Soc. Ec. Admin.*, **1,** 29.
    Kushlick, A. (1972) In *Approaches to Action.* p.81. Ed. McLachlan, G. London.
32. *Brit. med. J.* (1974) **1,** no. 5902, Feb. 16.
33. Warren, M. D. (1966) *Publ. Hlth*, **81,** 8.
34. Cochrane, A. L. (1972) *Effectiveness and Efficiency.* London.
35. *Evaluating a Community Psychiatric Service.* (1972) Ed. Wing, J. K. & Hailey, A. M. London.
36. Hulka, B. S. & Cassel, J. C. (1973) *Amer. J. publ. Hlth.*, **63,** 494.
37. *Report on Confidential Enquiries into Maternal Deaths in England & Wales.* (1972) HMSO, London.

Confidential Enquiry into Post-neonatal Deaths, 1964–1966. (1970) HMSO, London.
38. Hart, J. T. (1971) *Lancet*, **1**, 405; (1972) *Int. J. Hlth. Serv.*, **2**, 349.
Honigsbaum, F. (1972) *J. R. Coll. Gen. Practit.*, **22**, 429.
39. Lee, J. A. H. (1958) *Brit. med. J.*, **1**, 573.
40. Glover, J. A. (1950) *Mon. Bull. Minist. Hlth.*, **9**, 62.
41. *Update*, May 1971, 535.
42. Evans, H. E. (1968) *Clin. Pediat.*, **7**, 71.
Mawson, S. R., Adlington, R. A. & Evans, M. (1968) *J. Laryng.*, **82**, 963.
43. Heasman, M. A. & Carstairs, V. (1971) *Brit. med. J.* **1**, 495.
Ashley, J. S. A. (1972) *Brit. J. prev. soc. Med.*, **26**, 135.
44. Lee, J. A. H., Morrison, S. L. & Morris, J. N. (1957) *Lancet*, **2**, 785.
Lee, J. A. H., Morrison, S. L. & Morris, J. N. (1960) *Lancet*, **1**, 170.
Lipworth, L., Lee, J. A. H. & Morris, J. N. (1963) *Med. Care*, **1**, 71.
Nightingale, F. (1859) *Notes on Hospitals*. London.
45. Ashley, J. S. A., Howlett, A. & Morris, J. N. (1971) *Lancet*, **2**, 1308.
46. Butler, N. R. & Bonham, D. G. (1963) *Perinatal Mortality*. Edinburgh.
47. Goldberg, E. M., Mortimer, A. & Williams, B. T. (1970) *Helping the Aged*. London.
Palmer, T. B. (1973) *Social Work*, **18**, 2.
48. Klein, R. E. & Hall, P. (1974) *Caring for Quality in the Caring Services*. London.
49. *Report of the (Seebohm) Committee on Local Authority and Allied Personal Social Services*. (1968) HMSO, London.
50. Sorsby, A. (1973) *Hlth. Trends*, **5**, 7.
51. *The District General Hospital* (1967). Royal College of Physicians, London.
52. Klarman, H. E. (1965) *The Economics of Health*. New York.
53. Feldstein, M. S. (1967) *Economic Analysis for Health Service Efficiency*. North Holland.
54. *Accounting for Health* (1973) King Edward's Hospital Fund. London.
55. Susser, M. W. & Watson, W. (1971) *Sociology in Medicine*. London.
56. Grad, J. & Sainsbury, P. (1968) *Brit. J. Psychiat.*, **114**, 265.
57. Sainsbury, P. (1973) In *Policy for Action*. Ed. Cawley, R. & McLachlan, G. p. 129. London.
58. *Challenges for Change*. (1971) Ed. McLachlan, G. London.
59. Knox, E. G., Morris, J. N. & Holland, W. W. (1972) *Lancet*, **2**, 696.
60. Alderson, M. R. (1973). In *The Future — and Present Indicatives*. Ed. McLachlan, G. London.
61. Yates, J. M. *ibid.*
62. Adelstein, A. M. (1972) *Hlth Trends*, **4**, 2, 50.
63. Bodenham, K. E. & Wellman, F. (1972) *Foundations for Health Service Management*. London.
64. *Portfolio for Health*. 1 (1971); 2 (1973) Ed. McLachlan, G. London.
65. Doll, R. (1973) *Proc. R. Soc. Med.*, **66**, 729.

CHAPTER 4

1. Cohen, B. H., Lilienfeld, A. M. & Sigler, A. T. (1963) *Amer. J. publ. Hlth.*, **53**, 223.
2. Wynne Griffith, G. (1973) *Hlth. Trends*, **5**, 59.
Stein, Z., Susser, M. & Guterman, A. V. (1973) *Lancet*, **1**, 305.
3. Doll, R., Jones, F. Avery & Buckatzsch M. M. (1951) *Spec. Rep. Ser. med. Res. Coun. Lond.* No. 276.
4. Heady, J. A. & Barley, R. G. (1953) *Brit. med. J.*, **1**, 1105.
5. Morris, J. N. Heady, J. A. & Barley, R. G. (1952) *Brit. med. J.*, **1**, 503.
6. Morris, J. N. (1963) *Proc. R. Soc. B.*, **159**, 65.

7. *Road Accidents.* Annually, HMSO, London.
8. MRC Social Medicine Unit and Collaborators. Work in progress.
9. Doll, R. & Hill, A. B. (1952) *Brit. med. J.*, **2**, 1271.
10. Doll, R. & Hill, A. B. (1964) *Brit. med. J.*, **1**, 1399, 1460.
11. *Hospital in Patient Enquiry,* Annually, HMSO, London.
12. Böök, J. A. (1958) *Eugen. Quart.* **2**, 174.
13. Roberts, J. A. F. (1973) *An Introduction to Medical Genetics.* London.
14. Smith, C. (1972) *Brit. med. J.*, **1**, 495.
15. Parker, R. A. (1967) In *The Use of Predictive Methods in Social Work.* NISWT, London.
16. Mannheim, H. & Wilkins, L. T. (1954) Prediction Methods in Relation to *Borstal Training.* HMSO, London.
17. Morris, J. N., Kagan, A., Pattison, D. C., Gardner, M. J. & Raffle, P. A. B. (1966) *Lancet,* **2,** 553.
18. Morris, J. N. (1973) *Proc. R. Soc., Med.* **66,** 225.
19. *Build and Blood Pressure Study.* (1959) Society of Actuaries. Chicago, Ill.
20. Truett, J., Cornfield, J. & Kannel, W. (1967) *J. chron. Dis.,* **20,** 511.
21. Walker, S. H. & Duncan, D. B. (1967) *Biometr.,* **54,** 167.
22. Keys, A. (1972) In *Preventive Cardiology.* Ed. Tibblin, G., Keys, A. & Werkö, L. p., 21. Stockholm.
23. Gordon, T. (1974) *J. chron. Dis.,* **27,** 97.
24. Alberman, E. D. & Goldstein, H. (1970) *Brit. J. prev. soc. Med.,* **24,** 129.
25. Alberman, E. D. & Goldstein, H. (1972) In *From Birth to Seven,* Ed. Davie, R., Butler, N. & Goldstein, H. p., 180. London.
26. Fisch, L. (1957) *Arch. Dis. Childh.,* **32,** 230; (1967) *Lancet,* **2,** 1255.
27. Oppé, T. E. (1967) *Devl. Med. & Child Neurol.,* **9,** 13.
28. Roberts, C. J. & Khosla, T. (1972) *Brit. J. prev. soc. Med.,* **26,** 94.
29. Rogers, M. G. H. (1967) *Med. Offr.* **118,** 253.
30. Sheridan, M. D. (1962) *Mon. Bull. Minist. Hlth. Lab. Serv.* **21,** 238.

CHAPTER 5

1. Durham, R. H. (1966) *Encyclopaedia of Medical Syndromes.* New York.
2. Feinstein, A. R. (1967) *Clinical Judgment.* Baltimore, Md.
3. Scadding, J. G. (1967) *Lancet,* **2,** 877.
4. Mainland, D. (1968) *Notes on Biometry and Medical Research* V. A. Monog. 10–1, Suppl. 4. Washington, D.C.
5. Burkitt, D. P. (1972) *Lancet, * **2,** 1237.
6. Jennings, D. (1940) *Lancet,* **1,** 395, 444.
7. Morris, J. N. & Titmuss, R. M. (1944) *Lancet,* **2,** 841.
8. Doll, R., Jones, F. Avery & Bukatzsch, M. M. (1951) *Spec. Rep. Ser. med. Res. Coun. Lond.* no. 276.
9. Doll, R., & Buch, J. (1950) *Ann. Eugen. Lond.,* **15,** 135.
10. Doll, R., & Kellock, T. D. (1951) *Ann. Eugen. Lond.,* **16,** 231.
11. Clarke, C. A. (1962) *Genetics for the Clinician.* Oxford.
12. Morris, J. N., Heady, J. A. & Barley, R. G. (1952) *Brit. med. J.,* **1,** 503.
13. Morris, J. N. (1951) *Lancet,* **1,** 1, 69.
14. Morris, J. N. & Crawford, M. D. (1958) *Brit. med. J.,* **2,** 1485.
15. Morris, J. N. & Crawford, M. D. (1961) *Lancet,* **1,** 47.
16. Kuschlick, A. (1966) *Soc. Psychiat.,* **1,** 73. Personal communications.
17. Gruenberg, E. M. (1966) *Int. J. Psychiat.,* **2,** 78.
18. Roberts, J. A. Fraser (1952) *Eugen. Rev.,* **44,** 71; (1961) *Brit. med. Bull.,* **17,** 241.
19. Cooper, B. & Morgan, H. G. (1973) *Epidemiological Psychiatry.* Springfield, Ill.
20. Stein, Z. (1975) *Bull. N.Y. Acad. Med.,* **51,** 130.
21. Pickering, G. W. (1961) *The Nature of Essential Hypertension.* London.

22. Platt, R. (1959) *Lancet*, **2**, 55.
23. Miall, W. E. (1971) *Practit.*, **207**, 20.
24. Morrison, S. L. & Morris, J. N. (1959) *Lancet*, **2**, 864.
25. Lowe, C. R. & McKeown, T. (1962) *Lancet*, **1**, 1086.
    Ostfeld, A. M. & Paul, O. (1963) *Lancet*, **1**, 575.
26. Oberman, A. Lane, N. E., Harlan, W. R., Graybiel, A. & Mitchell, R. (1967) *Circulation*, **36**, 812.
27. Miall, W. E. & Lovell, H. G. (1967) *Brit. med. J.*, **2**, 660.
28. Miall, W. E., Bell, R. A. & Lovell, H. G. (1968) *Brit. J. prev. soc. Med.*, **22**, 73.
29. Feinleib, M., Halperin, M. & Garrison, R. J. (1969) Presented at Amer. Publ. Hlth. Assn. Philadelphia.
30. Jones, F. Avery (1957) *Brit. med. J.*, **1**, 719, 786.
31. Logan, W. P. D. (1950) *Popul. Stud.*, **4**, 132.
32. Registrar General, England and Wales (1927) *Dec. Suppt. Part II. Occupational Mortality for* 1921. London. HMSO.
33. Lee, J. A. H. (1961) *Lancet*, **2**, 815.
34. Harding, H. E. (1962) *Brit. med. J.*, **2**, 1028. (Appendicitis).
35. Lichtner, S. & Pflanz, M. (1971) *Med. Care*, **9**, 311.
36. Cochrane, A. L., Fletcher, C. M., Gilson, J. C. & Hugh-Jones, P. (1951) *Brit. J. industr. Med.*, **8**, 53.
37. Kreyberg, L. (1955) *Brit. J. Cancer*, **9**, 495.
38. Yesner, R., Gelfman, N. A. & Feinstein, A. R. (1973) *Amer. Rev. resp. Dis.*, **107**, 790.
39. Baird, D. (1957) *Brit. med. J.*, **1**, 1061. (1958) *Ibid*, **1**, 1477.
40. Elwood, P. C., Jacobs, A., Pitman, R. G. & Entwistle, C. C. (1964) *Lancet*, **2**, 716.
41. Cochrane, A. L. (1965) *Postgrad. med. J.*, **41**, 440.
42. Krivit, W. & Good, R. A. (1957) *Amer. J. Dis. Childr.*, **94**, 289.
43. *Statistical Report on the Health of the Army*, 1943-1945 (1948) HMSO, London.
44. Woolf, B. (1950) Personal communication.

CHAPTER 6

1. Morris, J. N. (1951) *Lancet*, **1**, 1. 69.
2. Crawford, M. D. & Morris, J. N. (1960) *Brit. med. J.* **2**, 1624.
3. I cannot trace this; sorry.
4. Gruenberg, E. M. (1961) In *Comparative Epidemiology of the Mental Disorders*. Ed. Hoch, P. M. & Zubin, J. New York.
5. Mackenzie, J. (1918) *Edin. med. J.*, **20**, 31.
6. Fremming, K. H. (1951) *The Expectation of Mental Infirmity in a Sample of the Danish Population*. Eugenics Society, London.
   Cooper, B. (1966) *Soc. Psychiatr.*, **1**, 7.
7. Gelfand, M. (1961) *Medicine in Tropical Africa*. Edinburgh.
8. De Haas, J. H. (1954) *Acta paediat.*, **43**, Suppl. 100, 374.
9. Morris, J. N. (1941) *Lancet*, **1**, 51.
10. Wedderburn, D. (1965) In Townsend, P. & Wedderburn, D. *The Aged in the Welfare State*. London.
11. Warren, M. D. (1974) *Report of Survey of the Impaired and the Handicapped in Canterbury*. City and County of Canterbury.
12. Kannel, W. B., Castelli, P. & McNamara, P. N. (1967) *J. occup. Med.*, **9**, 611.
13. Birmingham *Report of a Working Party appointed by the Royal College of General Practitioners*. (1962) *Brit. med. J.*, **1**, 1497; (1963) *ibid* **2**, 655; (1965) *ibid* **1**, 960; Crombie, D. L. personal communications.
14. *Present State and Future Needs of General Practice*. (1973) RCGP, London.
    Last, J. M. (1963) *Lancet*, **2**, 28.
    Fry, J. (1966) *Profiles of Disease*. Edinburgh.

15. *Medical Research. A Mid-Century Survey.* (1955) London.
16. Heasman, M. A. (1961) Mass Miniature Radiography. *Stud. med. Popul. Subj.* no. 17. HMSO, London.
    Brett, G. Z. (1968) *Thorax,* **23,** 414.
17. Shapiro, S., Strax, P & Venet, L. (1966) *J. Amer. med. Ass.,* **195,** 731; (1971) *ibid,* **215,** 1777.
    Shapiro, S. (1975) *Bull N.Y. Acad. Med.,* **51,** 80.
    Lowe, C. R. & MacMahon, B. (1970) *Lancet,* **1,** 153.
18. Heady, J. A., Morris, J. N., Kagan, A. & Raffle, P. A. B. (1961) *Brit. J. prev. soc. Med.,* **15,** 143.
19. Kilpatrick, G. S. (1961) *Brit. med. J.* **2,** 1736.
20. Hinchcliffe, R. (1961) *Brit. J. prev. soc. Med.,* **15,** 128.
    US Public Health Service (1968) National Center for Health Statistics, **11,** 32. Washington, D.C.
21. MRC Social Medicine Unit.
22. Logan, W. P. D. & Cushion, A. A. (1958) *Morbidity Statistics from General Practice.* HMSO, London.
    Pickering, G. W. (1955) *High Blood Pressure.* London.
23. Hughes, J. N. P. (1966) *Med. Offr.* **115,** 161.
    Alcohol Abuse (1970) Office of Health Economics. London.
24. Shepherd, M., Cooper, B., Brown, A. C. & Kalton, G. W. (1966) *Psychiatric Illness in General Practice.* London.
    Shepherd, M. personal communications.
25. Packman, J. & Power, M. J. (1968) In (Seebohm) *Report of the Committee on Local Authority and Allied Personal Social Services,* p.348. HMSO, London.
26. Morris, J. N. (1963) *Publ. Hlth Lond.,* **77,** 237.
27. Thomas, C. B., *et al. Collected Papers. The Precursors of Essential Hypertension and Coronary Artery Disease.* Vol. 1, 1948–59. Baltimore.
28. Cornfield, J. (1962) *Fed. Proc.* Suppl. no 11, 58.
29. Conn, J. W. & Fajans, S. S. (1961) *Amer. J. Med.,* **31,** 839.
30. Boyes, D. A., Fidler, H. K. & Lock, D. R. (1962) *Brit. med. J.,* **1,** 203.
    Knox, E. G. (1973) In *The Future—and Present Indicatives.* Ed. McLachlan, G. p. 17. London.
    McGregor, J. E. & Baird, D. (1963) *Brit. med. J.,* **1,** 1631.
31. Bullbrook, R. D. & Haywood, J. L. *Annual Reports* of the Imperial Cancer Research Fund. London.
32. Acheson, R. M. (1973) In *Serological Epidemiology,* p.177. New York.
33. Stromberg, V. (1962) *Acta ophthal. suppl.,* 69.
    Graham, P. A. (1967) *The Early Diagnosis of Visual Defects.* OHE. London.
34. Oliver, M. F. (1968) *The Early Diagnosis of Ischaemic Heart Disease.* OHE. London.
35. Fletcher, C. M. (1959) *Amer. Rev. resp. Dis.,* **80,** 483.
    Higgins, I. T. T. (1959) *Brit. med. J.,* **1,** 325.
36. Kass, E. H. (1962) *Ann. Intern. Med.,* **56,** 46; (1965) *Progress in Pyelonephritis,* Ed. Philadelphia.
37. Kunin, C. M., Zacha, E. & Paquin, A. J. (1962) *New Engl. J. Med.,* **266.** 1287,
38. Millar, M. (1963) *Models and Methods in Psychiatric Research.* Edinburgh.
    Baldwin, J. A. (1972) *The Statistician,* **21,** 325.
39. Acheson, E. D. (1967) *Medical Record Linkage.* London.
    Newcombe, H. H. (1966) *Brit. J. prev. soc. Med.,* **20,** 58.
40. Douglas, J. W. B. (1964) *The Home and The School.* London.
41. Davie, R., Butler, N. R. & Goldstein, H. (1972) *From Birth to Seven.* London.
42. Roberts, J. A. Fraser. (1973) *An Introduction to Medical Genetics.* London.
43. Slack, J. (1969) *Lancet,* **2,** 1380.
44. Slater, E. (1953) *Spec. Rep. Ser. med. Res. Coun., London.* No. 278.
45. Dukes, C. E. (1952) *Ann Eugen.* (Lond.), **17,** 1.

46. Tokuhata, G. K. (1963) *Publ. Hlth Rep. Wash.,* **78,** 121.
47. Lawrence, J. S., Laine, V. A. I. & De Graff, R. (1961) *Proc. R. Soc. Med.,* **54,** 454.
48. Hall, R., Owen, S. G. & Smart, G. A. (1960) *Lancet,* **2,** 187.
49. *Proceedings of the Conference on the Preventive Aspects of Chronic Diseases* (1951) Chicago, Ill.
50. Breslow, L. (1961) *Canad. J. publ. Hlth,* **52,** 375.
51. *Preventive Medicine.* (1967) Ed. Clark, D. W. & MacMahon, B. New York.
52. Harris, A. I. (1971) *Handicapped and Impaired in Great Britain.* HMSO, London.
    Gruenberg, E. M. (1969) *Lancet,* **1,** 721.
53. *Screening in Medical Care.* Reviewing the Evidence. (1968) London.
54. Wilson, J. M. G. & Junger, G. (1968) *Principles and Practice of Screening for Disease.* P. H. Papers, no. 34. WHO, Geneva.
55. *Mass Health Examinations* (1971) P.H. Papers, no. 45. WHO, Geneva.
56. Rose, G. A. (1971) *Brit. J. Hosp. Med.,* **6,** 647.
57. Cochrane, A. L. & Holland, W. W. (1971) *Brit. med. Bull.,* **27,** 3.
58. Bloom, H. J. G. (1965). *Brit. J. Radiol.,* **38,** 227.
59. *Screening for Inborn Errors of Metabolism.* (1968) *Wld. Hlth. Org. techn. Rep. Ser.* Geneva.
    Hudson, F. P. (1973) In *Treatment of Inborn Errors of Metabolism.* Ed. Seakins, J. W. T., Saunders, R. A. & Toothill, C. Edinburgh.
60. Keen, H. (1973) *VIII Confr. Internat. Diab. Fed. Proc.;* personal communications.
61. Chamberlain, J., (1973) *Proc. Roy. Soc. Med.,* **66,** 888.
    Garrad, J. & Bennett, A. E. (1971) *Brit. J. prev. soc. Med.,* **25,** 97.
    Isaacs, B. & Walkey, F. (1963) *Am. J. Psychiat.,* **120,** 173.
62. Milne, J. S., Maule, M. M., Cormack, S. & Williamson, J. (1972) *J. chron. Dis.,* **25,** 385.
63. Johnson, M. L. (1972) *Soc. Rev.,* **20,** 521.
64. Schilling, R. S. F. (1963) *J. Roy. Soc. Arts,* **111,** 933.
65. Veterans Administration Co-operative Study Group on Antihypertensive Agents. *J.A.M.A.* (1967) **202,** 1028; (1970) **213,** 1143.
    Wld. Hlth. Org. Tech. Rep. Ser. No. 469. Geneva.
66. Morris, J. N. (1973) *Lancet,* **2,** 1435.
67. Knox, E. G. (1968) In *Screening in Medical Care.* Reviewing the Evidence. London.
68. Breslow, L. & Hochstim, J. R. (1964) *Publ. Hlth. Rep.,* **79,** 107.
69. Suchman, E. A. (1964) *J. Hlth. soc. Beh.,* **8,** 197.
70. Fink, R., Shapiro, S. & Lewison, J. (1968) *Publ. Hlth. Rep.,* **83,** 479.
71. Auerbach, O., Stout, A. P., Hammond, E. C. & Garfinkel, L. (1961) *New Engl. J. Med.,* **265,** 253; (1962) **267,** 111, 119.
72. Kellerman, G., Shaw, C. R. & Luyten-Kellerman, M. (1973) *New Engl. J. Med.,* **289,** 934.
73. Barić, L. (1969) *Int. J. Hlth. Educ.* **12,** 24.

CHAPTER 7

1. Gavin, H. (1848) *Sanitary Ramblings.* London.
2. Clay, J. (1844) *Report of the Commission for Enquiry into the State of Large Towns and Populous Districts.* Appendix, p. 41. London.
3. Snow, J. (1855) *On the Mode of Communication of Cholera.* 2nd ed. Reprinted, 1936, with Appendix of 1856. New York.
4. Morris, J. N. (1969) *Lancet,* **2,** 811.
5. Susser, M. W. & Watson, W. (1971) *Sociology in Medicine.* London.
6. *Gender Differences.* (1972) Ed. Ounsted, C. & Taylor, D. C. Edinburgh.
7. Yerushalmy, J. (1963) *Amer. J. publ. Hlth.,* **53,** 148.
8. Karvonen, M. J. (1971) *Wld. Hlth.,* Jan., p. 3. WHO, Geneva.

9. Kraus, A. S. & Lilienfeld, A. M. (1959) *J. Chron. Dis.*, **10**, 207.
10. Abel-Smith, B. & Titmuss, R. M. (1956) *The Cost of the National Health Service in England and Wales*. London.
11. Ødegård, Ø. (1946) *J. ment. Sci.*, **92**, 35; (1953) *Acta psychiat. scand.* Suppl. **80**.
12. Benjamin, B. (1971) *J. biosoc. Sci.*, **3**, 61.
13. Kramer, M. (1969) *J. Roy. Stat. Soc.*, Ser. A (Gen.) **132**, 353.
14. *Crisis Intervention*. (1965) Ed. Parad, H. J. New York.
15. Registrar General. *Commentary*, 1965. HMSO, London.
16. Daw, R. H. (1971) *J. Inst. Actu.*, **97**, 17.
    Coates, B. E. & Rawstron, E. M. (1971) *Regional Variations in Britain*. London.
    Titmuss, R. M. (1938) *Poverty and Population*. London.
17. Daly, C. (1959) *Brit. J. prev. soc. Med.*, **13**, 14.
18. MRC Social Medicine Unit.
19. Buchanan, C. see *Listener,* March 16, 1967.
20. Benjamin, B. & Haycocks, H. W. (1970) *The Analysis of Mortality and Other Actuarial Statistics*. Cambridge.
    Kilpatrick, S. J. (1963) *Appl. stats.*, **12**, 65.
21. Vernon, H. M. (1939) *Health in Relation to Occupation*. London.
22. *Occupational Health Practice*. (1973) Ed. Schilling, R. S. F. London.
23. Alderson, M. R. (1967) *Brit. J. prev. soc. Med.*, **21**, 1.
24. Clarke, R. D. (1961) *J. Inst. Actu.*, **87**, 196; Personal communication.
25. Heady, J. A., Morris, J. N., Kagan, A. & Raffle, P. A. B. (1961) *Brit. J. prev. soc. Med.*, **15**, 143.
26. Montegriffo, V. M. E. (1968) *Ann. hum. Genet. Lond.*, **31**, 389.
27. *Diet and Coronary Heart Disease*. (1974) *Rep. Hlth. Soc. Subj.*, No. 7. HMSO, London.
    Garrow, J. S. (1974) *Energy Balance and Obesity in Man*. Amsterdam.
28. Morris, J. N., Kagan, A., Pattison, D. C., Gardner, M. J. & Raffle, P. A. B. (1966) *Lancet,* **2**, 553.
29. Mumford, L. (1968) *The Urban Prospect*. New York.
30. Morris, J. N. (1949) *Foundation* (S. Africa), **2**, 7.
31. Wolff, H. G. (1960) In *Stress and Psychiatric Disorder*. Ed. Tanner, J. M. Oxford.
    Hinkle, L. E. & Wolff, H. G. (1957) In *Explorations in Social Psychiatry*. Ed. Leighton, A. H., Clausen, J. A. & Wilson, R. N. New York.
32. Caudill, W. (1958) *Effects of Social and Cultural Systems in Reactions to Stress.* SSRC Pamphlet no. 14. New York.
33. Wolf, S. (1961). *Perspect. Biol. Med.* **4**, 288.
34. Lazarus, R. S. (1966) *Psychological Stress and the Coping Process*. New York.
35. Cassel, J. C. (1970) In *Cardiovascular Epidemiology in the Pacific*. CVD/70.6 WHO, Geneva.
36. Parkes, C. M. (1971) *Soc. Sci. & Med.*, **5**, 101.
37. *Society, Stress and Disease,* vol. 1. (1971). Ed. Levi, L. London.
38. *Psychophysiological Aspects of Cancer*. (1966) Ed. Weyer, E. M. *Ann. N.Y. Acad. Sci.,* **125**, Art 3, 773.
    Brit. med. J. (1971) **3**, 125.
39. Raab, W. (1962) *Cardiolog. Basel,* **41**, 10.
40. Rosenman, R. H., Friedman, M., Straus, R., Jenkins, C. D., Zyzanski, S. J. & Wurm, M. (1970) *J. chron. Dis.*, **23**, 173.
    Jenkins, C. D. (1972) In *Neural and Psychological Mechanisms in Cardiovascular Disease*. Ed. Bartorelli, C. Milan; in *Trends in Epidemiology*. Ed. Stewart, G. T. Springfield, Ill.
41. Roberts, J. A. F. (1957) *Brit. J. prev. soc. Med.*, **2**, 107; (1961) *Brit. med. Bull.*, **17**, 241.
42. Doll, R., Drane, H. & Newell, A. E. (1961) *Gut*, **2**, 352.
43. Mather, K. (1964) *Human Diversity*. Edinburgh.

44. *The Biology of Human Adaptability.* (1966) Ed. Baker, P. T. & Weiner, J. S. Oxford.
45. Allison, A. C. (1956) *Ann. hum. Genet.,* **21,** 67.
46. *Brit. med. J.,* (1969) **4,** 317; (1973) **1,** 1.
47. Thomas, M. & Job, C. K. (1972) *Brit. med. J.,* **3,** 390.
48. *Heredity and Society.* (1973) Ed. Baer, A. S. New York.
49. Engel, G. L. (1962) *Psychological Development in Health and Disease.* Philadelphia.
50. Lidz, T. (1968) The Person; His Development Throughout the Life Cycle. New York.
51. Churchill, W. S. (1948) *The Gathering Storm.* p. 601. London.
52. Kellerman, G., Shaw, C. R. & Luyten-Kellerman, M. (1973) *New Engl. J. Med.* **289,** 934.
53. Bodmer, W. F. & Bodmer, J. G. (1974). In *Tenth Symposium on Advanced Medicine.* Ed. Ledingham, J. C. G. p. 157. London.

MODERN EPIDEMIC

1. *Primary Prevention of the Atherosclerotic Diseases* (1972) *Circulation,* **42,** Dec. 1970. Revised, April 1972.
2. *Arteriosclerosis,* Vol. 2 (1971) HEW Publicn. No. (NIH) 72-219. Washington, DC.
3. Stamler, J. & Epstein, F. H. (1972) *Prev. Med.,* **1,** 27.
4. Morris, J. N. & Gardner, M. J. (1969) *Amer. J. Med.,* **46,** 674.
5. *Care and Prevention of Cardiovascular Diseases* (1974) Fejfar, Z., Strasser, T., Hatano, S. Ikeme, A. & Masironi, R. *WHO Chron.,* **28,** 55, 116, 190.
6. *Worldwide Cooperative Effort to Control Cardiovascular Diseases.* (1974) CVD/74.2. In preparation. WHO, Geneva.
7. *Prevention of Ischaemic Heart Disease: Metabolic Aspects.* (1973). Ed. Fejfar, Z. & Oliver, M. F. CVD/73.3. WHO, Geneva.
8. Slack, J. & Evans, E. A. (1966) *J. med. Genet.,* **3,** 239.
   Slack, J. (1974) *J. Roy. Coll. Phycns. Lond.,* **8,** 115.
9. Moynahan, E. J. (1961) *Lancet,* **1,** 673.
10. McKusick, V. A. & Murphy, E. A. (1963) In *Genetic Factors in the Etiology of Myocardial Infarction.* Ed. James, T. N. & Keyes, J. W. London.
11. Gershowitz, H. & Neel, J. V. (1970) In *Blood and Tissue Antigens.* Ed. Aminoff, D. p. 33. New York.
12. Morris, J. N. (1951) *Lancet,* **1,** 1, 69.
13. Morris, J. N. (1960) *Mod. Conc. cardiovasc. Dis.,* **29,** 625. ibid, **30,** 633.
14. Morris, J. N. & Crawford, M. D. (1958) *Brit. med. J.,* **2,** 1485.
15. Morris, J. N., Heady, J. A. & Barley, R. G. (1952) *Brit. med. J.,* **1,** 503.
16. Epstein, L. M., Miller, G. J., Stitt, F. W. & Morris, J. N. In the press.
17. Mitchell, J. R. A. & Schwartz, C. J. (1965) *Arterial Disease.* Oxford.
18. Rumball, A. & Acheson, E. D. (1963) *Brit. med. J.,* **1,** 423.
19. Rose, G. (1971) *Brit. J. hosp. Med.,* **6,** 647; (1974) Personal communication.
20. Gordon, T. & Kannel, W. B. (1970) In *The Community as an Epidemiologic Laboratory.* Ed. Kessler, I. I. & Levin, M. L. Baltimore; (1972) In *Trends in Epidemiology.* Ed. Stewart, G. T. Springfield, Ill.
21. Bronte-Stewart, B. & Krut, L. H. (1962) *J. Atheroscler. Res.,* **2,** 317.
22. Groen, J. J. (1958) *Ned. melk-en Zuiveltisdschr.,* **12,** 282.
23. *Coronary Heart Disease in Seven Countries.* (1970) Ed. Keys, A. AHA Monog. no. 29. New York.
24. Morris, J. N., Heady, J. A., Raffle, P. A. B., Roberts, C. G. & Parks, J. W. (1953) *Lancet,* **2,** 1053, 1111.
25. Morris, J. N. & Raffle, P. A. B. (1954) *Brit. J. industr. Med.,* **11,** 260.
26. Heady, J. A., Morris, J. N., Kagan, A. & Raffle, P. A. B. (1961) *Brit. J. prev. soc. Med.,* **15,** 143.

27. Registrar General, England and Wales. *Decennial Supplement on Occupational Mortality*. 1949–53. HMSO, London.
28. Kannel, W. B., Sorlie, P. & McNamara, P. (1971) In *Coronary Heart Disease and Physical Fitness*. Ed. Larsen, O. A. & Malmborg, R. O. p. 256. Baltimore.
29. Shapiro, S., Weinblatt, E., Frank, C. W. & Sager, R. V. (1969) *Amer. J. publ. Hlth.*, **59**, part 2, 18.
30. Cassel, J., Heyden, S., Bartel, A. G., Kaplan, B. H., Tyroler, H. A., Cornoni, J. C. & Hames, C. G. (1971) *Arch. intern. Med.*, **128**, 920.
31. Brunner, D., Manelis, G. & Modan, M. (1974) *J. chron. Dis.*, **27**, 217.
32. Chiang, B. N., Alexander, E. R., Bruce, R. A. & Ting, N. (1968) *Amer. Heart J.*, **76**, 760
33. Paffenbarger, R. S., Laughlin, M. E., Gima, A. S. & Black, R. A. (1970). *New Engl. J. Med.*, **282**, 1109.
34. Karvonen, M. J., Nygård, K. & Punsar, S. (1972) *Scand. J. clin. lab. Invest.*, **29**, suppl. 122, p.13.
35. Marr, J. W. (1973) *Hlth Trends*, **5**, 37.
36. Fox, S. M. & Naughton, J. P. (1972) *Prev. Med.*, **1**, 92.
37. Wyndham, C. H. (1974) *S. Afr. med. J.*, **48**, 571.
38. Blackburn, H. (1974) In *Controversy in Internal Medicine II*. Ed. Ingelfinger, F. J., Ebert, R. V., Finland, M. & Relman, A. S. p. 162. Philadelphia.
39. Oliver, R. M. (1967) *Brit. J. industr. Med.*, **24**, 181.
40. Alderson, M. R. & Yasin, S. (1966) In *Physical Activity in Health & Disease*. Ed. Evang, K. & Anderson, K. L. Oslo.
41. Yasin, S., Alderson, M. R., Marr, J. W., Pattison, D. C. & Morris, J. N. (1967) *Brit. J. prev. soc. Med.*, **21**, 163.
42. Yasin, S., (1967) In *Physical Activity and the Heart*. Ed. Karvonen, M. J. & Barry, A. J. p.372. Springfield. Ill.
43. Morris, J. N., Adam, C., Chave, S. P. W., Sirey, C., Epstein, L. M. & Sheehan, D. J. (1973) *Lancet*, **1**, 333.
    Epstein, L. M., Miller, G. J., Stitt, F. W. & Morris, J. N. In the press.
44. Morris, J. N. (1969) *Lancet*, **2**, 811; (1973) ibid, **2**, 1435; (1975) *Bull. N.Y. Acad. Med.*, **51**, 62.
45. *Preventive Cardiology*. (1972) Ed. Tibblin, G., Keys, A. & Werkö, L. Stockholm.
46. Werkö, L. (1971) *Ann. intern. Med.*, **74**, 276.
47. *Smoking and Health Now*. (1971) Royal College of Physicians. London.

EXPLORING ARTERIAL BLOOD PRESSURE

1. *The Epidemiology of Hypertension*. (1967) Ed. Stamler, J., Stamler, R. & Pullman, T. N. New York.
2. Pickering, G. W. (1974) In *Hypertension Manual*. Ed. Laragh, J.H. New York.
3. Grimley Evans, J. & Rose, G. (1971) *Brit. med. Bull.*, **27**, 37.
4. Ruiz, L. Personal communications.
5. Buchan, T. W., Henderson, W. K., Walker, D. E., Symington, J. & McNeil, I. H. (1960) *Hlth. Bull. Edinb.* **18**, 3.
6. Miall, W. E., Kass, E. H., Ling, J. & Stuart, K. L. (1962) *Brit. med. J.*, **2**, 497.
7. Miall, W. E. & Oldham, P. D. (1963) *Brit. med. J.*, **1**, 75.
8. Phillips, J. H., Jr. & Burch, G. E. (1959) *Amer. J. med. Sci.*, **238**, 97.
9. Gordon, T. (1964) *Natn. Center Hlth. Statist.*, Ser. 11, No. 5. HEW, Washington, DC.
10. Gordon, T. & Devine, B. (1966) *ibid*, no. 13.
11. Geiger, H. J. & Scotch, N. A. (1963) *J. chron. Dis.*, **16**, 1151.
    Scotch, N. A. & Geiger, H. J. (1963) *ibid*, 1183.
12. Hamilton, M., Pickering, G. W., Roberts, J. A. F. & Sowry, G. S. C. (1954) *Clin. Sci.*, **13**, 11.

13. Lovell, R. R. H., Maddocks, I. & Rogerson, G. W. (1960) *Australas. Ann. Med.,* **9,** 4.
    Maddocks, I. (1967) *Med. J. Austral.,* **1,** 1123.
14. Shaper, A. G. (1972) *Brit. med. J.,* **3,** 805.
15. Sinnett, P. F. & Whyte, H. M. (1973) *J. chron. Dis.,* **26,** 265.
16. Prior, I. A. M., Stanhope, J. M., Grimley Evans, J. & Salmond, C. E. (1974) *Int. J. Epid.,* **3,** 225.
17. Hamilton, M., Pickering, G. W., Roberts, J. A. F. & Sowry, G. S. C. (1954) *Clin. Sci.,* **13,** 273.
18. Miall, W. E. (1959) *Brit. med. J.,* **2,** 1204; personal communications.
19. Hamr, V. (1956) *Pracovnilékarstvi,* **8,** 126.
20. Myasnikow, A. L. (1961) In *Pathogenesis of Essential Hypertension.* Prague.
21. Cassel, J. C. (1970) *CVD/*70.6 WHO, Geneva.
22. Stamler, J., Berkson, D. M., Lindberg, H. A., Miller, W. A., Stamler, R. & Collette, P. (1967) In Ref. 1.
23. *Psychosomatics in Essential Hypertension* (1970) Ed. Koster, M., Musaph, H. & Visser, P. *Bibl. psychiat. neurol., no.* 144. Basle.
24. Stitt, F. W., Clayton, D. G., Crawford, M. D. & Morris, J. N. (1973) *Lancet,* **1,** 122.
25. Dahl, L. K. (1958) *New Engl. J. Med.,* **258,** 1152.
26. Dahl, L. K. (1972) *Amer. J. clin. Nutrit.,* **25,** 231.
27. Joossens, J. V. (1973) *Triangle,* **12,** 9.
28. Stamler, J. (1962) *Amer. J. Cardiol.,* **10,** 319.
29. *Build and Blood Pressure Study.* (1959) Society of Actuaries. Chicago, Ill.
30. Reid, D. D., Brett, G. Z., Hamilton, P. J. S., Jarrett, R. J., Keen, H. & Rose, G. (1974) *Lancet,* **1,** 469.
31. Wilber, J. A. & Barrow, J. G. (1972) *Amer. J. Med.,* **52,** 653.
32. Paul, O. (1974) *Mod. Conc. Cardiovasc. Dis.,* **43,** 99.
33. Neufeld, H. (1974) *Mod. Conc. Cardiovasc. Dis.,* **43,** 93.

MULTIPLE CAUSES

1. MacMahon, B. & Pugh, T. F. (1971) *Epidemiology.* Boston.
2. Knox, E. G. (1968) In *Recent Advances in Medicine.* Ed. Baron, D. N., Compston, N. & Dawson, A. M. London.
3. *Multiple Factors in the Causation of Environmentally Induced Disease* (1972) Ed. Lee, D. H. K. & Kotin, P. New York.
4. *Smoking and Health Now.* (1971) Royal College of Physicians, London.
5. Lee, J. A. H. & Morris, J. N. (1975) In *The Theory and Practice of Public Health,* Ed. Hobson, W. London.
6. Mackie, J. L. (1974) *The Cement of the Universe.* Oxford.
7. Galdston, I. (1954) In *Beyond the Germ Theory.* Ed. Galdston, I. New York.
8. Dubos, R. J. (1951) *Louis Pasteur,* chap. 9. London; (1953) *The White Plague.* London.
9. Greenwood, M. (1948) *Some British Pioneers of Social Medicine.* London.
10. Paul, J. R. (1966) *Clinical Epidemiology.* Chicago, Ill.
11. Winslow, C. E. A. (1944) *The Conquest of Epidemic Disease.* Princeton.
12. Steiner, G. A. (1965) In *The Creative Organisation.* Ed. G.A.S. Chicago.
13. Heasman, M. A. (1961) *Arch. Dis. Childh.,* **36,** 390.
14. Backett, E. M. (1965) *Domestic Accidents. Publ. Hlth. Pap. no.* 26. WHO, Geneva.
15. Susser, M. W. (1972) In *Trends in Epidemiology.* Ed. Stewart, G. T. Springfield, Ill.
16. Pond, D. A. & Bidwell, B. (1954) *Brit. med. J.,* **2,** 1520.
17. Kruse, H. D. (1954) In *Beyond the Germ Theory.* New York.

18. Von Haller, A. (1768). Quoted in Hanson, N. R. (1958) *Patterns of Discovery*. Cambridge. (Freely: In Nature, varied phenomena are linked into a network rather than a chain; but man can grasp only a chain of relationship because he cannot describe in words more than one relationship at a time.)
19. Burgess, A. & Dean, R. F. A. (1962) Ed. *Malnutrition and Food Habits*. London. *Nutrition, The Nervous System, and Behaviour*. (1972) Scient. Publicn. No. 251. PAHO, Washington, D.C.
20. Alvarez, A. (1971) *The Savage God: A Study of Suicide*. London.
21. Fox, W. (1962) *Lancet*, **2**, 413, 473; (1964) *Brit. med. J.*, **1**, 135. Tuberculosis Control Centre, Madras. *Bull. Wld. Hlth. Org.*, **21**, 51.
22. Morris, J. N., Kagan, A., Pattison, D. C., Gardner, M. J. & Raffle, P. A. B. (1966) *Lancet*, **2**, 553.
23. Morris, J. N. & Crawford, M. D. (1958) *Brit. med. J.*, **2**, 1485.
24. Epstein, L. M., Miller, G. J., Stitt, F. W. & Morris, J. N. In the Press.
25. Lasagna, L. (1964) *Perspect. Biol. Med.*, **7**, 457.
26. Harré, R. personal communication; Mackie, J. L. (1965) *Amer. Philosoph. Quart.* **2**, 245.
27. Heady, J. A. & Morris, J. N. (1959) *J. Obst. Gyn. Brit. Emp.*, **66**, 577.
28. Heady, J. A. & Heasman, M. A. (1959) *Social and Biological Factors in Infant Mortality*. HMSO, London. MRC Social Medicine Unit.

EPIDEMIOLOGY OF PERSONAL BEHAVIOUR

1. Sand, R. (1952) *The Advance to Social Medicine*. (English edition) London.
2. Schofield, M. (1973) *The Sexual Behaviour of Young Adults*. London.
3. Marr, J. W. (1973) *Hlth. Trends*, **5**, 37.
4. *Health, Culture and Community*. (1955) Ed. Paul, B. D. New York.
5. Read, M. (1966) *Culture, Health and Disease*. London.
6. *The Cross-Cultural Approach to Health Behaviour*. (1969) Ed. Lynch, L. R., Cranbury, N. J.
7. Williams, C. (1958) In *Matrix of Medicine*. Ed. Malleson, N. London.
8. Kirscht, J. P., Haefner, D. P., Kegeles, S. S., Rosenstock, I. M. (1966) *J. Hlth. hum. Behav.*, **7**, 248.
9. Becker, H. S. (1964) *Sociom.* **27**, 40.
10. Knutson, A. L. (1965) *The Individual, Society and Health Behaviour*. New York.
11. Mechanic, D. (1968) *Medical Sociology*. New York.
12. Johnston, M. L. (1972) *Soc. Rev.*, **20**, 521.
13. Susser, M. W. & Watson, W. (1971) *Sociology in Medicine*. London.
14. Suchman, E. A. (1967) *J. Hlth. Hum./Soc. Behav.*, **8**, 197.
15. Antonovsky, A. & Kats, R. (1970) *Soc. Sci. Med.*, **4**, 367. Steele, J. L. & McBroom, W. H. (1972) *J. Hlth. Soc. Behav.*, **13**, 382.
16. Wakefield, J. (1972) *Seek Wisely to Prevent*. HMSO, London.
17. Morris, J. N. (1969) *Lancet*, **2**, 811; (1973) *ibid* **2**, 1435; (1975) *Bull. N.Y. Acad. Med.*, **51**, 62.
18. *Symposium on Prevention of Artherosclerosis at the Pediatric Level*. (1973) Ed. Mitchell, S. C. *Amer. J. Cardio.*, **31**, No. 5, 539-594.
19. Seltzer, C. C. & Mayer, J. (1970) *Amer. J. Publ. Hlth.*, **60**, 679.
20. Burton, J. & Barić, L. (1975) In *The Theory and Practice of Public Health*. Ed. Hobson, W. London.

BRONCHITIS (CNSLD)

1. *Air Pollution and Respiratory Disease*. (1972) Ed. Holland, W. W. Westport, Conn.
2. *Air Pollution and Health* (1970) Royal College of Physicians, London.
3. Stuart-Harris, C. H. (1968) *Abst. Wld. Med.*, **42**, 649, 737.

4. Colley, J. R. T. (1971) *Brit. med. Bull.*, **27**, 9.
5. Fletcher, C. M. (1959) *Amer. Rev. resp. Dis.*, **80**, 483.
6. Higgins, I. T. T., Oldham, P. D., Cochrane, A. L. & Gilson, J. C. (1956) *Brit. med. J.*, **2**, 904.
7. Fletcher, C. M., Elmes, P. C., Fairbairn, A. S. & Wood, C. H. (1959) *Brit. med. J.*, **2**, 257.
8. Higgins, I. T. T. (1957) *Brit. med. J.*, **2**, 1198.
9. Higgins, I. T. T., Cochrane, A. L., Gilson, J. C. & Wood, C. H. (1959) *Brit. J. industr. Med.*, **16**, 255.
10. Medical Research Council (1960) *Brit. med. J.*, **2**, 1665.
11. Oswald, N. C. & Medvei, V. C. (1955) *Lancet*, **2**, 843.
12. Daly, C. (1954) *Brit. med. J.*, **2**, 687; (1959) *Brit. J. prev. soc. Med.*, **13**, 14.
13. MRC Social Medicine Unit.
14. Buck, S. F. & Brown, D. A. (1964) *Tobacco Research Council Paper* no. 7. London.
15. Lawther, P. J. (1958) *Proc. R. Soc. Med.*, **51**, 262.
16. Waller, R. E. & Lawther, P. J. (1957) *Brit. med. J.*, **2**, 1475.
17. Lawther, P. J., Martin, A. E. & Wilkins, E. T. (1962) *Epidemiology of Air Pollution* WHO, Geneva.
18. Reid, D. D. & Fairbairn, A. S. (1958) *Lancet*, **1**, 1147.
19. Fairbairn, A. S. & Reid, D. D. (1958) *Brit. J. prev. soc. Med.*, **12**, 94.
20. Lambert, P. M. & Reid, D. D. (1970) *Lancet*, **1**, 856.
21. Crofton, E. & Crofton, J. (1963) *Brit. med. J.*, **2**, 1161.
22. *Towards Cleaner Air* (1973); *Clean Air Today.* (1974) HMSO, London.
23. *Clean Air* (1974) **4**, 8.
24. Waller, R. E. (1971) *J. Roy. Coll. Phycns.*, **5**, 362.
25. Waller, R. E., Lawther, P. J. & Martin, A. E. (1969) *Proc. Clean Air Conf.* National Society for Clean Air, London.
26. Lawther, P. J., Waller, R. E. & Henderson, M. (1970) *Thorax*, **25**, 525.
27. Miller, F. J. W., Court, S. D. M., Walton, W. S. & Knox, E. G. (1960) *Growing Up in Newcastle upon Tyne.* London.
28. Colley, J. R. T. & Reid, D. D. (1970) *Brit. med. J.*, **2**, 213.
29. Gilson, J. C. (1970) *Proc. R. Soc. Med.*, **63**, 857.
30. Lowe, C. R., Campbell, H. & Khosla, T. (1970) *Brit. J. ind. Med.*, **27**, 121.
31. Reid, D. D. & Fletcher, C. M. (1971) *Brit. med. Bull.*, **27**, 59.
32. *Respiratory Disease in Europe* (1974) WHO, Copenhagen.
33. Holland, W. W., Halil, T., Bennett, A. E. & Elliott, A. (1969) *Brit. med. J.*, **2**, 205.
34. Colley, J. R. T., Douglas, J. W. B. & Reid, D. D. (1973) *Brit. med. J.*, **3**, 195.
35. Goldsmith, J. R. (1972) *Postgrad. Med.*, **51**, 93.

REDISCOVERY OF BYSSINOSIS

1. Schilling, R. S. F. (1974) Personal communications.
2. Hill, A. B. (1930) *Rep. industr. Hlth. Res. Bd. Lond.* No. **59**.
3. Schilling, R. S. F. (1956) *Lancet*, **2**, 261, 319.
4. McKerrow, C. B., Roach, S. A., Gilson, J. & Schilling, R. S. F. (1962) *Brit. J. industr. Med.*, **19**, 1.
5. Schilling, R. S. F. (1959) *J. occup. Med.*, **1**, 33.
6. Lammers, B., Schilling, R. S. F. & Walford, J. (1964) *Brit. J. industr. Med.*, **21**, 124.
7. Lévi-Strauss, C. Quoted in Douglas, M. (1973) *Natural Symbols*, p. 15. London.
8. Bouhuys, A., Heaphy, L. J., Schilling, R. S. F. & Welborn, J. W. (1967) *New Engl. J. Med.*, **277**, 170.
9. Schilling, R. S. F. (1964) *Yale J. Biol. Med.*, **37**, 55.

10. Bouhuys, A. (1974) *Breathing: Physiology, Environment and Lung Disease.* p. 416. New York.
11. El Batawi, M. A., Schilling, R. S. F. & Walford, J. (1964) *Brit. J. industr. Med.,* **21,** 13.
12. *British Medical Journal* (1974) **4,** 675.

CANCER IN THE REPORTS OF THE G.R.O.

1. Doll, R. (1967) *Prevention of Cancer: Pointers from Epidemiology.* London.
2. Waterhouse, J. (1972) In *The Pathological Basis of Medicine.* Ed. Curran, R. C. & Harnden, D. G. London.
3. Day, N. E. & Muir, C. S. (1973) In *Modern Trends in Oncology* — 1 Part 1: Research Progress. Ed. Raven, R. W. London.
4. *Cancer in the United States.* (1972) Ed. Lilienfeld, A. M., Levin, M. L. & Kessler, I. I. Cambridge, Mass.
5. Knox, E. G. (1968) In *Recent Advances in Medicine.* Ed. Baron, D. N., Compston, N. & Dawson, A. M. London.
6. Lee, J. A. H. (1972) *Postgrad. Med.,* **51,** Jan. 84. Personal communications.
7. Doll, R. (1971) *J. Roy. stat. Soc. Ser. A,* **134,** Pt. 2, 133.
8. Case, R. A. M. (1958) *Med. Press,* **240,** 640. (Adapted)
9. Case, R. A. M. (1966) In *Scientific Basis of Medicine Annual Reviews.* London.
10. Stocks, P. (1958) In *Cancer,* vol. 3. Ed. Raven, R. W. London.
11. De Waard, F. (1969) *Int. J. Canc.,* **4,** 577.
12. Shapiro, S., Strax, P., Venet, L. & Venet, W. (1973) *Seventh National Cancer Conference Proceedings.* p. 663.
13. Chamberlain, J. In preparation; LSHTM Dept. of Community Health.
14. Kodlin, D. (1972) *Meth. Inform. Med.,* **11,** 242.
15. Crofton, E. C. (1970) *Brit. J. prev. soc. Med.,* **24,** 110.
16. Stocks, P. (1936, 1937, 1939, 1957) *Reports of British Empire Cancer Campaign.* London.
17. Armstrong, R. W. (1972) In *Medical Geography.* Ed. McGlashan, N. D. London.
18. Terris, M., Wilson, F., Smith, H., Sprung, E. & Nelson, J. H. (1967) *Amer. J. publ. Hlth,* **57,** 840.
19. Hill, G. B. & Adelstein, A. M. (1967) *Lancet,* **2,** 605.
20. Beral, V. (1974) *Lancet,* **1,** 1037 (and subsequent correspondence).
21. Lowe, C. R. & MacMahon, B. (1970) *Lancet,* **1,** 153.
22. Acheson, E. D. (1968) *Proc. R. Soc. Med.,* **61,** 726.
23. Alderson, M. R. & Meade, T. W. (1967) *Brit. J. prev. soc. Med.,* **21,** 22.
24. Heasman, M. A. & Lipworth, L. (1966) *Accuracy of Certification of Cause of Death.* Stud, med. pop. Subj., No. 20. HMSO, London.
25. World Health Organization (1963) *Chron. Wld. Hlth. Org.,* **17,** 228.
26. Cole, P. (1975) *Bull. N.Y. Acad. Med.,* **51,** 75.

GEOGRAPHICAL PATHOLOGY

1. May. J. M. (1958) *The Ecology of Human Disease.* New York.
2. *World Health Statistics.* Annually. WHO, Geneva.
3. *Medical Geography.* (1972) Ed. McGlashan, N. D. London.
4. *Aspects of Medical Geography* (1974) Ed. Bain, S. M. & Herbertson, M. *J. biosoc. Sci.,* **6,** 185-293.
5. Puffer, R. R. & Wynne Griffith, G. (1967) *Patterns of Urban Mortality.* Pan American Health Organization, Scient. Publicn. No. 151. Washington, D.C.
   Puffer, R. R. & Serrano, C. V. (1973) *Patterns of Mortality in Childhood. ibid,* no. 262.

6. Neel, J. V. (1970) *Science,* **170,** 815.
7. Spillane, J. D. (1973) In *Tropical Neurology.* Ed. J. D. S. p. 3. London.
8. Zbinden, G. (1973) *Progress in Toxicology.* Vol. I, p. 66. Berlin.
9. *The Geographic Pathology of Atherosclerosis.* (1968) Ed. McGill, H. C. Baltimore; Strong, J. P. (1972) *Athero.,* **16,** 193.
10. *Cardiovascular Disease in the Tropics* (1974) Ed. Shaper, A. G., Hutt, M. S. R. & Fejfar, Z. London.
11. Shaper, A. G. (1972) *Brit. med. J.,* **3,** 683, 743, 805; **4,** 32.
12. Yerushalmy, J. & Hilleboe, H. E. (1957) *N.Y. St. J. Med.,* **57,** 2343.
13. Keys, A. (1967) *Acta. Med. Scand.* Ed. suppl. no. 460.
14. Doll, R. (1967) *Prevention of Cancer. Pointers from Epidemiology.* London.
15. *UICC Cancer Incidence in Five Continents.* Ed. Doll, R., Muir, C. S. & Waterhouse, J. (1970) Vol. II. UICC, Geneva.
16. Steiner, P. E. (1954) *Cancer, Race and Geography.* Baltimore.
17. MacMahon, B., Cole, P., Lin, T. M., Lowe, C. R., Mirra, A. P., Ravnihar, B., Salber, E. J., Valaoras, V. G. & Yuasa, S. (1970) *Bull. Wld. Hlth. Org.,* **43,** 209.
18. Cole, P. (1975) *Bull. N.Y. Acad. Med.,* **51,** 75.
19. Segi, M. (1963) *Trends in Cancer Mortality for Selected Sites in 24 Countries* 1950–1959. Sendai, Japan.
20. Gordon, T. (1957) *Publ. Hlth. Rep. Wash.,* **72,** 543.
21. Larsen, N. P. & Bortz, W. (1959) *Hawaii med. J.,* **19,** 159.
    Keys, A., Kimura, N., Kusukawa, A., Bronte-Stewart, B., Larsen, N. P. & Keys, M. H. (1958) *Ann. intern. Med.,* **48,** 83.
22. Higginson, J. (1968) *Proc. Eighth Canadian Cancer Conference.* Ontario.
23. Burbank, F., Fraumeni, J. F. (1972) *J. nat. Canc. Inst.,* **49,** 649.
24. *International Agency for Research on Cancer.* Ann. Rep. 1972–73. Lyon, France.
25. Burkitt, D. P. (1973) *Proc. Nutr. Soc.,* **32,** 145; *Brit. med. J.,* **1,** 274. Personal communication.
26. Painter, N. S., Cleave, T. L. & Campbell, G. D. (1969) *Diabetes, Coronary Thrombosis and the Saccharine Disease.* Bristol.
    Perry, H. M. (1973) *J. Am. Dietet. Ass.,* **62,** 631.
27. Robertson, J. (1972) *Nature,* **238,** 290.
28. Cutler, S. J. & Devesa, S. S. In *Host Environment Interactions in the Etiology of Cancer in Man.* Ed. Doll, R. & V. Vodopija, I. (1973) p. 15. Lyon.
29. Hill, M. J., Drasar, B. S., Aries, V., Crowther, J. S., Hawksworth, G. & Williams, R. E. O. (1971) *Lancet,* **1,** 95.
30. Hill, M. J. (1974) *Cancer,* **34,** 815.
31. Drasar, B. S. & Irving, D. (1973) *Brit. J. Cancer,* **27,** 167.
32. MacMahon, B. & Feinleib, M. (1960) *J. nat. Canc. Inst.,* **24,** 733.
33. World Health Organization (1959) Effect of Radiation on Human Heredity. *Wld Hlth Org. techn. Rep. Ser.* no. 166.
34. Marticorena, E., Ruiz, L., Severino, J., Galvez, J. & Penaloza, D. (1969) *Amer. J. Cardiol.,* **23,** 364.
35. Lapiccirella, V., Lapiccirella, R., Abboni, F. & Liotta, S. (1962) *Bull. Wld Hlth Org.,* **27,** 681.
36. Shaper, A. G. & Jones, K. W. (1962) *Lancet,* **2,** 1305.
    Mann, G. V., Shaffer, R. D., Anderson, R. S. & Sandstead, H. H. (1964) *J. Ather. Res.,* **4,** 289.
37. Toor, M., Katchalsky, A., Agmon, J. & Allalouf, D. (1957) *Lancet,* **1,** 1270.
38. *Patterns of Incidence of Certain Diseases Throughout the World* (1959) Opportunities for Research through Epidemiology. (Sixth Report) Washington, DC.
39. Cohen, A. M., Bavly, S. & Poznanski, R. (1961) *Lancet,* **2,** 1399.
40. Kurland, L. T., Mulder, D. W. & Westlund, K. B. (1955) *New Engl. J. Med.,* **252,** 649, 697.

41. Kachadurian, A. K. (1964) *Amer. J. Med.,* **37**, 402.
42. Koybayashi, J. (1957) *Ber.* Ohara. *Inst. landw. Forsch.,* **11**, 12.
43. Bennett, P. H., Burch, T. A. & Miller, M. (1971) *Lancet,* **2**, 125.
44. Davies, A. M. (1971) *"Geographical Epidemiology of the Toxaemias of Pregnancy"*. *Isr. J. med. Sci.,* **7**, 753.
45. Dacie, J. V. (1967) *The Haemolytic Anaemias*. p.1061. London.
46. Tuyns, A. J. & Massé, L. M. F. (1973) *Int. J. Epid.,* **2**, 241.
47. Kafuko, G. W. & Burkitt, D. P. (1970) *Int. J. Cancer.,* **6**, 1.
48. Morrow, R. H., Pike, M. C., Smith, P. G., Ziegler, J. L. & Kisuule, A. (1971) *Brit. med. J.,* **2**, 491.
49. World Health Organization (1962) *Second Report on the World Health Situation 1957-60*. WHO, Geneva.
50. Meneely, G. R., Paul, O., Dorn, H. F. & Harrison, T. R. (1960) *J. Amer. med. Ass.,* **174**, 1628.
51. Heady, J. A. (1973) *WHO Bull.,* **48**, 243.
52. Wing, J. K. (1970) In *Psychiatric Epidemiology*. Ed. Hare, E. H. & Wing, J. K. London.
53. *Report of the International Pilot Study of Schizophrenia* Vol. 1. (1973) WHO, Geneva.
54. Rose, G. & Blackburn, H. (1968) *Cardiovascular Survey Methods*. WHO, Geneva.
55. *Health, Culture and Community* (1955) Ed. Paul, B. D. New York.
56. Susser, M. W. & Watson, W. (1971) *Sociology in Medicine*. New York.
57. Cooper, B. & Morgan, H. G. (1973) *Epidemiological Psychiatry*. Springfield, Ill.
58. Mead, M. (1928) *Coming of Age in Samoa*. New York.
    Mead, M. (1931) *Growing Up in New Guinea*. London.
59. *Postgraduate Medical Journal,* Oct. 1965, **41**, 583–633.
60. *The Field Worker in Immigrant Health*. (1969) Ed. Dodge, J. S. London.
61. Moser, C. A. (1972) In *Social Trends* No. 3. p.20. HMSO, London.

ECOLOGY OF MENTAL DISORDERS

1. Cooper, B. & Morgan, H. G. (1973) *Epidemiological Psychiatry*. Springfield, Ill.
2. Reid, D. D. (1960) *Epidemiological Methods in the Study of Mental Disorders*. WHO, Geneva.
3. *Mental Disorders: A Guide to Control Methods*. (1962) APHA. New York.
4. *Causes of Mental Disorders* (1961) *Milb. Mem. Fd.,* New York.
5. Gruenberg, E. M. (1973) *Psychiat. Quart.,* **47**, 1.
6. Shepherd, M. & Cooper, B. (1964) *J. Neurol Neurosurg. Psychiat.,* **27**, 277.
7. Kramer, M. (1967) In *Psychiatric Research Report* 22. Amer. Psychiat. Assn., New York.
8. *Psychiatric Epidemiology*. (1970) Ed. Hare, E. H. & Wing, J. K. London.
9. Wing, J. K. (1971) *Brit. J. Hosp. Med.,* Jan, 53.
10. Faris, R. E. L. & Dunham, H. W. (1939) *Mental Disorders in Urban Areas*. Chicago, Ill.
11. Durkheim, E. (1897) *Suicide*. Ed. Simpson, G. (1951) Glencoe, Ill.
12. Sainsbury, P. (1973) *Proc. R. Soc. Med.,* **66**, 579.
13. Bagley, C. (1968) *J. Soc. Sci. Med.,* **2**, 1.
    Greer, S. & Bagley, C. (1971) *Brit. med. J.,* **13**, 10.
14. McCullough, J. & Philip, A. *Suicidal Behaviour*. Oxford.
15. Hagnell, O. (1966) *A Prospective Study of the Incidence of Mental Disorder*. Stockholm.
16. Wing, J. K. (1970) In *Psychiatric Epidemiology*. Ed. Hare, E. H. & Wing, J. K. London.
17. Goldberg, D. P., Cooper, B., Eastwood, M. R., Kedward, H. B. & Shepherd, M. (1970) *Brit. J. prev. soc. Med.,* **24**, 18.

18. *Report of the International Pilot Study of Schizophrenia Vol.* 1. (1973) WHO, Geneva.
19. Cooper, J. E., Kendell, R. E., Gurland, B. J., Sharpe, L., Copeland, J. R. M. & Simon, R. (1972) *Psychiatric Diagnosis in New York and London.* Maudsley Monog. no. 20. London.
20. Goldberg, E. M. & Morrison, S. L. (1963) *Brit. J. Psychiat.,* **109,** 785.
21. MRC Social Medicine Unit.
22. Shakow, D. (1973) *Psychiat.,* **36,** 353.
23. Wing, J. K. (1973) In *Biochemistry and Mental Illness.* Ed. Iversen, L. L. & Rose, S. P. R. London.
24. *The Transmission of Schizophrenia* (1968) Ed. Rosenthal, D. & Kety, S. S. New York.
25. Gottesman, I. I. & Shields, J. (1972) *Schizophrenia and Genetics.* New York.
26. Laing, R. D. (1959) The Divided Self. London.
27. Brown, G. W. & Birley, J. L. T. (1968) *J. Hlth. Hum. Behav.,* **9,** 203.
28. Brown, G. W., Sklair, F., Harris, T. & Birley, J. L. T. (1973) *Psychol. Med.,* **3, 74.**
29. *The Urban Condition.* (1963) Ed. Duhl, L. J. New York.
30. Fried, M. (1964) In *Urban America and the Planning of Mental Health Services.* G.A.P. New York.
31. Fried, M. (1969) In *Poverty and Health.* Ed. Kosa, J., Antonovsky, A. & Zola, I. K. Cambridge, Mass.
32. Parker, S. & Kleiner, R. J. (1966) *Mental Illness in the Urban Negro Community.* Glencoe, Ill.
33. Moynihan, D. P. (1967) *Commentary,* **43,** Feb., 31.
34. Hollingshead, A. B. & Redlich, F. C. (1958) *Social Class and Mental Illness.* New York.
35. Gray, J. L. & Moshinsky, P. (1930) In *Political Arithmetic.* Ed. Hogben, L. London.
36. Burt, C. (1946) *The Backward Child.* London.
37. Douglas, J. W. B. & Blomfield, J. M. (1958) *Children under Five.* London.
38. Douglas, J. W. B. (1964) *The Home and the School.* London.
39. Douglas, J. W. B. Ross, J. M. & Simpson, H. R. (1968) *All Our Future.* London.
40. Knobloch, H. & Pasamanick, B. (1966) *Merrill-Palmer Quart. Behav. Dev.,* **12,** 27.
41. Davie, R., Butler, N. R. & Goldstein, H. (1972) *From Birth to Seven.* London.
42. Wedge, P. & Prosser, H. (1973) *Born to Fail?* London.
43. *A Pattern of Disadvantage.* (1972) Ed. Donnison, D. London.
44. Bernstein, B. (1961) In *Economy, Education and Society.* Ed. Halsey, A. H., Floud, J. & Anderson, C. A. London.
45. *Educational Priority.* (1973) Ed. Halsey, A. H. HMSO, London.
46. Birch, H. G. (1972) *Amer. J. publ. Hlth.,* **62,** 773.
    Coleman, J. S. *et al* (1966) *Equality of Educational Opportunity.* DHEW. Washington, D.C.
47. Bone, M. (1973) *Family Planning Services in England & Wales.* HMSO, London.
48. Carstairs, G. M. (1963) *This Island Now.* London.
49. Bowlby, J. (1952) *Maternal Care and Mental Health.* WHO, Geneva.
    Ainsworth, M. D. (1962) In *Deprivation of Maternal Care: a Reassessment of its Effects.* WHO, Geneva.
50. Seeley, J. R., Sim, R. A. & Loosley, E. W. (1956) *Crestwood Heights.* Toronto.
51. Eisenberg, L. (1969) *Amer. J. Orthopsychiat.,* **39,** 389.
52. Wall, W. D. (1973) *Lond. Educ. Rev.,* **2,** No. 2, 3.
53. Rosen, G. (1959) *Milbank mem. Fd. Quart.,* **37,** 5.
54. Shepherd, M., Cooper, B., Brown, A. C. & Kalton, G. (1966) *Psychiatric Illness in General Practice.* London.

55. Jenkins, C. D., Rosenman, R. H. & Friedman, M. (1967) *J. Chron. Dis.*, **20**, 371.
Osler, W. (1910) *Lancet*, **1**, 696, 839, 974.
Marcus, S. (1964) *The Other Victorians*. p.149. New York.
56. Crick, B. (1974) *Crime, Rape and Gin*. London.
57. Becker, H. S. (1964) *Outsiders*. Glencoe, Ill.
58. Bynner, J. M. (1969) *The Young Smoker*. HMSO, London.
59. Lewis, A. J. (1953) *Brit. J. Sociol.*, **4**, 109.
60. Edwards, G. (1971) *Unreason in an Age of Reason:* Two Lectures on the Drug
Problem. RSM, London.
61. de Alarcón, R. & Rathod, N. H. (1968) *Brit. med. J.*, **2**, 549.
62. Gruenberg, E. M. (1957) In *Explorations in Social Psychiatry*. Ed. Leighton, A. H.,
Clausen, J. A. & Wilson, R. N. New York.
63. Revans, R. W. (1964) *Standards for Morale: Cause and Effect in Hospitals*.
London.

HYPOTHESES

1. MacMahon, B. & Pugh, T. F. (1970) *Epidemiology*. Boston.
2. Knox, E. G. (1968) In *Recent Advances in Medicine*. Ed. Baron, D. N., Compston,
N. & Dawson, A. M. London.
3. Susser, M. (1973) *Causal Thinking in the Health Sciences*. New York.
4. Lilienfeld, A. M. (1957) *Publ. Hlth. Rep. Wash.*, **72**, 51.
Cohen, M. R. & Nagel, E. (1939) *An Introduction to Logic and Scientific Method*.
5. Popper. K. R. (1963) *Conjectures and Refutations*. London.
6. Medawar, P. B. (1967) *The Art of the Soluble*. London.
7. Mackie, J. L. (1974) *The Cement of the Universe*. Oxford.
8. Lenz, W. (1962) *Lancet*, **1**, 45.
9. Schilling, R. S. F. (1956) *Lancet*, **2**, 261.
10. Wilkins, L. T. (1960) *Delinquent Generations*. HMSO, London.
11. Scott, E. (1960) *J. Coll. gen. Practit.*, **3**, 80.
12. Fraser-Roberts, J. A. (1961) *Brit. med. Bull.*, **17**, 241.
13. Clausen, J. A. & Kohn, M. (1954) *Amer. J. Sociol.*, **60**, 140.
14. Yerushalmy, J. & Hilleboe, H. E. (1957) *N.Y. St. J. Med.*, **57**, 2343.
15. Morrison, S. L. (1959) *J. ment. Sci.*, **105**, 999.
16. Morris, J. N., Crawford, M. D. & Heady, J. A. (1961) *Lancet*, **1**, 860; (1962)
ibid **2**, 506.
17. Crawford, M. D., Gardner, M. J. & Morris, J. N. (1968) *Lancet*, **1**, 827; (1971)
ibid, **2**, 327.
18. Gardner, M. J., Crawford, M. D. & Morris, J. N. (1969) *Brit. J. prev. soc. Med.*,
23, 133.
19. Farr, W. (1852) *J. Stat. Soc.*, **15**, 155.
20. Morris, J. N. (1961–2) *Yale J. Biol. Med.*, **34**, 359.
21. Miller, R. W. (1967) *J. Pediat.*, **71**, 455.
22. Good, R. A. (1968) *J. clin. Invest.*, **47**, 1466.
23. Stein, Z., Susser, M., Saenger, G. & Marolla, F. (1972) *Science*, **178**, 708.
24. *Smoking and Health* (1964) "The Surgeon-General's Report". PHS Publicn.
no. 1003, Washington, DC.
25. Cornfield, J. (1956) *Proc. 3rd Berkeley Symposium*, **4**, 135.
26. Hammond, E. C. & Horn, D. (1958) *J. Amer. med. Ass.*, **166**, 1159, 1294.
27. Yerushalmy, J. & Palmer, C. E. (1959) *J. chron. Dis.*, **10**, 27.
28. Doll, R. (1959) In *Medical Surveys and Clinical Trials*. Ed. Witts, L. J. London.
29. Greenberg, B. G. (1969) *J. Amer. Stat. Assn.*, **64**, 739.
Sterling, T. D. (1971) *ibid*, **66**, 251.
30. Yerushalmy, J. (1972) *Amer. J. Obst. Gyn.*, **112**, 277.
31. Pasamanick, B. & Knobloch, H. (1966) *Merrill-Palmer Quart. Behav. Dev.*, **12**, 7.
Knobloch, H. & Pasamanick, B. *ibid*. 29.

32. Buoisson, M. (1859) *Montpell. med.,* **2,** 539; **3,** 19.
33. *Epidemiology: A Guide to Teaching Methods.* Ed. Lowe, C. R. & Kostrzewski, J. IEA, London.
34. White, C. & Bailar, III, J. C. (1956) *Amer. J. publ. Hlth.,* **46,** 35.
35. Ludwig, E. G. & Collette, J. C. (1971) *JAMA,* **216,** 493.
36. Goldberger, J. (1914) *Publ. Hlth. Rep.,* **29,** 1683.
37. Hill, A. B. (1953) *New Engl. J. Med.,* **248,** 995.
38. Cochran, W. G. (1965) *J. Roy. statist. Soc.* Ser. A, **128,** Prt. 2, 234.
39. Blalock, H. M. (1964) *Causal Inference in Non-Experimental Research.* Chapel Hill.
40. Morris, J. N. & Heady, J. A. (1955) *Lancet,* **1,** 343.
41. Heady, J. A., Daly, C. & Morris, J. N. (1955) *Lancet,* **1,** 395.
42. Morrison, S. L., Heady, J. A. & Morris, J. N. (1959) *Arch. Dis. Childh.,* **34,** 101.
43. Heady, J. A. & Morris, J. N. (1959) *J. Obstet. Gynaec. Brit. Emp.,* **66,** 577.
44. Heady, J. A. & Heasman, M. A. (1959) *Social and Biological Factors in Infant Mortality.* HMSO, London.
45. MRC Social Medicine Unit.
46. Morris, J. N., Kagan, A., Pattison, D. C., Gardner, M. J. & Raffle, P. A. B. (1966) *Lancet,* **2,** 553.
47. Gardner, M. J., Kagan, A., Meade, T. W. & Morris, J. N. In preparation.
48. Purola, T. (1972) *Med. Care,* **10,** 373.
49. Lewin, K. (1951) *Field Theory in Social Science.* New York.
50. Maruyama, M. (1963) *Amer. Scient.,* **51,** 164.
51. *Modern Systems Research for Behavioural Scientists.* (1968) Ed. Buckley, W. Chicago.
52. Feldstein, M. S., Piot, M. A. & Sundaresan, T. K. (1973) *Resource Allocation Model for Public Health Planning.* Suppl. to Vol. 48. *Bull. Wld. Hlth. Org.* Geneva.
53. Cole, P. (1975) *Bull N.Y. Acad. Med.,* **51,** 75.
54. Clayton, D. C. In preparation.
55. Levin, M. L. (1953) *Acta. Un. Internat. Cancer,* **9,** 531.
56. Morris, J. N., Adam, C., Chave, S. P. W., Sirey, C., Epstein, L. M. & Sheehan, D. J. (1973) *Lancet,* **1,** 333.
57. Clayton, D. C., Epstein, L. M., Stitt, F. W. & Morris, J. N. In preparation.

EXPERIMENTAL EPIDEMIOLOGY

1. Goldberger, J. (1914) *Publ. Hlth. Rep.,* **29,** 1683.
2. Goldberger, J. Waring, C. H. & Tanner, W. F. (1923) *Publ. Hlth. Rep. Wash.,* **38,** 2361.
   Goldberger, J. & Wheeler, G. A. (1920) *Bull. U.S. hyg. Lab.* No. 120. US Public Health Service, Washington, DC.
3. McCollum, E. V., Orent-Keiles, E. & Day, H. G. (1939) *The Newer Knowledge of Nutrition.* New York.
4. McGonigle, G. C. M. (1933) *Proc. R. Soc. Med.,* **26,** 677; McGonigle, G. C. M. & Kirby, J. (1936) *Poverty and Public Health.* London; Kuczynski, R. R. (1936) *Eug. Rev.,* **28,** 137.
5. Tizard, J. (1967) *Survey and Experiment in Special Education.* London.
6. Hill, A. B. (1962) *J. Inst. Actu.,* **88,** Part II, No. 379, 178.
7. *Trigger for Community Conflict: The Case of Fluoridation* (1961) *J. soc. Iss.,* **17,** No.4. Ed. Paul, B. D., Gamson, W. A. & Kegeles, S. S.
   Mitchell, G. E. (1964) In *Economic Benefits from Public Health Services.* PHS Publicn. no. 1178. Washington, DC.
8. Frank, M. & De Vries, A. (1966) *Arch. environ. Hlth.,* **13,** 625.
9. Corry Mann, H. C. (1926) *MRC Spec. Rep. Ser.* no. 105. HMSO, London.

10. Terris, M. (1962) *Amer. J. publ. Hlth.*, **52**, 1371.
11. Wilner, D. M., Walkley, R. P., Pinkerton, T. C. & Tayback, M. (1962) *The Housing Environment and Family Life*. Baltimore.
12. Saev, S., Dorossiev, D., Venov, D. & Fitchev, N. (1969) *Proc. IV Symp. Anaesthes. Internat.* Varna.
13. Cochrane, A. L., Miall, W. E., Clarke, W. G., Jarman, T. F., Jonathan, G. & Moore, F. (1956) *Brit. med. J.*, **1**, 1193.
14. Cornfield, J. & Mitchell, S. C. (1969) *Arch. environ. Hlth.*, **19**, 382.
    Halperin M., Cornfield, J. & Mitchell, S. C. (1973) *Lancet*, **2**, 438.
15. Oliver, M. F. (1972) Paper presented at WHO Symposium on Prevention of Ischaemic Heart Disease: Metabolic Aspects. WHO/CVD/73.3, Geneva.
16. Morris, J. N. (1975) *Bull N.Y. Acad. Med.*, **51**, 62.
17. Stamler, J. (1967) *Lectures in Preventive Cardiology*. New York.
18. Rose, G. (1970) *Trans. Soc. Occup. Med.*, **20**, 109.
19. Blackburn, H. (1972) In *Trends in Epidemiology*. Ed. Stewart, G. T. Springfield, Ill.
20. *Methodology of Multifactor Preventive Trials*. (1973) WHO, Copenhagen.
21. Puska, P. (1973) *WHO Chron.*, **27**, 55. (See Fig. VII. 9, Karelia.)
22. Marks, H. H. (1960) *Bull N.Y. Acad. Med.*, **36**, 296.
23. Himsworth, H. P. (1961) In *Clinical Aspects of Genetics*, p.129. Ed. Jones, F. Avery. London.

THREE WAYS OF LEARNING

1. *Lead Poisoning*
   Baker, G. (1767) *Essay Concerning the Cause of the Endemial Colic of Devonshire*. London. Reprinted. Delta Omega, 1958.
   Simon, J. (1890) *English Sanitary Institutions*. London.
   Charles, J. A. (1961) *Research and Public Health*. London.
   Lancet, (1971) **1**, 278.
   Waldron, H. A. (1973) *J. R. Coll. Phycns., Lond.*, **7**, 177.

2. *Occupational Cancer*
   Pott, P. (1775) Reproduced in "*Percival Pott's Contribution to Cancer Research*, Potter, M. (1963) Nat. Canc. Inst. Monog. no.10. Washington, DC.
   Cook, J. W., Hieger, I., Kennaway, E. L. & Mayneord, W. V. (1932) *Proc. R. Soc. B.*, **111**, 455.
   Kennaway, E. L. (1955) *Brit. med. J.*, **2**, 749.
   Vernon, H. M. (1939) *Health in Relation to Occupation* London.
   Henry, S. A. (1946) *Cancer of Scrotum in Relation to Occupation*. London.
   Butlin, H. T. (1892) *Brit. med. J.*, **1**, 1341; **2**, 166.
   Wade, L. (1864) *Arch. env. Hlth.*, **9**, 364.
   Fisher, R. E. W. (1965) *Trans. Assn. industr. med. Offrs.*, **15**, 122.

3. *Cancer of Bladder*
   Case, R. A. M., Hosker, M. E., McDonald, D. B. & Pearson, J. T. (1954) *Brit. J. industr. Med.*, **11**, 75.
   Case, R. A. M. & Pearson, J. T. (1954) *Brit. J. industr. Med.*, **11**, 213.
   Hueper, W. C. (1942) *Occupational Tumors and Allied Diseases*. Springfield, Ill.
   Case, R. A. M. (1966) *Ann. RCS Eng.*, **39**, 213.
   Case, R. A. M. (1969) *Proc. R. Soc. Med.*, **62**, 1061.
   Cole, P. (1974) In *Cancer Epidemiology and Prevention* Ed. Schottenfeld, D. Springfield, Ill.
   Brit. med. j. (1971) **i**, 517.

4. *Cancer of Breast*
Hoffman, F. L. (1915) *The Mortality from Cancer Throughout the World.* Newark.
MacMahon, B. & Feinleib, M. (1960) *J. nat. Canc. Inst.,* **24,** 733.
Lowe, C. R. & MacMahon, B. (1970) *Lancet,* **1,** 153.
Bulbrook, R. D., Hayward, J. L. & Spicer, C. C. (1971) *Lancet,* **2,** 395.
MacMahon, B., Cole, P. & Brown, J. (1973) *J. Nat. Canc. Inst.,* **50,** 21.
De Waard, F. (1969) *Int. J. Canc.,* **4,** 577.

5. *Rubella Malformation*
Gregg, N. M. (1941–2) *Trans. opthal. Soc. Aust.,* **3,** 35.
Ministry of Health (1960) *Rubella and other Virus Infections during Pregnancy.*
Ed. Manson, M. M., Logan, W. P. D. & Loy, R. M. Rep. publ. Hlth. med.
Subj. Lond. no. 101. HMSO.
Jackson, A. D. M. & Fisch, L. (1958) *Lancet,* **2,** 1241.
Lancaster, H. O. (1951) *Brit. med. J.,* **2,** 1429.
Lancaster, H. O. & Pickering, H. (1952) *N.Z. med. J.,* **51,** 184.
Stevenson, A. C. (1956) *Ulster med. J.,* **25,** 101.
Stevenson, A. C. & Fisher, O. D. (1956) *Brit. J. prev. soc. Med.,* **10,** 134.
Woollam, D. H. M. (1962) *Brit. med. J.,* **2,** 236.
Rubella Symposium. (1965) *Am. J. Dis. Child.,* **110,** 345.
Forbes, J. A. (1969) *Am. J. Dis. Child.,* **118,** July, 5.
Horstmann, D. M. (1971) *J. infect. Dis.,* **123,** 640; (1974) Personal communications.

6. *Goitre*
Clements, F. W. & Wishart, J. W. (1956) *Metabolism,* **5,** 623.
Clements, F. W. (1960) *Brit. med. Bull.,* **16,** 133.
Gibson, H. B., Howeler-Coy, J. F. & Clements, F. W. (1960) *Med. J. Aust.,* **1,** 875.
Clements, F. W., Gibson, H. B. & Howeler-Coy, J. F. (1968) *Bull. Wld. Hlth. Org.,* **38,** 297.
Clements, F. W., Gibson, H. B. & Howeler-Coy, J. F. (1970) *Lancet,* **1,** 489.
Connolly, R. J., Vidor, G. I. & Stewart, J. C. (1970) *Lancet,* **1,** 500.
Hetzel, B. S. (1974) Personal communication.

POSTSCRIPT

1. Morris, J. N. (1973) *Proc. R. Soc. Med.,* **66,** 225.
2. Godber, G. E. (1971) *J. R. Soc. Hlth,* **91,** 165.
3. Ashley, J. S. A., Howlett, A. & Morris, J. N. (1971) *Lancet,* **2,** 1308.
4. Fries, E. D. (1970) *Bull. Internat. Soc. Cardiol.,* 11/4, p.6.
5. *World Health Organisation Tech. Rep. Ser.* (1971) No. 469. Geneva.
6. Hodes, C., *et al.* In preparation.
7. Morris, J. N. (1975) *Bull. N.Y. Acad. Med.* **51,** 62.
8. Nordin, B. E. C. (1972) *Brit. med. J.,* **2,** 287.
9. Tracey, M. V. (1971) *Search,* **2,** 357.
10. Waterlow, J. C. (1971) In: *Metabolic Adaptation and Nutrition.* PAHO Scientific Publ. No. 22, p. 76, Washington, DC.
11. Shaper, A. G., Marr, J. W., Heady, J. A. & Morris, J. N. (1972) *Brit. Ht J.,* **34,** 202.
12. Casdorph, H. R. (1971) Ed. *Treatment of the Hyperlipidemic States.* Springfield, Ill.
13. Ariés, P. (1960) *Centuries of Childhood.* Paris.
14. Fiedler, L. A. (1965) *Partisan Rev.,* **32,** 505.

15. Birren, J. E. (1964) *The Psychology of Aging*. Englewood Cliffs, N.J.
    Blau, Z. S. (1973) *Old Age in a Changing Society*. New York.
16. Russell, M. A. H. (1971) *Brit. J. med. Psychol.*, **44**, 1.
    McKennell, A. C. & Thomas, R. K. (1967) *Adults' and Adolescents' Smoking Habits and Attitudes*. HMSO, London.
17. Seebohm *Report of the Committee on Local Authority and Allied Personal Social Services*. (1968) Cmnd 3703. HMSO, London.
18. Brown, G. W. & Birley, J. L. T. (1970) In *Psychiatric Epidemiology*. Ed. Hare, E. H. & Wing, J. K. p.321, London.
19. Hinkle, L. E. (1967) *Soc. Sci. and Med.*, **1**, 129.
20. Rahe, R. H. & Lind, E. (1971) *J. Psychosom. Res.*, **15**, 19.
21. Duhl, L. J. (1963) Ed. *The Urban Condition*. New York.
22. Roth, M. (1972) In *Patient Doctor Society*. Ed. McLachlan, G. p.113, London.
23. Goodman, P. (1969) *N.Y. Rev. Books,* Nov., 20.
24. Harvard University *Program on Technology and Society* 1964–1972, A Final Review (1972) Cambridge, Mass.
25. Morris, J. N. (1969) *Lancet,* **2**, 811.

Index of Subjects

The first page of a main reference is in **heavy type**; passing reference is
indicated by *pass.*